The Harvard Medical School
Health Letter Book

the HARVARD MEDICAL SCHOOL

Health Letter Book

EDITED BY

G. Timothy Johnson, M.D.
Stephen E. Goldfinger, M.D.

HARVARD UNIVERSITY PRESS
Cambridge, Massachusetts
London, England 1981

Drawings by Harriet Greenfield

Copyright © 1981 by the President and Fellows of Harvard College
All rights reserved
Printed in the United States of America

Library of Congress Cataloging in Publication Data
Main entry under title:

The Harvard Medical School health letter book.

Includes index.
1. Health. 2. Medicine, Popular. I. Johnson, G. Timothy. II. Goldfinger,
Stephen E. [DNLM: 1. Medicine—Collected works. WB 5 H339]
RA776.H32   613   80-27215
ISBN 0-674-37725-7

Foreword

Six years ago, the Harvard Medical School made a commitment to support a publication designed to provide the public with accurate and timely health information. The result was the *Harvard Medical School Health Letter,* which reaches over 300,000 subscribers each month.

It is with great pride that we now present *The Harvard Medical School Health Letter Book*—a completely up-dated synthesis of information that has appeared in the *Health Letter.* Together, the *Harvard Medical School Health Letter* and the *Health Letter Book* are the Harvard Medical School's principal effort to inform the general reader about human health and disease. On behalf of the Faculty of Medicine, I want to congratulate Drs. Timothy Johnson and Stephen Goldfinger and their colleagues for these superb contributions to learning in medicine. I hope that they will help you, the reader, to care more effectively for your own health.

Daniel C. Tosteson
Dean
Harvard Medical School

Contents

Staying Healthy

Hazards of Living

Reproduction and Child Care

Diseases Mainly of Adulthood

Some Problems of Aging

You and the Doctor

Preface

The last word on health hasn't been written—and so much the better for all of us. New knowledge is always appearing. Some of it will make us healthier. Some of it just makes the world, not to mention our bodies, a more interesting place to live in.

But, last word or not, there is no shortage of words—often confusing and sometimes misleading—about medical subjects. Medical misinformation is dangerous—and becoming more so as we enter an era when people are expected to assume a great deal of responsibility for their own health. Short of going to medical school, how can people learn what they need to know in order to take advantage of the right information at the right time?

The doctor who cares for a patient is the best person to answer specific questions. But let's face it: a busy family doctor, let alone a surgeon, back specialist, or radiologist, cannot always sit down to talk over the host of legitimate questions about general health that a patient may want to ask. The *Harvard Medical School Health Letter* was begun late in 1975 as one way to serve this need. Appearing monthly, it carries general essays, short articles, interviews, and notes on topics of current or perennial interest. Its major emphasis has always been placed on ways to prevent disease or detect it early, rather than on details of treatment.

As the *Harvard Medical School Health Letter* completed its fifth year of publication, demand was growing for a book that would put the information in its various issues all together. Here it is. We have brought everything up to date, dropped a few pieces that seemed dispensable, combined essays and notes that originally appeared at various times, and arranged the material according to a few important themes. What we have *not* done is to write an encyclopedia pretending to cover everything medical. Instead, we've tried to round out the book with information that we judge to be of interest to the general public. We won't hit the mark for everyone, all the time, but we hope we're on target often enough to serve your needs and your family's.

So, this isn't the last word, or all the words, but it is our best effort to give you a good selection of the right ones. We've tried to avoid mistakes, but as new knowledge appears we'll be correcting ourselves in future issues of the *Harvard Medical School Health Letter*.

From its inception, the *Health Letter* has been written mainly by Dr. Johnson (recently with some assistance from Dr. William Bennett), who may call on any of the faculty at Harvard Medical School for consultation on facts and interpretation. The first draft is then sent to all members of the Advisory Board and to any additional experts whose opinion is needed. Each member of the Board reads and comments on the draft within seven days. Then the copy is edited by Dr. Goldfinger and Dr. Johnson to take account of the Board's reactions and their own second thoughts. This process has been the same from the first issue, which was mailed to some 7,800 subscribers, until the latest, which went to more than 300,000.

The staff of the *Harvard Medical School Health Letter* and the Advisory Board join us in wishing you many years of good health, and we hope this book contributes its share to that goal.

G. Timothy Johnson, M.D., M.P.H.
Stephen E. Goldfinger, M.D.

Harvard Medical School Advisory Board

The Harvard Medical School
Health Letter Book

Staying Healthy

*Food is a lot more
fattening if you eat
it late at night.*

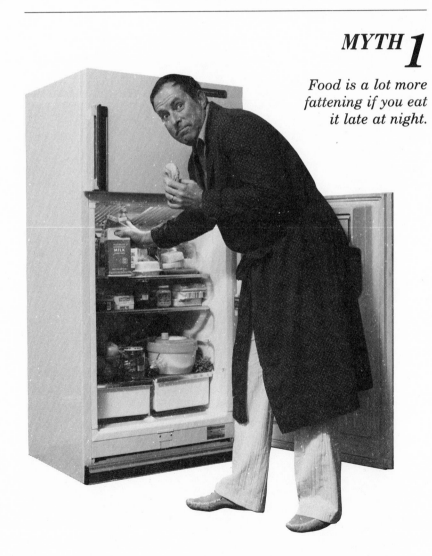

Exercise

The word "exercise" has become provocative. Many people praise exercise as a vital—even joyful—part of their lives. Others register dismay and describe guilt feelings when confronted by the word. Some doctors promote exercise as though it were the answer to all health problems. Others cynically point out that there is no final evidence that exercise accomplishes all the benefits often ascribed to it.

The fundamental question in any discussion about exercise is this: *Does it pay?* Obviously, the answer depends on what is meant by "pay." Few would minimize the psychological value of exercise—the "feel good, look good" benefits. And even though exercise is a very inefficient way to lose weight (it takes about 15 minutes of continuous jogging to use up the calories in *one* martini), exercise does shift the balance from fat to lean tissues in our bodies. There is also good evidence that regular exercise results in better appetite control. But *the pay that most people have in mind is the prevention of heart attacks;* the answer to this question is somewhat complicated.

THE GOAL   Though there are many forms of exercise, that which enhances cardiovascular fitness and stamina (versus strength or skill) must be a form of exercise that can significantly *increase the pulse rate for a prolonged period of time.*

(1) The goal of such exercise is a physiological one—that is, *a sustained increase* in heart activity and oxygen consumption—rather than a specific physical goal such as muscle building or skill development. Types of exercise that achieve such sustained activity include jogging, swimming, rope jumping, stationary bike riding—anything that can be done without slowing down or stopping.

3

Tennis, bowling, and golf do not offer continuously strenuous exercise and therefore do not qualify for this type of exercise program, though they have many other benefits in terms of pleasure and skill development.

(2) The measure of cardiovascular exercise is an *appropriate increase in pulse rate*—not fatigue or sweat or muscle aching or anything else.

SOME SPECIFICS   The full details of an individualized exercise program are beyond the scope of this essay; such information can be obtained by writing or calling the nearest chapter of the American Heart Association. However, the following general points can be made:

(1) A cardiovascular fitness exercise program involves three phases: a warm-up period, the actual exercise period during which the pulse rate is increased, and a cool-down period. *All three are important* and should be tailored to the individual and the particular kind of exercise involved.

(2) The actual pulse rate and amount of exercise will vary with each person according to *age* and *physical condition.* In general, the *maximal heart rate* for a healthy person is about 220 minus his or her age; the *exercise heart rate* (the pulse rate to be sustained during exercise) is approximately 75% of this maximal rate. A *rough* guide would be:

Age range	Exercise pulse rate (average)
30–40	140
40–50	130
50–60	125
60–70	115

Exercise at less than 70% of the maximal pulse rate for a given individual loses some of its value in developing cardiovascular fitness; exercise at more than 85% of the maximal heart rate introduces unnecessary stress and adds no benefit.

(3) The actual amount of such exercise needed for benefit is a matter of debate among experts. In general, however, the recommendations suggest sustained exercise for *at least twenty minutes*

(after a warm-up period) *at least three times per week. And this program should be achieved gradually over a period of weeks*—even months for those who previously have not been physically active.

THE DANGERS   Now come the all-important qualifications. As is true of all health recommendations, any exercise program must be tailored to the individual. In the case of exercise with the *expressed purpose of stressing the heart,* it is imperative that significant heart disease be ruled out before such a program is undertaken. This does *not* mean that a person with heart disease cannot and should not exercise under the careful direction of a physician. It *does* mean that there is a danger in the kind of exercise described above—especially for anyone with heart disease. In fact, there are some relatively rare forms of heart disease where even milder exercise could be dangerous.

Ideally, one should have a complete physical examination—including a stress electrocardiogram—before beginning any exercise program. However, from a practical and financial point of view, such a recommendation is not very helpful. In general, *a person under age 35 with no current health problems and no past history of disease* can undertake an exercise program if it is done gradually and stopped at the earliest sign of any problem—chest pain, dizziness, shortness of breath to the point of inability to speak while exercising, and so on. *Over age 35, hidden heart disease becomes more likely* and a physician's check-up before undertaking an exercise program is highly recommended.

IN SUMMARY   We are now in a better position to answer the question posed earlier—does appropriate exercise (the kind described above) "pay" in preventing heart attacks? The only honest answer to that question is that *there is yet no evidence to answer that question conclusively.* However, several lines of suggestive evidence have emerged in recent years to "explain" the possible benefits of cardiovascular exercise. For example, several studies have now documented that exercise of the level described above leads to higher levels of HDL—or "good"—cholesterol, the kind that protects against coronary heart disease (see p. 178). More recently, researchers have discovered that persons who exercise regularly may have an increased ability to destroy blood clots which might cause serious blockage in the arteries supplying blood to the heart or brain. Again, final evidence is not in. But we endorse the position of the American Heart Association—that it is "prudent" to exercise regularly.

A "Running Commentary"

Come spring—at least in Boston—a young man's fancy is as apt to turn to running as anything else. For all would-be marathoners, or others interested in less ambitious types of running, we have asked Dr. Rob Roy McGregor, a podiatrist and expert in sports medicine, to answer some basic questions.

Is there a difference between running and jogging?

It's really a matter of semantics. The person who runs the six-minute mile may look upon the eight-minute miler as a jogger, yet that eight-minute miler is running as fast as he can. Perhaps a fairer definition would be that those who run for competition are *runners* and those who run for fitness are *joggers*.

How should a first-time jogger "break into" the activity?

A new jogger will do best by alternately walking and jogging for one mile until that distance can be covered by continuous jogging. The same procedure should be followed for two, three, and four miles— or as many as are intended. This gradual approach allows the runner to escape most, if not all, of the aches and pains of the conditioning process.

Is it really important to warm up before jogging?

Yes—and there are two basic steps to a warm-up. First, it is important to stretch and loosen muscles, especially those of the lower extremities. Unless this is done, the jogger will sooner or later develop pains due to tightness of joints or contraction of muscles. Some exercises for this are as follows:

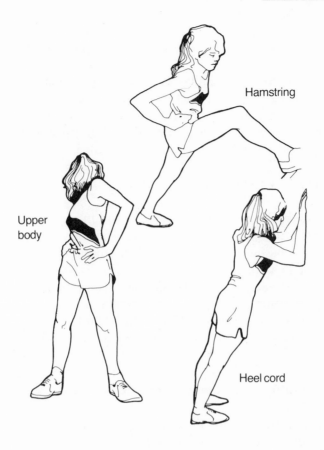

Hamstring

Upper body

Heel cord

To limber the upper body: Stand legs astride, hands at hips, and rotate the upper trunk.

To stretch the hamstring muscle (behind the thigh): With one leg on a table top, lean into that leg, hold for thirty seconds, and repeat; do the same for the other leg.

To stretch the heel cord: With feet parallel, stand back about 18 inches from the wall, lean forward into it with knees and hips straight until you feel a slight pull behind the knee or leg. (Don't do this in the presence of pain.)

Once basic exercises are done, actual jogging should begin at a slow pace until the body is warmed up—about six to nine minutes.

Is it really necessary to do heel-cord stretch exercises?

Yes. The heel cord (or Achilles' tendon) joins two major muscles of the back of the leg to the back of the heel bone. In long-distance running there is a tendency for this heel cord to become contracted. If this happens, several symptoms may result (such as tendonitis, heel pain) which can be prevented by stretching.

Is it necessary to wear running shoes?

No. However, the more (or longer) you run in regular sneakers or tennis shoes, the greater the chance that your feet will hurt so that running will become a literal pain. A dramatic difference will be noted after switching to running shoes—that is, shoes designed for running only. Such shoes have special construction features that provide extra cushioning on impact and also minimize the twisting received by the foot. Anyone can spot this difference by checking the ease with which a regular tennis shoe can be twisted—versus a true running shoe.

Are there differences among running shoes?

The *racing* shoe is usually light and without much support or cushioning, whereas the *training* shoe is heavier as a consequence of the protective and supportive features built into it. There are also "look-alike" training shoes, usually less expensive, that tend to be stiffer and have less cushioning. As such, they may fall short of the desired or necessary goal of comfortable, protected running. As with all shoes, it is important that the shoe fit comfortably—though running shoes should be initially fitted to feel slightly tighter than a regular dress or casual shoe.

Is it better to run on soft ground or track—versus pavement?

Probably. However, there are several problems. Soft ground often has hidden irregularities which can cause an ankle or foot to twist. Also, soft ground or paths may not be readily available. Tracks can be boring and therefore don't lend themselves to interesting long-distance running.

Can "runner's knee" be caused by foot problems?

Runner's knee is probably the same as "jumper's knee," "hiker's knee," "skier's knee," and "skater's knee." In other words, it's a common expression for a generalized pain in the knee. It's a descriptive and not a diagnostic term and it doesn't tell us much.

The two most common causes of knee pain in runners are muscle imbalance and abnormal foot placement. For the former, the answer lies in stretching the contracted muscles and strengthening the weak ones. If pain is caused by the latter, it is usually necessary to balance the foot by some mechanical support, meaning shoe inserts.

What are orthotic devices? Does everyone need them?

An orthotic device is a custom-made shoe insert prescribed by a doctor. One might think of it as similar to glasses for the eyes. Just as glasses permit clear vision, orthotic devices permit pain-free foot function. However, not everyone needs them.

What is a heel spur? Can you run with it?

A heel spur is a projection of bone either on the bottom or back of the heel. It usually arises because of a constant abnormal pull of tendons or muscles which attach to the bone. Indeed, one can run with a heel spur. In fact, many people who have heel spurs don't know it and run without any symptoms.

Strength-Building Programs

The recent proliferation of exercise equipment—for both personal and professional purposes—has led to overall questions about the benefits of strength-building programs. It should be pointed out that there are three basic kinds of such exercise:

(1) *Isometric* exercise involves muscle contraction but no movement of the body part that is stressed; pushing against a wall is a good example.

(2) *Isotonic* exercise involves movement; weight-lifting is the

classic example. A modern version of this theme is "dynamic variable resistance"—the varying of resistance throughout the range of motion (versus concentrating the contraction in a sudden burst of energy). The popular Nautilus equipment is designed for this kind of exercise.

(3) *Isokinetic* exercise involves resistance by muscular effort to equipment that moves at a fixed speed, such as pushing and pulling against a moving lever.

None of these exercises qualifies as cardiovascular exercise designed to improve heart and lung efficiency. Cardiovascular fitness programs require sustained body movement that increases oxygen consumption and pulse rate. In fact, some experts stress that strength-building exercises can even be dangerous to the heart in rare circumstances. To state it briefly, a magnificent physique is no guarantee of a strong heart—or one free of coronary disease. And for those who still wish to emulate Arnold Schwarzenegger, there is no good evidence that any one form of strength-building exercise (or any one kind of equipment) is clearly superior to another—though many strong opinions can be found among devotees.

Safety Note

In an issue of *The Physician and Sportsmedicine,* Dr. James Bennett of the Baylor College of Medicine called attention to the danger of wearing rings during sports activities. The most common problem is the ring's snagging on an immovable object (usually during an accidental fall), thus forcing the weight of the body to pull the finger out of the ring in a manner that severely damages the finger. Sometimes the finger is completely pulled off. Solution? Simple: Take your rings off during sports activities.

Weight Control

An estimated twenty million Americans are on a "serious" diet at any given time; yet Americans on the average are reported to be gaining weight. If there were easy formulas for appetite control or weight loss, the record should be a little better. The fact that it isn't should make you very suspicious of special diets, highly visible commercial products, and hard-sell programs offering to make you into an instant sex symbol in just a few easy weeks (and with more than a few of your hard-earned dollars).

Here are a few observations that may be useful if you are contemplating an attack on your own waistline.

HOW MUCH IS TOO MUCH?   There is no satisfactory definition of obesity, although many have been offered. According to some of them, as many as a third or more of adult Americans are "overweight." In fact, it is hard to be sure what "overweight" means. Past insurance company studies suggest that life expectancy is better for skinny people and gets less with each added pound above the bare minimum. But several epidemiological studies on more representative populations indicate that both the very fat and the very thin have an increased mortality rate; in between, a few pounds here or there may not mean very much.

To be sure, for certain people, extra pounds are a clear and present danger. People with diabetes or high blood pressure suffer more complications if they are very fat, and they benefit from losing weight. Massively obese people experience ill health as a result of their extra adipose tissue. In these cases, weight loss is definitely a way to improve health—although it is often a *very* difficult achievement for the people affected.

For many, though, being thin is a cosmetic rather than a health goal—which is fine for people who are naturally svelte. But human beings come in a variety of shapes and sizes. It is unreasonable to expect that everyone will conform to a single, ultra-thin standard. A lot of people (especially women) who are not by any reasonable definition overweight are subjected to discrimination and pressure to change their basic body type. This pressure should be resisted, difficult as it is to do so. Rather than trying to trim their bodies to fit this year's fashions, many individuals should probably cut their clothing more appropriately to their figures.

MYTHS   Few subjects have accumulated as much misleading and potentially dangerous folklore as the subject of weight control. Here are some of the fallacies:

"It's better to smoke than be fat": False. The few pounds that you may keep off because of a cigarette habit have little or no significance to your health. The cigarettes, on the other hand, are deadly. There's just no comparison.

"Calories don't count": Meaningless. The only thing that counts is calories—more specifically, the balance of calories (energy) in the food you eat *versus* the energy (calories) that you use up every day. To gain a pound of fat, you must eat 3,500 more calories than you use up. What kind of food the calories come from doesn't matter.

But it's also true that consciously counting calories is very difficult. Just 100 extra calories a day will add 12 pounds to your body in a year's time. And yet no one, not even a professional nutritionist, can accurately estimate a day's intake to within 200 or 300 calories. So obsessive calorie counting can be used for weight *loss*—by guaranteeing that you undershoot every day—but not for keeping in balance.

"Some foods, such as boiled eggs or grapefruit, burn up calories": Wrong. Digestion of food does consume some energy, but there is no particular kind of food that costs so much energy to digest that eating it favors weight loss. (There are diets so disgusting, though, that people just don't eat very much of them.) Some individuals do seem to burn up more energy when they eat pure protein, but it is impossible to live on pure protein, and many people don't show the effect anyway.

On the other hand, you can pick your foods to get the maximum nutritional value (vitamins, minerals, and other essential substances) for the minimum number of calories. Vegetables, whole-grain products, and fruits are particularly desirable in this regard. Red meat, on the other hand, is not a particularly low-calorie item; three ounces of roast beef contain more calories (270) than three slices of white bread (190).

"A crash diet is a good way to begin a weight loss program": A bad idea. Crash diets, especially when they are low in carbohydrate, produce rapid fluid loss in the first week or so. (This fluid loss has nothing to do with how much liquid is drunk; it is a change in the body's ability to hold fluid.) Many dieters, fooled by the scales, think their fat is "melting off." It isn't. Fat is coming off, slowly, but it is easily regained when the diet is abandoned—and most crash diets, because they are so extreme, are soon abandoned. Also, not only fat but protein can be lost during an extreme diet or a fast, and when weight is regained it is regained first as fat. So, indeed, the crash dieter may wind up with more fat than he or she started with.

"Exercise is a relatively unimportant factor in weight control": Probably the reverse of the truth. Regular physical activity can make a tremendous difference. Even though exercise seemingly burns few calories, the point is that it burns up those *extra* ones, which add the fat. There also are indications that appetite is better regulated in people who are physically active. They may eat more than they would if they were completely indolent, but not enough more to keep them fat. Also, exercise may change metabolism in a way that favors weight loss. And, finally, exercise contributes to good health (lowering blood pressure, improving the cholesterol picture, lowering blood sugar, and so on) even if the person exercising does not lose appreciable amounts of weight.

"If you eat more in the morning than in the evening, you won't get fat as easily": There may be a slight difference in the way the body handles its food between morning and night, but there's no evidence as yet that the difference has any practical significance.

"Everyone gains weight with equal ease": Not so. There clearly are differences between people in how easily they add or shed pounds, but the ways in which fat and thin people differ from each other are still poorly understood; and just as there is no magic key, there is not, as a rule, any "medical" secret to weight loss.

RECOMMENDATIONS In light of the above misconceptions, what constitutes a sensible approach to weight loss? Obviously there are no easy answers. But it is important to begin by learning to live with the body you have. Appreciate its good features and ask yourself whether you have realistic expectations for it. Set modest goals and be prepared to take a while in reaching them. In addition, you should be aware of the following points:

(1) High-pressure dieting can lead to episodes of compulsive "binge" eating. Eat enough to keep yourself comfortable most of the time. Focus on foods that are not chock-full of calories, but don't try to live on grapefruit, lettuce, and iced tea. It just won't work in the long run for most people.

(2) Behavior modification programs were touted as the answer to overweight a few years ago. It is now clear that these are not as effective as one might wish. Even so, a combination of behavior modification and group support seems to offer some encouraging results. Behavior modification involves changing the *way* people eat so that they'll spontaneously eat less, and it seems to work a little better than brute dieting.

(3) Exercise is a valuable part of any weight-loss program. To be effective in terms of weight loss an activity must *feel* like exercise—it should make you sweat a little—and it should take place at least every other day. Don't kid yourself that strolling or leisurely bicycling is burning up those calories. Calisthenics won't do the trick either. On the other hand, brisk walking—brisk enough to make you breathe faster—can be very good exercise, as is jogging or swimming. Some people respond to daily brisk walking by losing weight spontaneously—without any effort to diet. Heroics aren't necessary or desirable. Start out with a program you can manage—say ten minutes of effort—and build it up gradually. But be sure you do something *at least every other day,* and be prepared to increase the amount (without cutting back on your other, usual physical activities, of course) up to at least twenty-five to thirty minutes a day. If you have any doubts about your health, you should check with your doctor before starting strenuous activity.

(4) Preventing weight gain is ultimately the best defense against obesity. Once gained, pounds tend to stick to the ribs. A change in lifestyle that leads to more sedentary habits (such as buying an automobile) is often the beginning of a spare tire. Keep up activity levels and cut back on desserts when you notice yourself adding a

few pounds. Focus on *not gaining* rather than slimming down for a summer on the beach.

(5) Evidence on the significance of weight gain *in children* is not as clear as it seemed a few years ago. Although very fat children tend to be fat adults, the reasons are not completely understood. Putting infants on strict diets appears to be both impractical and of uncertain value; harm might even result.

(6) People who suffer from massive, uncontrollable obesity are particularly likely to seek drastic forms of therapy. Most of these methods have proved to be dangerous or unrewarding and have been abandoned after a while as the complications became known. Two approaches are currently receiving the most attention:

> *The protein-sparing modified fast* is, in essence, a medically supervised, very low-calorie diet. Whether the diet should be predominantly protein or a mixture of protein and complex carbohydrate is a matter of debate, though it seems that some carbohydrate should be eaten. What is clear is that, although these diets are effective for a while, they don't guarantee long-term weight loss; many people eventually regain the weight they lose.
>
> *Various forms of surgery on the digestive tract* have been tried a good deal in the past few years. One operation, which bypasses much of the intestine, has led to serious complications and is not generally recommended any more. A less radical procedure, which makes the stomach smaller, seems safer and perhaps just as effective. But the answers are not all in, and much more experience is required before a final judgment can be made.

IN CONCLUSION   Much remains to be learned about appetite and weight control. Not even the experts know very much. And a lot of charlatans are all too happy to exploit people's ignorance and unhappiness to sell them "miracles" that are worthless and even dangerous.

Vitamin and Mineral Supplements

A daily vitamin pill has become a ritual for tens of millions of Americans, and a particular source of strength for many pharmaceutical corporations. In the first part of this chapter, Dr. Judith Wurtman, a member of the Department of Nutrition at the Massachusetts Institute of Technology, answers some questions concerning the real value of vitamins and mineral supplements.

How do vitamin and mineral supplements compare with what's in food?

Supplements contain the vitamins known to be necessary for good health, and many of them also provide key minerals, such as calcium, iron, and zinc. A varied, balanced diet ordinarily provides a full complement of vitamins and minerals. As a rule, children and adults in good health get all the vitamins they need if they eat dark green vegetables (spinach, romaine lettuce, broccoli), yellow vegetables (carrots, squash, sweet potatoes) or fruits (peaches, cantaloupe), whole grains or cereals (whole wheat bread), and a source of vitamin C (citrus fruits, baked potatoes, strawberries, green peppers, parsley). A diet that includes dairy products for calcium; red meat, lentils, or beans (such as kidney beans), brown rice, or peanuts for iron; and shellfish or meat for zinc provides adequate amounts of these and other needed minerals.

Supplemental vitamins and minerals are available in pills or certain breakfast cereals that provide 100% of the recommended dietary allowance per serving. "Natural" vitamins are no better than synthetic ones; the body can't tell the difference. And if you do take a daily supplement, don't assume you can now eat empty calories for the rest of the day. These vitamin preparations contain only the nu-

16

trients for which recommended intakes have been established. There are many other nutrients in food that haven't been incorporated into supplements.

When is an otherwise normal adult likely to run short of vitamins and minerals?

People who restrict their diets for one reason or another risk deficiency. Minerals are more often a problem than vitamins, though both can be missing from abnormal diets. Here are some examples:

"Casual" vegetarians: These are people who aren't committed to a vegetarian diet but don't eat meat because they "feel better not eating meat," don't like the bother of cooking it, or are saving money. Likewise, because of price or lack of time or interest, they don't eat fish or shellfish and don't cook kidney beans or other legumes and brown rice, which are good sources of iron. Eggs and cheese become the main protein sources, and the intake of iron becomes inadequate because these foods, compared to the neglected protein sources, are low in iron.

Single eaters: People who take most of their meals alone may become indifferent to their diets or find that it is too much trouble to stock a variety of foods in the house.

People who restrict their diet for religious or ideological reasons: Some cult diets are quite deficient in one or another nutrient. Traditional (kosher or Hindu) restrictions may create a problem for people who are traveling or otherwise unable to get a full diet that is acceptable to them.

Others: People on extreme reducing diets, those with limited food preferences, and heavy drinkers who eat poorly are also at risk.

Who has a special need for vitamins and minerals?

Women during pregnancy and lactation: It is possible for a pregnant woman to eat with such care and devotion that all her added needs for vitamins and minerals are met, but the necessary eating changes may be too difficult. For example, requirements for folic acid (a vitamin) and iron double during pregnancy. These needs can be met by eating lots of parsley and liver, for example, but a supplement may be more practical. To get enough calcium, the pregnant or nursing mother must eat extra dairy products or else take calcium supplements.

During the first few weeks after her baby is born, a nursing mother often lacks the time and energy to plan and provide an adequate diet for herself. She may do well to continue her supplement until she is back in a normal routine, say six weeks to two months later. (If the pediatrician doesn't ask about a nursing mother's diet, she should raise the issue. In the shift from obstetrician to pediatrician, communications can sometimes become a bit shaky.)

The newborn infant: If the baby is receiving breast milk from a well-nourished mother, only vitamin D is likely to be insufficient, and this should be supplemented with oral drops. (Supplements containing vitamins A and C as well as D tend to be prescribed because they are more readily available than plain vitamin D preparations. There is no danger of excess if they're used as directed.) Since virtually all of the small iron content of breast milk is absorbed, no supplement is needed during the first four months of life. Thereafter, if breast milk remains the exclusive food, an iron supplement should be considered. In areas where fluoride in the drinking water is less than 0.3 parts per million, infants and children should receive a supplement. (See pp. 216–217.)

Infants fed with formula receive all the vitamins they need, but if the formula does not contain iron, this mineral should be provided in drops or with weaning foods, such as dried cereals. Again, fluoride supplementation depends on the local water supply.

The child after weaning: Small children often go through periods of diminished appetite, or they can get very finicky. Sometimes, a combination of circumstances—illness, dietary quirks, ignorance—can lead to slight or even marked deficiency of a nutrient. When a child changes his or her relative position on the height and weight charts, it's time to look for illness, dietary deficiency, or both. But there is no automatic reason to have a healthy child on vitamin supplements—and starting large doses without a doctor's guidance can be dangerous. If the question of a deficiency comes up, the mother should keep a careful record of what the child eats for several weeks before a check-up and ask the pediatrician whether the diet is adequate.

The elderly: For a host of reasons, older people may be deterred from eating a diet with all the vitamins and minerals they need. Meats are expensive. Whole grains and dark green, leafy vegetables can be hard to chew and digest. Poor vision, arthritis, or other disability may interfere with food preparation. Living alone diminishes interest in food. Yet, because they do not absorb vitamins and minerals as well as before, the elderly need to take in more of them, not less. Deficiencies of the B vitamins and folic acid can contribute to mental confusion or changes in emotional or intellectual behavior; an insufficiency should be considered as one factor contributing to premature loss of faculties.

Patients with certain diseases, such as malabsorption: Their doctors should guide the selection and dosage of vitamin supplements.

What about the use of vitamins to treat diseases?

Vitamins, as we ordinarily think of them, are needed in the diet in rather small amounts. The only diseases they treat, as a rule, are the disorders that result from deficient intake or absorption. When vitamins are recommended in doses a hundred to a thousand times the usual level, they must be regarded as drugs, with the potential for toxicity and complication that any drug presents (see below). So far, there is no persuasive evidence that vitamins hold much promise for improving cancer survival or reversing mental illness. Approximately doubling the recommended dose of vitamin C has been reported by some to reduce slightly the severity of colds; however, larger doses have no added benefit and do not prevent colds.

Vitamin Therapy

The issue of whether or not consumers should be allowed to take large amounts of vitamins without medical supervision has become a source of contention in this country. Given the known dangers of excessive doses of vitamins A and D in particular, the Food and Drug Administration attempted to regulate them by making amounts greater than 10,000 IU (international units) and 400 IU (A and D respectively) available only by prescription. Health-food advocates, rallying against this regulation, succeeded in getting the courts to eliminate it, as of a Court of Appeals decision in June 1977.

VITAMINS A AND D DANGERS   Vitamins A and D are of particular concern because excessive amounts remain in the body (in fat tissue) rather than being excreted. Recently, three Yale pediatricians reported in the *Journal of the American Medical Association* the case of a four-year-old boy with so-called minimal brain dysfunction (an ill-defined diagnosis that often includes learning disabilities or hyperactivity) who had allegedly been treated with large amounts of vitamin A by his grandmother, the owner of a health-food store. The child evidenced some of the classic signs of vitamin A poisoning—irritability, fever, and bone pain. (Those of vitamin D include lethargy, loss of appetite, and kidney stones or kidney failure.) The Yale pediatricians pointed out that about 10% of the children they see with minimal brain dysfunction have been "treated" with large amounts of vitamins. In an accompanying editorial, a nutritionist from the American Medical Association suggested that "the lid is off" for those who wish to use potentially toxic amounts of these vitamins.

Two issues underlie concern about such vitamin therapy. One is the question of effectiveness versus potential hazards. In the opinion of our Advisory Board, there is no good scientific evidence that extra amounts of vitamins—beyond the recommended daily allowance (RDA)—improve health or effectively treat disease *except* in specific cases of malabsorption or vitamin deficiencies. *In the case of vitamins, at least, more is not necessarily better.*

The other issue is a deeper one, concerning the role of regulation in individual consumer decisions. Does anyone or any government have the right to protect us from ourselves? Some would argue that we should be allowed to choose our own poison—whether it be the certain dangers of cigarettes or the less certain, but clearly possible dangers of excess vitamins.

At present, at least in the matter of vitamins, the courts have decided on a "hands off" policy that means "buyer beware."

VITAMIN A AND CANCER   During recent months, several articles have appeared in the public press suggesting that extra amounts of vitamin A might be helpful in preventing—or even treating—

some cancers. As so often is the case, these stories are usually exaggerated, though they contain a kernel of truth. It has long been known that minimal amounts of vitamin A are essential for the normal growth of epithelial tissues (such as lung, pancreas, prostate) and that a deficiency of vitamin A can lead to abnormal tissue growth resembling cancer. Laboratory studies have also indicated that retinoids (the name applied to vitamin A-type derivatives) can inhibit such abnormal tissue growth in some animals. However, the problem is that it is difficult to extrapolate from laboratory and animal studies to human cancers. There are some pieces of suggestive evidence from human studies—for example, persons who develop lung cancer may have lower levels of vitamin A than persons who don't. But many gaps in our knowledge remain—gaps which are now the subject of intensive research. In the meantime, it would be wrong to recommend that consumption of large amounts of vitamin A—a potentially dangerous nutritional practice—might prevent cancer. However, several cancer experts have proposed that no harm—and possibly some good—could come from taking a daily minimal supplement of vitamin A if one's diet lacks the usual vitamin A contained in foods such as carrots, sweet potatoes, apricots, orange squash, cheese, and milk.

VITAMIN E   This vitamin actually consists of four varieties of a substance more formally named "tocopherol." Vitamin E, like vitamins A and D, is oil soluble and easily stored in fat tissues. It is plentiful in many common dietary components, particularly vegetable oils. This fact, plus its slow elimination by the body, make true vitamin E deficiency almost unheard of in normal humans. Vitamin E deficiency can occur in newborns—particularly "premies"—and in persons with gastro-intestinal problems (malabsorption diseases, surgical removal of stomach or intestines, and so on.)

Controversy begins, however, with claims for the benefits of taking extra vitamin E for the following diseases or conditions:

(1) Aging: Claims made for vitamin E as an "anti-aging agent" are intriguing and are based on interesting theory. Vitamin E can be classified as an "anti-oxidant"—meaning that it inactivates those products of oxidation processes known as "free radicals." Free radicals interact with protein to form "aging pigments" which *may* have

something to do with aging. All of this theory is in a *very early stage* of development. There are no human data to prove the value of vitamin E as an agent effective in preventing or slowing aging. Mouse studies have shown a reduction in aging pigments following supplemental vitamin E, but there was *no change* in the important endpoints—namely, death rates or the "normal" decline of performance due to aging.

(2) Pollution protection: Rat experiments have shown that vitamin E *may* provide protection against lung damage caused by certain components of air pollution.

(3) Intermittent claudication: This common medical problem (see p. 391) is best described as calf pain that develops during normal activities such as walking. It is related to vascular insufficiency of lower extremities. Evidence proposed for the usefulness of vitamin E in combating this condition has not received widespread acceptance.

(4) Sexual vitality: Vitamin E was first discovered as a substance that helped rats produce healthy offspring. Since then it has gained an undeserved reputation as a sexual stimulant. There is no sound evidence to support any beneficial effects of extra vitamin E in the sexual performance of humans (although it may have a very welcome "placebo effect" in this regard).

(5) Other claims: There is no good evidence to support often-made claims for the beneficial effects of vitamin E in heart disease, muscular dystrophy, or cancer, or that vitamin E enhances athletic performance.

The controversy concerning vitamin E must also take into account potential dangers from the use of supplementary amounts. Such possible dangers have precedent, since two other important fat-soluble vitamins, A and D, can produce serious health problems when taken in excessive amounts; however, to date no such effects have been documented for vitamin E.

To summarize, most of the claims made for vitamin E are either excessive or false. However, much remains to be learned about this vitamin and there is enough suggestive evidence for some benefits to merit further research.

More Notes
on Nutrition

MILK—NATURE'S PERFECT FOOD? Attacking milk used to be like attacking motherhood and apple pie. Yet, milk has come under scrutiny—if not actual attack. Specifically, since milk contains cholesterol and saturated fats, many advocates for low-fat, low-cholesterol milk have appeared. Some have even suggested that adults do not need milk—a far cry from the milk industry's slogan "Everybody Needs Milk."

In this particular nutritional controversy, the truth lies in the middle. The following statements summarize sound information concerning milk:

(1) Milk is an excellent food—an excellent source of calcium (about 3/4 of calcium available to Americans comes from milk products), vitamins D and B-12, and quality proteins. Indeed, most vegetarians rely on milk products for some of these essentials.

(2) Most adults do not need the cholesterol and fats of milk. Skimmed or low-fat milk makes sense. However, *this may not be true for children*. Indeed, the American Academy of Pediatricians has warned against using low-fat, low-cholesterol milk routinely in children.

(3) "Milk intolerance"—caused by inability to digest the lactose of milk—has received wide publicity. While it is true that some people, especially non-Caucasians, have a true deficiency of the enzyme necessary to digest lactose, the problem is not universal. *Before rejecting milk*—an economical source of important nutrients—specific guidance from a nutritionist or physician should be sought.

(4) Finally, just how much milk should an individual drink? In part that will depend upon the individual situation. Adults need less milk than children. Pregnant and breast-feeding women need extra

23

milk products. But, in general, about 3 glasses of milk per day is sufficient for most of us and the low-fat, low-cholesterol variety is probably best for adults.

CAFFEINE   Caffeine is one of those substances that periodically "make the news." Most recently, the concerns have been birth defects and cystic breast disease. And in the past, caffeine has been linked with everything from heart disease to ulcers. No wonder that Americans—who consume 35 million pounds of caffeine *per year*—are continually curious about the possible health hazards of this substance so widely utilized as a "non-prescription stimulant."

That's a good place to begin. Caffeine certainly qualifies as a drug and has several effects in the body. For example, caffeine acts to promote urination (it has a "diuretic" effect) and any experienced coffee drinker knows better than to consume a large amount of coffee or tea before a long meeting from which there is no escape. But the most pronounced effect of caffeine is its stimulant activity; indeed, pharmacology texts classify caffeine as a "central nervous system stimulant." As such it can produce widely varying effects, from mild irritability to severe insomnia—and those effects can vary remarkably from one individual to another. (The "dose" of caffeine is about 100mg in an average cup of coffee, and about 50mg in a typical serving of a cola drink or tea.) There is also little doubt that some people become addicted to the stimulant effect of coffee—and experience withdrawal symptoms (most typically a headache) without their usual "dose." Fortunately, of course, the "addiction" and "withdrawal" are not life-threatening, but the jitteriness and jumpiness produced by even small amounts of caffeine in some people can be a serious problem.

However, the health issues that most people think about in relation to caffeine are more "spectacular"—and include the following:

(1) Birth defects: Recently, the Food and Drug Administration issued a warning about the possible effects on the developing fetus of caffeine consumed by pregnant women. That action came largely from the efforts of a Washington group (called the Center for Science in the Public Interest) which has been promoting this concern for several years. Most scientists feel the question deserves attention but point out that the data supporting this possible linkage are

largely from small animal studies (using very large amounts of caffeine) and that there are no good studies to support the claim of danger in humans.

(2) Cystic breast disease: The word "cyst" is often used loosely to describe benign cysts or lumps in the breast which can be disfiguring and/or painful. Cysts are usually of greatest concern because they can be confusing during self-examination and they often need to be biopsied in order to be distinguished from cancer. Furthermore, women with cystic (or lumpy) breasts are thought to be at somewhat higher risk for the development of breast cancer. For all these reasons, there has been keen interest in the recent suggestion (largely proposed by one physician, an Ohio surgeon, Dr. John Minton) that women can reduce or minimize breast cysts by eliminating methylxanthines (caffeine is the most common substance in this family of chemicals) from the diet. *This suggestion needs to be carefully studied by others,* as interest will undoubtedly continue in the possible link between methylxanthines and breast cysts.

(3) Heart disease and high blood pressure: Several years ago, some Boston researchers suggested that heavy coffee drinkers were at higher risk for heart attacks; however, more recent and better-constructed studies have not confirmed this association. But others have demonstrated that a daily dose of 250mg of caffeine (about 2–3 cups of coffee) could cause a rise of about 10 points in both systolic and diastolic blood pressures. There is also no doubt that caffeine can produce temporary heart rhythm problems in some people.

(4) Other disease links: Over the years, caffeine has been linked to other diseases such as ulcers, diabetes, and bladder cancer. However, to date there is no firm evidence proving that caffeine causes any of these disorders, though it may aggravate existing problems (such as ulcers) in some people.

So what is the final word on the beloved cup? Though it sounds like a cop-out, our ultimate advice has to be that of "moderation." Clearly some people—those who are exquisitely sensitive to caffeine's stimulant effects—should not consume any. And since our advice has always been to avoid any drug during pregnancy unless absolutely necessary, we would be consistent in suggesting that pregnant women avoid caffeine if possible. It would also be reasonable for a woman with cystic breast disease to eliminate caffeine and other methylxanthines from her diet just to see what effect such a change might have. But one or two cups of coffee per day probably will cause little harm to most of us.

HEALTH FOODS AND REMEDIES Health-food products are apparently not easily checked or regulated and, *in some instances,* may not be as healthy as assumed. For example, several cases of lead poisoning from "health foods" have now been cited—one from *bone meal* imported from England and the other from *herbal health pills* imported from Hong Kong. Various *herbal tea* preparations have caused serious liver problems. An article in the *New England Journal of Medicine* reported a case of acidosis (when the blood becomes more acid than it should be) from ingestion of *"flowers of sulfur"*—a 99.5% pure sulfur product that can be purchased without prescription and that is apparently widely used as a folk remedy for bowel and breathing problems. And in the *Journal of the American Medical Association* Dr. Ronald Siegel of the UCLA Medical Center has suggested that long-term users of large amounts of the popular herb *ginseng* can develop what he describes as GAS—the Ginseng Abuse Syndrome. This includes high blood pressure, sleeplessness, nervousness, skin eruptions, and morning diarrhea. Since 5 to 6 million persons use ginseng in this country, these side effects may be much more common than one might guess.

NUTRITION AND THE ATHLETE Many athletes (weekend or otherwise) believe that certain nutritional practices can enhance their performance. As discussed by authors from the Milton Hershey Medical Center in Pennsylvania (October 1979, *The Physician and Sportsmedicine*), some of these common beliefs are false—and even potentially dangerous. Among the concepts singled out for debunking in their review are the following:

(1) "Fluid intake during competition is dangerous": In fact, the opposite is true. Restriction of fluid during competition can lead to dangerous dehydration. Athletes should be allowed to satisfy their thirst during competition; they will not become "water-logged" or develop muscle cramping.
(2) "Sugar drinks provide quick energy": If an adequate amount of food is eaten three to four hours before competition, there

is little to be gained by gulping special sugar drinks during the contest. Theoretically, such a practice might actually cause the gastrointestinal tract to delay absorption.

(3) "Extra proteins help build muscles": Assuming a balanced diet that is adequate in calories, the only practice that really helps to build muscles is the exercise of those muscles. Given the cost of steak, that may be good news for athletic department budgets.

(4) "Extra vitamins are needed for energy": Again, just not so. Normal amounts of vitamins are essential for us all, but athletes need no more than the rest of us if their diets are well-balanced.

In short, persons engaged in strenuous athletics require more total calories and fluids than those who are sedentary, but such increases need only be balanced to be effective. Fancy concentrates and special vitamin supplements do not give an "edge," they only thin the wallet.

The "Bran Hypothesis"—A Grain of Truth?

It doesn't look very appetizing, tastes about the way it looks, and is, in actuality, almost thoroughly indigestible once swallowed. Yet more and more people are turning to bran to relieve what's ailing them—and to prevent what isn't. As the most popular of all dietary fiber products, bran in particular has become "the answer" to many of life's problems. For persons with constipation, it's the simplest way of remaining "regular." For others with long-standing diverticular disease, bran may serve as a reminder to maintain a healthy skepticism of medical advice: the standard instruction of a decade ago to avoid fiber has now been discarded in favor of high fiber intake as *therapy*. And for those who like to act on wishful thinking when evidence is insufficient, bran has become a daily ritual to ward off bowel cancer, atherosclerosis, varicose veins, hemorrhoids, and sundry other afflictions of humankind. The purpose of this essay is to take a careful look at dietary fiber—why it's been touted as "healthy" and what the evidence shows to date.

DIETARY FIBER—WHAT IT IS AND WHAT IT DOES   A simple definition of dietary fiber is that portion of food which cannot be broken down by our intestinal juices and which therefore passes through the bowel undigested. The cellulose, hemicellulose, gum, pectin, and lignin components of vegetables, cereals, and fruits are the main sources of dietary fiber (which averages 10 to 30 grams daily in the typical Western diet). Vegetarian and "high fiber" diets contain about twice this amount, and the predominantly maize diets of some Africans may have 90 grams of total fiber daily. Nutritional chemists have brought some confusion to the numbers game by introducing the concept of "crude fiber"—which refers to that residue which remains after treating food with a variety of chemicals. Crude fiber determinations usually underestimate total dietary fiber by at least 50%. As suggested by its definition, the one thing dietary fiber assuredly does is make the stool larger and softer by virtue of the increased water trapped within the fiber. The daily stool of an African averages 400 grams—more than twice that of a person on a Western diet high in refined foods. Transit time through the bowel is also reduced by increased fiber; the bulkier stools are passed by defecation at an earlier time.

THE BRAN HYPOTHESIS   Nearly ten years ago, Drs. Painter and Burkitt noted the very low incidence of diverticulosis of the colon in rural Africa where high fiber diets are the rule. They suggested that the near epidemic of diverticular disease in Western society observed since 1900 is a consequence of refining flour and sugar, which removes much of the fiber from these products. It was thus proposed that colon diverticula—outpouchings of the wall of the large bowel that may become inflamed—are actually a disease of "dietary fiber deficiency." Other medical problems common in Western society and rare in Africa were also attributed to fiber deficiency—including colon cancer, appendicitis, ulcerative colitis, duodenal ulcers, gallstones, hernias, atherosclerosis, diabetes mellitus, varicose veins, and hemorrhoids. As might be expected, many have criticized the highlighting of a single factor as an explanation for a difference in disease rates when numerous *other* differences (genetic, chemical and infectious exposures, other dietary components) also exist between such populations. Moreover, the cause of many of these diseases is complex, poorly understood, and certainly not apt to be due to any single factor. Given these many uncertainties, a perspective on dietary fiber is needed—and the following represents our current understanding in respect to specific medical problems:

(1) Constipation: Whether in the form of natural foods (unprocessed cereal, raw, unskinned fruits and berries, or root vegetables) or more expensive extracts (such as Metamucil prepared from seed husks), dietary fiber helps routine constipation and, unlike many other bowel "therapies," carries no danger when taken on a long-term basis.

(2) Diverticular disease: Though the original concept that the advent of food processing produced the explosion of diverticular disease in Western society has been challenged (on the basis of contrary evidence from other population studies as well as a reassessment of total fiber content now deriving from fruits and vegetables), there is much to suggest that dietary fiber is useful in preventing the formation of diverticula. These outpouchings of the colon are believed to be caused by increased pressure within the bowel; it is known that a high fiber diet will protect from such a buildup of pressure. Moreover, there is excellent evidence that symptoms of diverticular disease improve when high fiber diets are begun—though it may take as much as two months (and enduring a brief period of increased bloating and flatulence) before such benefits are realized.

(3) Irritable bowel syndrome: Even though many have suggested that the irritable bowel syndrome—intermittent bloating, pain, gas, variable constipation and diarrhea—may be a forerunner of diverticular disease, careful trials with dietary fiber treatment have not shown consistent improvement in symptoms beyond those offered by a placebo. Thus, the recommendation of high fiber diet is based more on theory than on observation at this time.

(4) Bowel cancer: The "bran hypothesis" argues that bowel cancer—which is uncommon in rural Africa—is due to chemical carcinogens that cause the cells lining the colon to become malignant; the theory is that dietary fiber not only binds these chemicals to make them inactive but also promotes earlier defecation, thus reducing their contact time with the bowel wall. However, recent studies of bowel cancer in human populations and in experimental animals have pointed away from the fiber hypothesis as an important factor. The correlation of bowel cancer with the animal fat and protein contained in red meat is receiving increasing attention and could be another possible explanation for the low incidence of such cancers in rural Africa.

(5) Inflammatory bowel disease (ulcerative colitis, Crohn's dis-

ease): There is nothing to suggest that lack of dietary fiber causes these diseases—and fiber treatment has no important advantage. In fact, fiber can be hazardous when bowel narrowing is present, as is the case in some patients with Crohn's disease.

(6) Other diseases: Whether high fiber diets really do reduce the occurrence of atherosclerosis, gallstones, diabetes, dental caries, hernias, hemorrhoids, ulcers, and other diseases is still a matter of conjecture. In some instances, theories can be advanced for a causal link (for example, that decreased straining on defecation may be beneficial for those prone to hernias or hemorrhoids). The arguments are more tenuous for such problems as diabetes or atherosclerosis, where other factors such as heredity and excessive caloric intake are more likely culprits than insufficient fiber. In other words, the lower incidence of many of these diseases in rural Africa is probably due to a host of genetic and environmental differences and not just dietary fiber.

IN SUMMARY   Bran is not the magic for all that ails or might ail you. It is not even unique as a source of dietary fiber; fruits and vegetables are a more nutritious alternative. There is good evidence that dietary fiber will help constipation and the symptoms of diverticular disease. The preventive role of fiber in regard to the other diseases cited above is largely speculative. Fortunately, there is no real hazard to eating more fiber and it is a relatively simple way to "have an edge" on any possible risk factors for those who are willing to accept a recommendation that does not make any promises. How do you know how much is enough? Fortunately, each of us has a direct "bottom line" signal—the frequency, comfort, and bulk of bowel movements—that can serve as a guide in answering that question. Some will suffer from gas and bloating while increasing their dietary fiber, but most of us can do so with little or no discomfort.

The Skin Trade

Most of us are bewildered by the variety of non-prescription skin-care products and their even larger variety of claims. Therefore, in the first part of this chapter Dr. Kenneth A. Arndt, Associate Professor of Dermatology at the Beth Israel Hospital, Harvard Medical School, will discuss some of the common OTC (over-the-counter) skin-care products in terms of their effectiveness and dangers—and will guide us through the various chemicals listed on their labels. After Dr. Arndt's discussion, we'll turn to the causes and treatment of one of the most common and bothersome skin problems, especially among teenagers—acne. That essay will be followed by three short items on steroid skin creams, shaving bumps, and skin rashes.

Soaps

Soaps help to dissolve (really to "emulsify") greasy or oily substances in water; thus they remove oils and foreign particles from the skin. Their detergent and alkaline properties, however, can be irritating; the hallmark of soap damage is "chapping"—rough, red, dry, and cracked skin. Until recently, no published study had compared different commercial soaps for their safety and irritant potential. Soaps have been called "mild" on the basis of their manufacturers' beliefs, wishes, or commercial interests. But a study in the *Journal of the American Academy of Dermatology* (July 1979) measured the irritant effect of eighteen well-known toilet soaps and showed that Dove was by far the "mildest," whereas Zest, Camay, and Lava were most harsh. Between the extremes were many products whose irritant properties bore no relationship to such characteristics as cost, transparency, or the label's description of them as "neutral," "superfatted," or "for dry skin."

31

Dry-skin products

Skin that is repeatedly exposed to soaps—or solvents or disinfectants—becomes dry and chapped. These agents can damage the skin's ability to serve as a barrier to the loss of body water, thus allowing water to escape at 75 times the normal rate. Other factors leading to deficient moisture in the skin are certain skin diseases (psoriasis, eczema, ichthyosis); aging of skin on sun-exposed areas; dry air (from heating of cold, dry winter air); and exposure to dry, cold winds, which literally "pull" water from the skin. Protective clothing (gloves and mittens), the use of humidifers, and avoidance of excessive washing all help to prevent dry skin.

Three things must be done to repair dry skin: (1) the moisture level must be raised; (2) once raised, it must be kept up; and (3) the outer layer of skin must be restored to its normal texture. The most effective means to correct dryness and add protection is to soak the dry area in water for five to ten minutes, then apply a greasy ointment such as petrolatum (Vaseline) or lanolin, or somewhat lighter preparations (for example, hydrophilic petrolatum, Eucerin). Less oily but still effective are oil/water emulsions (for example, Keri, Lubrex, Lubriderm, or Nutraderm creams or lotions; Nivea cream). After they are applied, the water evaporates, leaving a thin film of oil on the skin.

Urea and lactic acid, it is claimed, have a softening and moisturizing effect, and they may increase the skin's capacity to bind water. Aquacare HP, Carmol Ten, and Nutraplus contain 10% urea; Carmol has 20% urea. Lacticare lotion and Purpose Dry Skin Cream contain lactic acid. U-lactin lotion has both.

Bath oils are added to tub water on the theory that the skin absorbs a portion of the oil in conjunction with a surfactant also in the fluid. The oil makes the skin feel smooth and may prevent water from evaporating. Bath oils come in two types: those dispersed in the water (Alpha-Keri, Domol, Lubath, Jeri-bath), and those that lie on the surface to coat the body as one steps out (Surfol). Paradoxically, some people feel more itchy after they've taken a bath with one of these products.

A person may need to experiment to find the product that works best; products with fancy names, high prices, and exotic ingredients are no more effective than many others. Furthermore, excessive use of moisturizers on the face may lead to an acne-like condition.

Also, products containing lanolin or any of the many other ingredients in these preparations may cause allergic reactions.

Products for skin infections

Skin infections, such as impetigo and folliculitis, which are superficial and caused by bacteria, may be treated with topical ointments—either antibiotics (such as bacitracin) or antiseptics (such as the iodine-polymers Betadine or Efudine). Neomycin-containing ointments are also effective, but they often cause a contact allergy. *Before* using one of these ointments, it is helpful first to soak the area and then gently remove crusts and debris. If the infection is angry-appearing or widespread, antibiotics by mouth or injection may be necessary and medical attention should be sought.

Fungal infections are most common in hot, humid areas where the skin is kept moist with sweat. Usually on the feet or between the toes (athlete's foot) or in the groin ("jock itch"), these infections may also affect the scalp, trunk, hands, and nails. Thorough drying after bathing, use of a talcum powder, and wearing of sandals and absorbent clothing help to prevent and cure fungal infections. Treatment with non-prescription agents is often quite effective. Most commonly recommended is tolnaftate (Tinactin and other brands) in powder, cream, or solution. Powders and ointments containing undecyclenic acid (such as Desenex) have long been used and are as effective as tolnaftate.

No effective drug is available to treat the most common viral infections of skin—oral and genital herpes simplex (cold sores, fever blisters), herpes zoster (shingles), and warts. Preparations recommended for herpes may decrease discomfort, but they have no effect on healing time and do not delay recurrence. The callus covering a wart can be reduced and sometimes the wart itself eliminated slowly by remedies containing skin-softening agents. Sold for removal of calluses, corns, and warts, such products include Compound W and various corn-plasters.

Antiperspirants and deodorants

Many people are troubled by sweating from their armpits because it stains their clothing or they find the odor unpleasant. Either heat or emotions stimulate armpit glands to produce sweat, and the two combined cause the most intense perspiration. When sweating is felt to be a problem, it can be inhibited with antiperspirants. Aluminum compounds are reasonably effective for this purpose, and they are the main ingredient of all over-the-counter antiperspirants. Even so, the armpit sweat glands are relatively resistant to antiperspirants; agents that reduce sweating by 100% on most areas of the body achieve only a 50% reduction in the armpits.

Commercial antiperspirants work reasonably well for most people, but there is no published study which compares the various brands. People who are particularly troubled by armpit sweating may need to take more drastic measures. A saturated solution of aluminum chloride in alcohol, kept in place overnight under an airtight wrap, can almost eliminate sweating for a few days. The preparation, known as Drysol, requires a prescription. Occasionally, mild tranquilizers help. For people who have an uncontrollable problem with excess sweating, the best course may be surgical removal of the armpit skin that contains sweat glands—a relatively simple procedure. Unfortunately, drugs to inhibit the nerves that stimulate sweat glands are sometimes recommended; whether applied to the skin or taken by mouth, these drugs are usually ineffective.

Odor in the armpit is not caused by sweat itself so much as by bacteria that grow in the warm, moist environment it provides. Successful deodorants, then, must prevent the bacteria from growing. The aluminum compounds in antiperspirants are moderately effective against bacteria and thus reduce odor by diminishing both the output of sweat and the growth of bacteria. Some people who cannot tolerate the usual antiperspirants or deodorants may be helped by antibacterial soaps such as chlorhexidine (Hibiclens) or solutions such as povidone-iodine (Betadine, Efudine), or by topical antibiotics such as Neosporin cream (which requires a prescription) or ointment (which does not).

Acne, a Treatable Disease

There is probably no disease more frustrating for teenagers (and their parents) than acne. Unfortunately, folk remedies or procrastination often replace the use of treatment which can greatly reduce cosmetic damage. It is the purpose of this essay to review the most important treatment methods now available—and to put in perspective new and more dramatic therapy.

CAUSES   The basic problem in acne starts in small skin structures known as "pilosebaceous follicles"—which are found in large numbers on the face, back, and chest. Each follicle consists of a tiny but active sebaceous gland (which secretes a waxy substance known as *sebum*) in association with a hair remnant and a narrow channel leading to the skin surface. Acne occurs when these channels either leak or become plugged with sebum, causing the follicles to expand into visible lumps known as *comedones*. If a comedo stays closed at the skin surface, it becomes what is called a "whitehead"; if it opens, exposed pigment causes the comedo to become a "blackhead," a discoloration that is *not* caused by dirt. If excessive pressure within comedones produces leakage into surrounding skin, disfiguring cysts and abscesses can form. The important question, of course, is why all of this happens. Final answers are not in—though the following factors are known to be important:

(1) *Hormone stimulation:* Acne is almost unheard of until the age of puberty when increased levels of male hormones (androgens) stimulate secretion by sebaceous glands; females produce less of these hormones, but they do produce some in their adrenal glands, which explains why girls also get acne—though usually less severely than boys.

(2) *Bacteria:* While their exact role is not understood, there is evidence that certain normal skin bacteria contribute to inflammation by causing the breakdown of skin fats into irritating chemicals. The effectiveness of antibiotics (see below) in treatment tends to confirm the importance of bacteria in causing acne.

(3) *Other factors:* While hormone stimulation and bacterial action are thought to be the major themes in the development of acne, other factors may contribute to the process—including excessive humidity, various cosmetics, exposure to oils or greases which may plug up skin ducts, and medications such as steroids, iodides, and Dilantin. Birth control pills can work in either direction, depending upon the constituents of the particular pill. They may cause acne in some women and improve the skin of others; some women will develop acne after they stop the pill.

It has been well established that chocolate, colas, and emotions do *not* cause acne. However, if any particular factor seems to contribute to acne in a given individual, common sense suggests avoiding that item—even for peace of mind.

TREATMENT Although the exact causes of acne are unknown, making prevention impossible, excellent treatment methods are now available. Adequate control of acne should be expected in the majority of cases. The following methods of therapy are listed in the usual order of use as the severity of acne increases:

(1) General measures: As indicated above, special dietary measures are usually not helpful or necessary; indeed, some "health" foods—such as iodide-containing kelp tablets—may cause or aggravate acne. Oily facial creams and moisturizers should be avoided, as they may block off skin ducts; some contain chemicals which induce whiteheads and blackheads to form. Most lubricants are tested for their blackhead-forming potential prior to marketing. So-called "hypoallergenic" cosmetics are less likely neither to cause contact allergies nor to cause acne problems than regular cosmetics. Tight-fitting clothing articles—such as head bands and turtleneck sweaters—may block glands. Although washing when the skin feels oily is advisable, compulsive scrubbing with soap and water can make acne worse. Contrary to myth, hair length does not affect acne unless it contributes to oily skin. Ultraviolet lighting (including sunlight, of course) can be very helpful in milder forms of acne.

(2) Benzoyl peroxide: Though many so-called peeling agents have been tried in the treatment of acne, most dermatologists prefer benzoyl peroxide (Benoxyl, Oxy-5, Oxy-10, Persadox, and others)—which apparently acts both by reducing bacterial activity and by promoting the healing of comedones. Initial treatment usually consists of once-a-day application of a 5% gel—but other preparations are available as needed. In many cases, benzoyl peroxide will be the only treatment necessary. In a small number of persons, it will cause a contact sensitivity reaction requiring discontinuation.

(3) Retinoic acid: In more severe cases, this substance (also known as vitamin A acid or tretinoin) can be very effective—either alone or in combination with benzoyl peroxide. Unlike benzoyl peroxide, retinoic acid often requires very careful physician supervision

because of the potential for excessive skin irritation. Initially, all other facial applications must be stopped *and excessive exposure to ultraviolet light must be avoided.* It is also important to apply retinoic acid only to thoroughly dried skin. But in patients with acne not responsive to benzoyl peroxide alone, retinoic acid (used alone or with other topical agents) can make a dramatic difference.

(4) Antibiotics: Most authorities feel that antibiotics should never be given as the sole form of treatment for acne. However, when the above measures fail to control acne—or especially when acne is inflammatory with the development of pustules, abscesses, and scarring—antibiotic therapy can be very effective. The most commonly used drug today is low-dose tetracycline, which has been very adequately studied for long-term effectiveness and safety. Tetracycline should not be used by pregnant women because of its effects upon the fetus.

(5) Estrogens: In women with severe acne not responsive to the above measures, estrogens (given as birth control pills) may be useful in counteracting the effects of male hormones. The use of estrogens in men is not possible because of unacceptable side effects.

(6) Surgical measures: Various procedures to drain and remove acne skin lesions can be helpful *in carefully selected cases.* Most dermatologists rely on non-surgical treatment except for very large pustules or abscesses. Dermabrasion techniques are used only for severe scars left by old acne, and *should never be directed to active, inflammatory areas.* Steroid injections into acne lesions can also be useful.

More recently, the media has featured the success of a "new" pill for acne. However, the promise of this medication—a synthetic member of the vitamin A family (described above) known as "13-*cis*-Retinoic Acid"—has been known for several years within dermatology circles and its potential value is new only to the media and the general public. It is expected that several more years of testing for safety will be necessary before release for general use. Even then, many observers expect that it will be used only for the relatively small number of acne patients who do not respond to the treatment measures outlined above. It is also expected that this pill may not be generally available to women because it is likely to cause birth defects. Because of all the recent publicity about vitamin A for acne, doctors are concerned that sufferers will turn to self-medication with excessive amounts of natural vitamin A pills—a practice that could lead to serious side effects including liver damage.

IN SUMMARY   Though complete eradication of acne should not be expected, the vast majority of acne sufferers can achieve great improvement by appropriate treatment. Such treatment is not difficult in milder cases, but the expertise of a skin specialist can be invaluable in more severe ones.

Steroid Skin Creams— Without Prescription

Drugs derived from the adrenal family of hormones (steroids like cortisone and prednisone) can produce dramatic relief in a wide variety of human ailments: their powerful anti-inflammatory effects find application in many catastrophic diseases. However, these drugs can also produce powerful side effects. Therefore, steroids have been available only by prescription; even so, too many physicians still prescribe them for mild conditions that could be managed in other ways.

When these drugs are applied to the skin as topical medication, they are much less likely to produce systemic (body-wide) side effects. Thus, there has been increasing pressure to make mild versions of steroid skin medications available without the cost and inconvenience of obtaining a prescription. Recently, the Food and Drug Administration has supported such use, and several products of one particular steroid, hydrocortisone, are now being marketed as more powerful "over-the-counter" skin medications. And while this availability should prove useful for many minor skin problems, several words of caution are in order:

(1) Since steroids act to cut down on the body's inflammatory response (which is why they usually relieve the itching and irritation that accompany most inflammatory reactions), adequate doses of steroids should predictably produce initial improvement in almost any skin problem. However, if an underlying bacterial or fungal infection is the problem, such improvement may be short-lived, and

interfering with the body's appropriate response could be counter-productive. Indeed, using steroids on herpes simplex infections may lead to dramatic worsening of the problem, and since herpes infections can lead to blindness, such creams should not be used for infections near the eye unless approved by a competent physician.

(2) The doses approved for use by the FDA—only up to 0.5% strength—may be strong enough only for very mild problems. Indeed, the 0.25% strength used in some preparations may be no more effective than placebo preparations. It should be pointed out that topical steroids of any type are seldom effective against poison ivy; in severe cases of poison ivy, oak, or sumac, oral steroids must be used for significant relief.

In short, more experience with these "weaker" (vs. prescription) skin medications will be needed before their benefits for general use can be clearly established.

"Shaving Bumps"—Treatment vs. Mistreatment

"Pseudofolliculitis barbae"—a facial skin problem—has become a subject carrying unfortunate racial overtones in the armed services, and the cause for a civil discrimination suit before the United States Supreme Court. In plain English, the disease can be described as an inflammatory skin reaction caused by hairs which, sharpened by shaving, pierce the skin and cause an irritative reaction known popularly as "shaving bumps." This phenomenon is more likely to occur in black males because their facial hair tends to grow at a more acute angle compared to others. The initial treatment for shaving bumps is to avoid shaving—but growing a beard often flies in the face of certain civilian and armed services regulations. Since recommended therapy has been interpreted by some to "favor" blacks, bitter feelings have been generated—particularly in the armed services; sadly, some black military personnel have felt compelled to suffer the consequences of shaving rather than jeopardize their careers. While not in a position to solve this very real problem, we do feel it necessary to stress that growing a beard is appropriate therapy for shaving bumps.

High-Intensity Lamps and Skin Rashes

A fascinating case of medical detective work reported by the New Jersey Department of Health stemmed from the sudden development of skin rashes and eye irritation in 69 of 81 girls on the basketball team of a New Jersey high school. The problem was traced (within 24 hours) to a hole in a high-intensity mercury vapor lamp in the gym of another high school in which the girls had played the day before. These commonly used lights have an outer glass envelope to reduce the ultra-violet light exposure produced by the inner arc lamp. The hole allowed excessive exposure on the girls who were sitting in the stands. Moral: check high-intensity mercury lamps regularly for breakage in the protective glass envelope.

Hair Care

Given the concern that most of us have about the covering on our scalp (or the lack thereof), we have asked Dr. Kenneth A. Arndt, Associate Professor of Dermatology at the Beth Israel Hospital, Harvard Medical School, to answer the following questions about hair.

Could you describe normal hair growth?

The hair follicle, residing just below the skin surface, is the essential growth structure (see diagram). If a hair follicle is destroyed, no new hairs can form. If hair is plucked or cut but the follicle remains, new hair *will* grow. The total number of hair follicles in an adult has been estimated at about five million, of which about 100,000 are in the scalp. The number of hair follicles decreases with age. As dividing cells at the bottom of a hair follicle are pushed upward, they eventually die and become the visible product we know as "hair." It is important to emphasize that each hair we see above the skin is dead protein tissue; the follicle, lying deeply within the skin, is the essential growing part of the hair.

In humans, each follicle grows hair in cycles and the duration of the cycle is different in each part of the body. In the scalp, for instance, each hair grows steadily and continuously for 3 to 5 years; growth then stops and after 3 months the hair is shed. After another 3 months of a resting phase, a new hair starts to grow from the same follicle. On the eyebrows, however, the growing phase is only about 10 weeks and thus the hairs can never grow very long. Scalp hair grows about one-third millimeter each day (one centimeter per month, one inch in 2–3 months). Since there are about 100,000 scalp hairs, this growth produces about 100 feet of practically solid protein each day (seven miles per year). People who tend to grow long hair

41

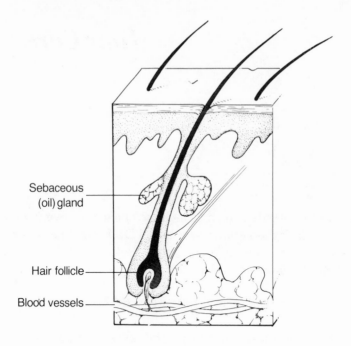

Sebaceous (oil) gland

Hair follicle

Blood vessels

have long growth periods (6–8 years), but their hair does not grow any faster than others.

People often complain about their hair falling out. Is this normal?

Normally, about 90% of scalp hairs are growing and 10% are resting. The resting hairs stay in place for several months, but when a new hair is formed and begins its own growth cycle, the old one is pushed up and out. We normally lose 50–100 scalp hairs per day as old hairs are shed to make room for their successors.

Many events can cause a definite change in the hair cycle. A temporary increase in the rate of shedding may occur 3–4 months after childbirth, or following a high fever, major illness, major surgical procedure, blood loss, or severe emotional stress. It has also been seen recently in association with rapid weight-loss diets involving severe restriction of calories (less than 800 per day) or protein. In these situations, hair will literally come out by the handful, but it always regrows some months later. Various drugs can also cause hair shedding. In other instances, hair loss is not increased but replacement is inadequate. This can occur as a result of thyroid disease, cancer, iron deficiency, and some cases of diabetes.

What causes common baldness and what can we do about it?

So-called "male-pattern" hair thinning, the all-too-familiar receding hairline seen earliest at the temples and over the top of the scalp, is very common in men. It may also occur in women, in whom it normally appears 15–20 years later than in their male relatives. The age of onset, degree of thinning, and ultimate hair pattern are determined by male hormone (androgen) stimulation and by heredity. In other words, the eventual development of male-pattern thinning is a normal and inevitable response to the same stimuli (androgens) which promote normal sexual development. Although seborrhea (oiliness) and dandruff are sometimes associated with this type of hair loss, treating these conditions does *not* influence the regrowth of hair.

In women, genetic hair thinning is more difficult to diagnose with certainty at an early age, but it seems to be quite common. The hair loss is more diffuse and less patterned. If one can exclude other common causes of hair loss, if there is a family history of the condition, and if the onset is gradual and not associated with irregular menstrual periods or excessive growth of hair elsewhere on the body (hirsutism), it is likely that this hair loss is a normal event.

Familial (or genetic) hair thinning has never been shown to be helped by local applications or injections, by radiation, or by any other physical treatment in either sex. There are no foods or vitamins which will specifically help hair growth—though good health and nutrition are generally important.

What about hair transplantation—and other methods of hair replacement?

Hair transplantation depends on the fact that if you take hair-bearing skin from one site and put it at another, the hair will continue to grow with the same characteristics as if it had never moved. The most common form of hair transplantation uses four millimeter "plugs" of hair-bearing skin taken from the rear scalp fringe and transplanted to the front. It takes about 200–250 plugs to fill in a normal receding hairline. Most plugs "take," with 3–5 hairs growing from each one.

Several recent reports warn against the terrible problems that develop after *synthetic* hair implants—not to be confused with the technique of transplanting one's own hair just described. Synthetic implants are rejected by the scalp, leaving a battlefield of scarring and infection which often requires extensive hospitalization and even scalp removal.

One should consider both wigs and sutured ("sewn-in") hair pieces. The former are made out of various combinations of artificial and real hair and are kept in place on the scalp by adhesives. With the sutured types, stitches are actually put permanently into the scalp and the hair piece is woven into place. Although the results are often good, whenever a foreign object is left in place, such as a suture, there is always the possibility that a chronic skin infection will occur.

What about protein-containing rinses and shampoos?

Physical and chemical injury to the hair is by far the most common cause of hair abnormalities in our culture. Hairs are exposed to sunlight, to the physical trauma of brushing and combing and curling, to heat and tension, and to a variety of chemical insults. These can result in brittle and unmanageable hair, with a rough, irregular surface. Protein-containing rinses temporarily fill in the defects on the surface of the hair shaft, making it smoother and thicker. For some people, these products are of benefit in caring for their hair, but they do not cause hair to grow.

How can excessive hair be removed?

Hair growing excessively, or in the "wrong" places, often troubles people. Usually the only significance is cosmetic, and the cause is genetic—a "family tendency." But very occasionally, an unusual growth of hair signals a hormonal or other medical problem which should be attended to.

Fine hair can be *bleached* to make it less obvious. The most common preparation is 6% hydrogen peroxide (commonly known as "20-volume peroxide"). Adding about 10 drops of ammonia to an ounce of peroxide immediately before it is used will make the bleaching action more intense.

There are several ways to remove hair. *Plucking* is painful but effective. Since each pluck starts another growing cycle in the hair root, this is not a permanent method. *Wax epilation* is essentially widespread plucking. Warm wax is placed on the skin, allowed to dry, and then peeled off—with the hairs attached. *Shaving* is quick, easy, and effective, and it does *not* cause hair to grow back more abundantly or rapidly. However, it does leave the cut shaft of hair in place. *Rubbing with a pumice stone* or other mild abrasive also removes fine hair.

Depilatories cause hair to disintegrate but leave the roots, thus permitting regrowth. By disintegrating chemical bonds in the hair shaft, they turn it into a gelatinous mass, which is then wiped away. Because these agents dissolve protein, they also affect the skin and can irritate it if left on too long. Two types of depilatory are available. The sulfide types (such as Magic Shaving Powder and Royal Crown Shaving Powder) are more effective, but their odor is pungent and they are more irritating. The thioglycollate types (such as Better Off, Nair, Neet, and Sleek) must be left on longer, but they are more easily perfumed and are not so irritating.

Electrolysis is the only permanent method of hair removal. With this procedure, the hair bulb is destroyed by an electric current so that hair cannot regrow. However, electrolysis may be complicated by temporary irritation from the procedure or, later, by pitlike scarring. Also, incompletely destroyed hair may grow back. As with everything, the quality of the results depends on the skill of the operator; both cost and skill vary but not necessarily together.

Are there any significant differences among the types of shampoo available?

The many commercial varieties on display usually advertise themselves as being for dry, normal, or oily hair, but clinical trials reveal that these fine distinctions are meaningless. Also, there is little or no connection between the cost of a shampoo and its usefulness as a cleansing agent.

People with scaling disorders of the scalp, such as dandruff or seborrheic dermatitis, often find medicated shampoos useful. In these conditions, the skin is replacing itself too rapidly, so excess cells are shed from the scalp. Medications that control (not cure) these conditions usually work by slowing down cell division to a near normal rate. The most effective shampoos are those containing 2½% selenium sulfide (available only by prescription). Then, in descending order of effectiveness, are those containing zinc pyrithione (for example, Danex, Head and Shoulders, Zincon); salicylic acid and sulfur (Ionil, Sebulex, Vanseb); tar shampoos (Ionil-T, Sebutone, Pentrax, Zetar); and finally, any non-medicated shampoos, particularly those containing surfactants (detergents), if used at least every other day.

Contact Lenses

We have asked Dr. George Garcia, Assistant Clinical Professor of Ophthalmology, Harvard Medical School, an expert on contact lenses, to take a hard look at soft contact lenses and to talk about the future of contact lenses.

What kinds of contact lenses are available today, and what are their advantages?

Three main types of lenses are now in use: hard, soft, and gas-permeable.

(1) Hard lenses: The first successful contact lenses, developed about forty years ago, were made of plastic and were quite large; techniques for fitting them were cumbersome and successes were few. Then, in the late 1940s, contact lenses that covered only the cornea (the transparent membrane at the very front of the eye) were introduced. These early *hard* lenses were all made of PMMA (*poly-methylmethacrylate*), and the greater success with them resulted from modifications in design. Hard lenses continue to be widely used because they offer good vision (especially when the patient has astigmatism), ease of care, durability, and low cost. However, in the past ten years, new materials have been introduced into contact-lens manufacture. Lenses made with these substances have not only increased the success rate of fitting, but also have allowed more people to use contact lenses.

(2) Soft lenses: Lenses made from plastics such as HEMA (*hydroxyethylmethacrylate*) are more flexible than the older PMMA lenses. As a result, they are more comfortable than hard lenses, and

they require very little time for adaptation. They can be worn for many hours without producing edema (swelling) of the cornea. Soft lenses have some valuable advantages, but they also have limitations. Vision is frequently not as sharp as with conventional glasses or hard lenses. Because bacteria can grow on the surface of soft lenses, they must be disinfected with a heating unit or antiseptic and rinsing solutions, which add to potential complications and to expense. Many ophthalmologists believe that, even with proper cleaning, soft lenses carry a slightly higher risk of causing eye infection. Soft lenses can be damaged in more ways than hard lenses, so they require fairly frequent replacement.

(3) *Gas-permeable lenses:* A new generation of lenses is being made from plastics such as cellulose acetate butyrate (CAB), silicone, or a third polymer (plastic) made by linking silicone with PMMA. This last substance is usually just called "Polycon." The CAB and "Polycon" lenses resemble hard lenses in their high optical quality, durability, and ease of care, but they permit more oxygen and carbon dioxide to pass through them. This is important because the cornea must "breathe" directly from the air. In addition, CAB lenses are more flexible than hard lenses and thus allow for better pumping of tears across the eye's surface. They also transmit heat more readily—a property that may have some advantages during long-term wear. Silicone lenses resemble soft lenses in their optical properties, but they are more easily cared for and are more durable.

These newer materials have solved many problems of contact-lens technology, and now more patients than ever can be successfully fitted. But failures still occur, and every patient should be thoroughly evaluated before a fitting and then advised what type of lens is best in his or her situation. This evaluation should include a thorough examination of the entire eye to discover any abnormality that might make wearing lenses hazardous.

Are there any advantages to wearing contact lenses other than convenience and cosmetic preference?

Most people who wear contact lenses wear them for the sake of appearance. There are circumstances, however, in which contact lenses offer greater optical advantages than conventional glasses. An obvious one is that contact lenses correct eyesight through the full extent of the visual field. Certain problems are particularly suitable for contact lenses. *Keratoconus,* for example, is an unusual hereditary disease in which the cornea gradually thins, protrudes, and acquires fine scars; eventually the diseased cornea may have to be replaced by a transplanted one. Glasses do not correct the visual defect, whereas contact lenses usually work very well (unless the condition is severe), thus postponing or even eliminating the need for a transplant. For the patient who has had cataract surgery, contact lenses can provide vision very close to normal, whereas the thick lenses of cataract glasses result in magnification, distortions, and limitation of peripheral vision, all of which can be very annoying. An injury to the cornea can produce irregular scarring for which spectacles are of no value, but with contact lenses it may be possible to correct vision.

What are some of the more common problems encountered by people wearing lenses?

The most common one is disappointment when their lenses don't come up to expectations, as when there is a persistent awareness of the lenses or a sense of discomfort. Chemical irritation from the solutions used to clean and moisten the lenses, or an allergic reaction to them, is fairly frequent. With soft lenses, blurred vision is not uncommon, and wearers of hard lenses frequently complain that lights appear streaked or surrounded by halos. In some cases replacing lost or damaged lenses can become very costly.

Fortunately, relatively few serious problems are associated with contact lenses. Irritation from the "overwearing syndrome" that occurs with hard lenses is temporary and heals completely—albeit with considerable discomfort. It can be prevented by wearing gas-permeable or soft lenses. Warping of the cornea (the development of an irregular curve on the surface of the eye) rarely occurs in a patient who is properly fitted and followed. Blood vessels are not normally present in the cornea (where they could interfere with clarity of vision), but they may grow in if the cornea is deprived of oxygen for a long time. Contact lenses can have this effect, but it is extremely rare with proper fitting and follow-up. The most serious complication of contact lenses is infection. Once begun, an infection may lead to corneal ulceration, a condition in which the outermost surface of the eye becomes eroded and swollen. Corneal ulcers can be painful and difficult to treat; they may result in permanent scarring with resultant loss of vision. *A red, painful eye signals the need for immediate evaluation in any circumstance, but particularly in a patient wearing a contact lens.*

What is coming in the future?

In the short term, people who have undergone cataract surgery can expect considerable improvement. The uncorrected vision of these patients is so poor that they have great difficulty preparing, inserting, and removing contact lenses. Also, their vision with spectacles is so different from that with contact lenses that switching back and forth creates problems. One solution is to implant an artificial lens at the time the diseased one is removed—a procedure still under investigation. Space doesn't allow the pros and cons to be discussed here (see the chapter on cataracts), but the bottom line is that surgical implantation of a lens within the eye carries a definite risk, which is warranted in some instances but not in many others. In our judgment, a safer alternative is to devise a contact lens suitable for extended wear—one that doesn't have to be removed every night. Two types of lenses are currently under development for this purpose: gas-permeable lenses and soft lenses with a high water content. Results to date have been very promising; the lenses currently available are successful in 80% or more of patients.

New materials offer exciting prospects for the future. For example, we can foresee the appearance of inexpensive lenses that can be worn for a month or so and then simply thrown away.

And here is a more speculative possibility: instant contact lenses. Imagine a liquid polymer (plastic) available in a range of different viscosities. Conceivably, if we knew the curvature of a patient's cornea and the power of the lens required (easy information to obtain), we could select the appropriate polymer, put a drop of the material onto the eye, and watch it flow and harden into the shape of the desired lens.

On Surgery for Nearsightedness

The most common eye problems in this country involve so-called refractive errors—meaning that the front parts of the eye (cornea and lens) do not bend light rays correctly so as to focus them on the retina, the "film" at the back of the eye. If rays focus in front of the retina, the person tends to bring objects in closer and is said to be nearsighted; if rays focus behind the retina, the person will hold objects farther away and is labeled far-sighted.

Fortunately, both of these common problems are easily corrected with additional bending power placed in front of the cornea—either in the form of glasses or contact lenses. However, some are dissatisfied with these corrective approaches—because of vanity or inconvenience or strict occupational requirements for uncorrected vision. And in recent years, several operations to reshape the cornea—and thus to avoid the need for lenses—have been devised.

The operation recently introduced in this country for those who are nearsighted is known as a *radial keratotomy*—which involves making sixteen cuts in the cornea like spokes in a wheel pointing to the center. If all goes well, the cornea will flatten in the center as it heals, resulting in less bending of light rays and thereby correcting nearsightedness. However, most ophthalmologists—and several official study groups—have urged great caution in accepting this procedure on a widespread basis *until* long-term safety and effectiveness are established. And given the option of safe and effective alternatives, we agree with that caution.

Summer and Winter Safety

Lest we be accused of focusing on good-weather health problems out of a Boston-based envy of those who enjoy the warm out-of-doors year-round, we hereby go on record unequivocally as praising the health benefits that usually stem from recreation in the fresh, warm air. However, we gently and respectfully call your attention to a few tips to help ensure summertime health.

EXCESSIVE SUN EXPOSURE   Many a vacation has been ruined by over-exposure to the sun—not to mention that chronic ultraviolet light is a cause of premature skin aging and the development of skin cancers. Effective sunscreens retard these processes. Opaque white and tinted creams with titanium dioxide or zinc oxide are most effective and may be useful for particularly vulnerable areas such as the nose or lips, but most people prefer a cosmetically more attractive product. Many agents, all available without prescription, contain one or more light-absorbing chemicals. To be most effective, they should be applied one to two hours before exposure and then generously reapplied, particularly after swimming or sweating. Compounds containing glyceryl PABA (para-aminobenzoic acid) may cause rashes, and various PABA compounds may stain clothing.

Look for SPF (sun-protection factor) ratings on commercial sunscreens. The SPF is the time required to produce redness when the product is used *divided by* the time required when it is not used. SPF ranges from 2 (minimal protection) to 15 or more (super protection). Among the highly effective products currently available are Super Shade 15, Piz Buin Exclusiv Extrem Creme, and Total Eclipse (SPFs between 10 and 15); Eclipse, Pabanol, Piz Buin 6, and Pre-Sun have SPFs in the range of 6 to 12.

HEAT DISORDERS Truly excessive heat may pose specific problems. When exposed to excessive heat, the healthy person responds by sweating; the evaporation of sweat actually serves as our major cooling system. In addition, the blood vessels near the surface of the body automatically dilate to allow increased blood flow where surplus heat can be radiated to the outside world. Both of these events—sweating plus diversion of blood to skin vessels—can result in circulatory problems. Loss of salt and water through excessive sweating reduces overall blood volume. This, along with diversion of blood from vital organs (heart, brain, and kidneys) to the skin, can lead to dizziness and fainting. However, as long as the body contains enough fluid to sweat, it can withstand very high temperatures. *Therefore, the most important preventive step against heat disorders in the healthy person—aside from common-sense measures such as avoiding excessive activity and exposure during peak midday temperatures—is to drink plenty of fluids and sensibly increase the intake of salty food;* salt *tablets* should be considered only in the rare circumstance of heavy exertion by a person who has not been able to adjust to very hot, humid weather.

It is important to stress that some persons are at higher risk of developing problems during excessive heat—namely, the very young (who should not be overly wrapped in hot weather), the elderly, and those with certain chronic diseases such as diabetes and hardening of the arteries. Such persons must be especially careful about maintaining adequate salt and fluid intake. At the same time, it's worth pointing out that this can be tricky business for some patients with heart or kidney disorders—where salt and fluid supplementation should be planned with one's physician. Finally, the importance of acclimatization—gradually "breaking-in" to physical exertion in a hot environment—should be emphasized.

Typically, heat disorders fall into three categories which may overlap somewhat. These problems are likely to occur in the initial days of a heat wave before the body can adjust to the sudden rise in temperature. In order of increasing danger, they are:

(1) Heat cramps: These painful muscle spasms usually follow strenuous activity. While their exact cause is uncertain, the fact that such cramps respond to (and can be prevented by) salt and water intake strongly suggests that a chemical imbalance sets off the spasms.

(2) Heat exhaustion: Also known as "heat prostration," this condition can take several forms. Most typical is a fainting spell in the presence of profuse sweating—usually occurring when persons not acclimated to the heat stand for prolonged periods. (The classic example is the soldier who suddenly collapses while standing guard.) Other symptoms include headache, nausea, and tiredness. While persons who faint under any circumstances may temporarily appear to be seriously ill, those with heat collapse soon recover when placed head down and feet up in a cool place. Most important, persons suffering from heat exhaustion continue to sweat, indicating that their temperature control system is still intact.

(3) Heat stroke: Unlike the above, this rare occurrence represents a dire emergency that demands prompt treatment to prevent death. The underlying problem is gross malfunction of the heat regulation system of the body—as evidenced by the *absence of sweating*—which in turn leads to dangerously high internal body temperatures. Heat stroke almost always occurs when the humidity is high, and may be regarded as an end stage of prolonged heat exhaustion—with prior symptoms of dizziness, faintness, confusion, and abdominal upset. When collapse occurs, delirium, seizures, or prolonged unconsciousness may be observed. The very young and the elderly are most likely to be victims of heat stroke. *Persons found in a state of collapse and not sweating during hot weather should be brought immediately to an emergency room for treatment with intravenous fluids and ice water immersion.* Dousing with cold water or ice should occur en route, if possible.

Most persons who are healthy and who take common-sense precautions and increase salt and fluid intake should not experience serious difficulty during hot weather. Among the problems that can arise in others, the one requiring urgent attention is heat stroke—which should be suspected when collapse is accompanied by the absence of sweating.

INSECTS   These can be annoying at best—and potentially life-threatening at worst. More than twice as many persons are killed every year in this country by bites from hymenopterous insects (bees, wasps, hornets, and fire ants) as by snake bites. The vast majority of such deaths are caused by allergic reactions which usually occur within minutes. *Persons who have experienced serious aller-*

gic reactions to stings from such insects should have desensitiza-tion treatment from a competent allergist and should carry emer-gency sting kits (containing injectable epinephrine) during all times of possible exposure. Such kits should also be available for im-mediate use in places of public gathering—swimming pools, beach areas. Also, practical measures of insect avoidance should be prac-ticed—including wearing shoes, avoiding perfumes or other scented preparations, avoiding bright-colored objects or wool, suede, or leather-like apparel, using insect repellents for exposed body areas, and disposing of food and other items which might attract the little pests.

FOOD POISONING   Bacteria thrive and multiply in the presence of warmth plus food that they find nourishing. The latter is roughly equatable with "food that spoils." Custard, whipped cream, and but-ter are but a few of the many items that should either be kept cold or not brought along on picnics where they'll be sitting for many hours in the hot sun.

Another word on picnic foods: The Consumer Products Safety Commission reports that 32,000 persons were treated for pop bottle injuries during 1974. The Commission recommends the following preventive measures: storing pop (soda, tonic, soft-drink) bottles in cool places and on lower shelves; avoiding shaking or hitting bottles together; and pointing the cap away from the body or face when opening it.

LIGHTNING   The chances of lightning injury can be minimized by avoiding open areas and seeking indoor shelter or the inside of a closed car. Hiding under trees increases the chance of being struck—as does contact with metal objects. (Golfers beware!) If un-avoidably caught in the open, curl on the ground or squat with feet close together. (The reason for keeping the feet close together is to avoid something known as "stride potential"—the difference in elec-trical energy that might develop between legs when lightning strikes nearby—which produces electrical current between the two legs.) Best of all, pay attention to impending thunderstorms.

SWIMMER'S EAR   Medically known as "otitis externa," this trou-blesome problem is well-known during summertime when increased exposure to moisture causes maceration of the ear canal lining, a setting in which inflammation and infection easily occur. Treatment with appropriate ear drops is usually successful, though at times slow. More important is the prevention of such a problem—or its all too common recurrence. While all kinds of home remedies have been suggested for *preventing* swimmer's ear, we think the following advice is sound: after getting water in the ear—as during swimming or showering—put several drops of glycerin (obtained without prescription at a drugstore) in each ear and put in a small bit of cotton which should be removed after an hour. This will keep the canal dry in a non-irritating manner and decrease the possibility of infection for those chronically troubled with outer ear infections. (Eardrops should be avoided in the presence of a perforated eardrum.)

DIVING   Paralysis due to injury of the spinal cord in the neck—so frequently caused by diving in shallow water—is a tragedy that could usually be prevented by attention to the following common-sense rules:

(1) Never dive into unfamiliar water and don't assume that familiar lakes, rivers, and swimming holes have not changed water levels; always check by jumping *feet first* into the water before diving.

(2) Remember that a raft can be dangerous if it can drift; the anchor and cable holding the raft may be in the diving area.

(3) Remember that dangerous objects can be hidden by cloudy water.

(4) Avoid alcoholic beverages before swimming; alcohol can impair judgment.

WATERSKIING   A letter in a recent issue of the *New England Journal of Medicine* is entitled "The Water-Skier Seer Syndrome" and describes three cases of severe injury to persons assigned to a boat to watch the water skier. Looking backward from the front of the boat, these spotters could not see upcoming waves and were thrown overboard by unexpected bumps. Each sustained a propeller injury when the boat's driver instinctively turned it away from the side of the fall—which drove the blades directly into the victim. Moral: hang on when you look to the rear.

SURFBOARDING   A recent report from the University of Hawaii Medical School indicates that the risk of injury in surfboarding is approximately one per 17,500 surfing days, an incidence far below most sports—and another reason why we should all consider moving to Hawaii to take up surfing.

SCUBA DIVING   An issue of the *Journal of the American Medical Association* reported that there are about 4 million scuba divers in the U.S. and about 100 of them die of injuries each year. The most common contributing factor to serious injury stems from panic among the inexperienced—and the best safeguard by far is to use the buddy system.

HANG GLIDING   The same journal reported that hang gliding is far more hazardous for its much smaller group of devotees than is scuba diving. One survey reports 81 deaths during a recent three-year period.

SKATEBOARDING   The U.S. Consumer Product Safety Commission reports that skateboard injuries decreased by 38%—from 140,000 emergency room visits in 1977 to 87,000 in 1978. Good news for once. (But maybe it's because people have switched to roller skates?)

BIKING   Bicycles and shoulder bags can combine to produce a serious problem: if the person with the shoulder bag bends over the handlebars and the bag swings forward to get caught in the spokes, the rider can go head over heels. If a bag must be used, it should be safely secured to the body or bike.

In a letter to the *New England Journal of Medicine,* Dr. Thomas Converse of Minneapolis described a personal medical problem that developed during a bicycle tour—namely, the development of numbness, muscle weakness, and coordination loss in both hands. Dr. Converse's problem was ultimately traced to pressure on the ulnar nerve branches coursing through the palm of the hand—and the cycling doctor points out that some simple preventive measures might help avoid the problem. They are: using gloves, padding bike handlebars, changing hand positions frequently, and riding in the upright position (versus the bent-over racing position) to relieve palm pressure. This is one problem where the answer may indeed reside in the palm of our hand (our comment, not his).

TENNIS   Tennis balls hit at high speeds may cause serious eye damage. Recent reports describe various injuries (including detached retinas) from such a blow to the eye. Persons so afflicted should have a prompt and thorough eye exam by a competent specialist (followed by lessons from a competent teacher on how to play net). Also, special glasses are available to protect the eyes.

In the Good-Ol' Wintertime

Since we've included a section on summertime health problems, we feel it only fair to include a section on several winter problems that are potentially life-threatening.

ACCIDENTAL HYPOTHERMIA   The words literally mean low body temperature secondary to accidental exposure to cold temperatures—as might occur in a person trapped in a snowstorm. However, they have also come to refer to a situation where someone— usually an elderly person—reacts to only a moderate lowering of heat by developing an abnormally low body temperature. In many cases, there is clear evidence that the body's temperature-regulating system is not working correctly; on exposure to cold, such people do not shiver or turn pale (because of surface blood vessel constriction) as do most people. The problem may be further compounded in the elderly by the use of alcohol and phenothiazine tranquilizers.

The diagnosis of hypothermia has been traditionally hampered by two factors. First, the symptoms of hypothermia in the elderly— confusion, drowsiness, dizziness—may be easily misinterpreted to mean heart problems or a stroke. And second, until recently, body thermometers that record low temperatures were not readily available. Once hypothermia is diagnosed, it is critically important to treat it with gradual rewarming under carefully controlled medical supervision.

In brief, *when an elderly person exposed to cool temperatures (even in the low 60°sF) does not feel well or act right, think of the possibility of accidental hypothermia—a unique winter hazard for the senior citizen.*

FROSTBITE   Frostbite need not occur given common-sense prevention. And prevention is still best summarized by the adage known to every seasoned mountain climber: "Keep warm, keep moving, and keep dry." Outdoor warmth is best achieved by several layers of clothing topped with a windproof outer garment—as severe winds can make even above zero temperatures very dangerous.

The initial symptoms of mild frostbite are numbness, prickling, and itching. These symptoms are best treated by returning to a source of indoor heat as soon as possible. Under the rare circumstance of severe frostbite (no sensation, skin appears white or yellow), rewarming by immersion in water heated to no more than 108°F is advised. *Under no circumstances should damaged tissues be rubbed.*

Rewarming a frozen part can be hazardous if refreezing is likely, as the result can be even greater tissue damage. For example, the frostbitten mountain climber should be warmed definitively when shelter has been reached, not at the site of rescue. Medical attention should be sought as soon as possible.

SKIING   In *The Physician and Sportsmedicine,* Dr. Robert Mack, a team physician for the U.S. National Ski Team, decribed a method for testing binding release at home. Here it is, somewhat paraphrased:

For the toe release: With the ski boot on and inserted into the binding, you should bend your knee forward and inward, thus trapping the inner edge of your ski. You should then be able to cause your toe to release with further forceful internal rotation of the lower leg—that is, continuing to turn your knee inward.

For the heel release: With the ski flat on the floor and someone standing on the tail of the ski, you should be able to step forward with the other leg (no ski on) and pull the heel being tested upward enough with your own muscle strength to effect a heel release.

Since about 40% of ski injuries to the lower extremities are caused by faulty release of bindings, the time it takes to check them out would seem well spent.

CHOPPING WOOD   The U.S. Consumer Product Safety Commission indicates that about 50,000 persons are treated each year for chain-saw injuries and points out that the number of such injuries seems to be increasing as more and more persons turn to wood as a source of energy.

Travel Tips

Be it business or pleasure, Americans travel extensively to other countries. We have asked Dr. Peter Braun, a specialist in infectious disease and a member of our Advisory Board, to answer the most common health questions related to travel outside the United States.

What are the risks of intestinal illness during foreign travel?

Much depends on *where a person goes* and *what he or she consumes.* In some places, the incautious person has a good chance of developing diarrhea or other intestinal symptoms. Picturesque names, such as Delhi Belly, Montezuma's Revenge, and Aztec Two-Step, often characterize the problem and the region. Fortunately, the vast majority of these illnesses subside fairly quickly without any specific treatment. Only a small number of persons who develop diarrhea in a foreign country are infected with parasites, such as amebae, or dangerous bacterial organisms such as typhoid, but the diagnosis of these infections may require a level of laboratory expertise that is not available everywhere.

How can intestinal infections be prevented?

There is no one vaccine that can protect against the great variety of micro-organisms—bacterial, viral, and parasitic—that can cause diarrhea. We have vaccines for only a few of these, such as typhoid and cholera, and they are only partially effective. There is recent evidence suggesting that both doxycycline (one form of tetracycline) and Pepto Bismol are effective in preventing diarrhea caused by strains of the bacterium *E. coli,* known to be responsible for many

61

cases of travelers' diarrhea. *The most important point regarding protection is that all of the various infectious agents are destroyed by thorough cooking, and they are not apt to contaminate commercially bottled carbonated beverages.* Therefore, to be as safe as possible, one should stick to well-cooked foods, avoiding salads, raw vegetables, and unskinned fruits. If the quality of the drinking water is uncertain, it should not be used for brushing teeth or for making ice cubes that might be put into an otherwise safe drink. All these precautions should help, although in the end, there's no absolute guarantee.

How should diarrhea be treated if it occurs?

The best treatment is rest plus fluids, such as juices, carbonated beverages, and salt-containing clear soups to avoid dehydration. Stick to simple foods, such as toast and biscuits, until symptoms subside. For severe diarrhea, paregoric or tincture of opium can prove very useful, despite the theoretical concern that the infecting micro-organisms are not shed from the body as rapidly. For truly debilitating diarrhea, high fevers, or bloody stools, medical attention should be sought.

What about immunizations?

It is not generally realized that national public health regulations are primarily designed to keep certain diseases from entering various countries, rather than to protect the traveler from diseases already *in* those countries. Thus, the vaccinations may do more to "immunize" against delay at the borders than to protect against the health hazards one is likely to encounter. As most people now know, smallpox has been eradicated worldwide since the last case was recorded in October 1977 in East Africa. Smallpox vaccinations are no longer required in most parts of the world—including the United States. Complete and up-to-date information on immunizations is available in "Health Information for International Travel" from the Superintendent of Documents, U.S. Government Printing Office, Washington, D.C. 20402.

Is malaria still a problem?

Yes, the risk of malaria for unprotected travelers still exists in many parts of the world. Most of the infections are acquired in Africa, Asia (primarily India and Southeast Asia), Central America, and northern South America. There were approximately 500 cases of malaria, some of them fatal, brought into the United States from abroad in 1978. Ironically, there are no travel regulations here or in foreign countries which protect the traveler. Detailed information on specific risks—not only by location but by time of year—can be obtained in the publication described above. This can be vital because there *is* effective and easy preventive drug treatment for malaria that should be used. One must be aware that it is the mosquito that spreads the disease, and persons likely to have significant exposure (those camping out of doors in tropical regions, for example) should use insect repellent, protective clothing, and mosquito netting. But these measures can never be relied upon as foolproof prophylaxis. The Center for Disease Control recommends that the exposed traveler take chloroquine phosphate (which requires a physician's prescription) once a week beginning one week prior to arrival and continuing for six weeks after departure. Since malaria resistant to chloroquine is present in certain regions, especially Southeast Asia, Panama, and northern South America, travelers to these areas should consult a physician or the Center for Disease Control for more specific recommendations.

In summary, what should a traveler do in preparation for foreign travel?

The traveler who thinks about it far enough ahead of time can get a great deal of useful information from such publications as "Health Information for International Travel." Naturally, legal vaccination requirements must be met. In addition, anyone traveling to a developing or primitive region should be certain that he or she has been properly immunized against poliomyelitis, since the virus is still present in many parts of the world. I would recommend typhoid vaccine for persons going to areas where sanitation is poor. Similarly, there is a risk of acquiring hepatitis in areas where water and food purity is substandard; injections of gamma globulin are recommended for protection against this risk. In countries where it is recommended but not required, cholera vaccine should be given to persons who travel under primitive conditions where the disease is endemic. Most important, one should be prepared to limit one's intake to safe food and drink.

Finally, it's a good idea for a traveler to have a first aid kit with a few simple preparations. These include insect repellent and sunscreens or other skin preparations for those who are going to have significant outdoor exposure. Antihistamine drugs are very helpful for suppressing motion sickness. These antihistamines may also be quite useful for persons highly allergic to insect bites. Paregoric, Lomotil, or tincture of opium are recommended for diarrhea control. Persons with a cold who fly may develop very painful blockage of the ears, which can be prevented in many instances by decongestants.

Jet Lag and Body Rhythm

Scientific study clearly supports the fact of circadian (from the Latin *circa dies* meaning "about a day") body rhythms—that is, variations in many body functions during a 24-hour light/dark cycle. And, as anyone who has made a transcontinental flight or experienced an abrupt change in a job shift knows, it may be very difficult to adapt to a new light/dark cycle that varies by only a few hours.

The most obvious aberration of body rhythm usually occurs during sleep. Presumably, disruption of the REM (rapid eye movement) stage of sleep results in the tired, irritable feeling so well dramatized by TV ads. Unfortunately, sleeping pills often do not restore REM sleep and, therefore, are not terribly helpful. Other body functions, such as variation in body temperature (lowest at night, highest during day), heart rate, breathing rate, urination, hormone secretions, and so on must also adapt to a new time pattern.

The general rule (with enormous individual variation) is that it takes about a day of adaptation for each hour of time-zone change; thus, flying from one coast to another results in about three days of mild discombobulation for most people. If you are disciplined—and can accomplish it—you might "pre-adapt" for several days by going to bed an hour earlier for each hour lost going east—or an hour later for each hour gained going west. Persons with unusual medical problems or those taking special medications should check with their doctors regarding any particular precautions needed.

By the way . . . have a good time!

First Aid

First aid has often been presented as a complicated and technical subject to be mastered by a select few. "Critical care" of the seriously sick and injured *does* involve great skill and knowledge. But the basic principles of true first aid—the "treatment" literally given until further help can be obtained—can and should be reduced to a minimum that all can remember.

Collapse

The word "collapse" refers to situations in which people lose consciousness. The immediate cause of collapse is usually a diminished oxygen supply to the brain due to less oxygen in the blood or decreased blood flow. Decreased blood flow, in turn, may be the result of severe bleeding or trouble with the pumping system—the heart and blood vessels. Collapse is often the result of one of the following conditions:

(1) Fainting spell: This is the most common cause of collapse and occurs when the body responds to stimuli (usually emotional) with less blood flow to the brain. In this case, falling to the ground helps the situation by increasing blood flow to the brain (as does raising the person's legs). Spontaneous recovery should occur within minutes.

(2) Heart attack: A massive heart attack renders the heart muscle unable to pump blood to all parts of the body, including the brain. Interference with normal heart rhythm may lead to the same result.

(3) Stroke: This term refers to disruption of blood flow to the

66

brain due to problems (blockage or rupture) in a blood vessel in the neck or head. The net result is brain damage. Most strokes do not cause collapse but lead to less severe and more localized evidence of brain damage, such as loss of movement or speech.

(4) *Seizure:* Seizures are unique in this listing in that the dramatic loss of consciousness associated with some seizures is caused by internal "electrical" problems in the brain rather than decreased oxygen to the brain. However, prolonged seizures may interfere with oxygen delivery to the brain.

The above listing is only partial but indicates the kinds of events that can lead to collapse.

THE APPROACH   The key question in this simplified presentation is this: How can a non-medical person intelligently respond to a situation of collapse when there are so many possible causes? Fortunately, a diagnosis of the cause of collapse is not necessary to administer appropriate *first* aid. The major responsibility of anyone who encounters a collapsed individual is to *determine if the vital functions of unobstructed breathing and circulation are present.* If breathing or circulation are compromised, further action is necessary immediately since brain damage due to lack of oxygen can occur within minutes. So the next obvious question is this: *How can one determine the presence of adequate breathing and circulation in a collapsed individual?*

(1) *Breathing:* Often the sight of chest movement or the sound of air movement will provide the needed reassurance. However, if there is any question, breathing can be confirmed by the feel of exhaled breath against a hand held close to the mouth and nose. If gurgling noises are heard, an attempt should be made to clear the mouth of any obstructing material—secretions, dentures, and so on. (Choking requires special action and will be discussed in the next section.)

(2) *Circulation:* Determining whether the heart is pumping requires feeling a pulse beat—and that can be tricky in the collapsed individual. The best place to feel for the carotid artery pulse is in the neck on either side of the voicebox (see diagram). The technique involves gentle pressure with the middle three fingers placed vertically in the groove that runs up and down in the neck on either side of the

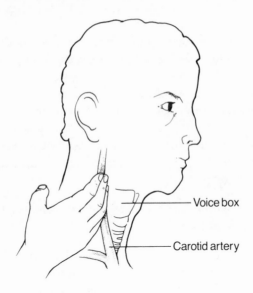

Adam's apple. Practice on yourself or a willing partner so you'll know how to do it in an emergency.

If unobstructed breathing and circulation are present, no further treatment is necessary other than the following measures:

(1) If the collapsed person is not horizontal (for example, remains slumped in a chair or toilet area), he or she should be moved to a flat position to improve circulation of blood to the brain. Raising the legs will also help to improve circulation to the brain.

(2) The collapsed person should also be rolled onto his side or stomach. Such a position prevents inhaling of vomitus into the lungs should vomiting occur—as it often does in situations of collapse. One easy way to accomplish the "rolling over" of even a large person is to "roll" one of the legs over the other.

If there are other signs of distress or prompt recovery does not occur, safe transportation to the nearest emergency room should be arranged. But as long as unobstructed breathing and circulation are intact, immediate action is not required.

THE TREATMENT   *If adequate breathing and circulation are absent,* cardio-pulmonary resuscitation (CPR) must be instituted without delay to prevent permanent brain damage. CPR is a specific method to provide ventilation to the lungs and at the same time keep blood circulating by repeated chest compression. This can be accomplished by a single person who has mastered CPR. The actual technique is relatively simple but *does require practice* on a mannequin under the tutoring of a qualified instructor. Local chapters of the American Heart Association offer courses for lay persons. Many studies now indicate that *lay people can make the difference between life and death* if they know how to give CPR.

CHOKING   Choking occurs when food or some other object gets stuck in the back of the throat or windpipe. *The hallmarks of choking are agitation and attempted speech but the inability to make voice sounds.* Often the person will point to his mouth or throat. In contrast, a person experiencing a heart attack may be agitated but is usually able to speak unless totally felled by the attack. One common set-up for choking is the person who is eating while drinking alcoholic beverages; the lessened coordination makes choking on food more likely—especially for the person with false teeth.

   Most choking incidents do not involve total blockage of the air passage. If the individual can be calmed down enough to breathe slowly, adequate air can be moved in and out to "buy time" to reach a hospital. If total blockage has occurred and the person turns blue and proceeds to total collapse, immediate action is necessary. This may include any or all of the following:

   (1) Sharp *back blows* with the heel of the hand are directed at the level of the spine between the shoulder blades. As many as 4 such blows are recommended; if possible, the victim's head should be below his chest so that gravity's force will help extrude the obstructing material. If the victim has become unconscious, he should be placed on his side (with his chest propped against the rescuer's thigh) before the back blows are delivered.

   (2) The *Heimlich Maneuver* has become the method of choice in most choking incidents (see diagram). The procedure involves standing behind the victim and applying up to 4 rapid squeezes (directed with a clenched fist) in an upward and inward direction to the center of the upper abdomen (below the lower-most tip of the breastbone). This pushes air out of the lungs with a sudden burst of pressure—thus attempting to pop out the blocking material much

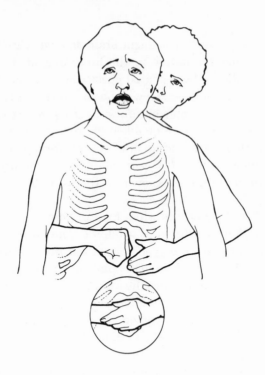

like a cork from a champagne bottle. This same pressure may be produced in someone lying on the ground by pushing forcefully in an inward and upward direction on the upper part of the abdomen. Theoretically, a person who is choking could perform this maneuver if alone by "throwing" his upper abdominal area against the edge of a table or other stable object.

(3) Devices to remove material from the back of the throat can be life-saving in trained hands. Many restaurants have such devices available. *However, blind and frantic attempts to reach into the back of the throat* should be avoided; too often such attempts merely serve to push the blocking material further down into the air passage.

Poisoning

Ingestion of harmful substances is an emergency that usually could have been prevented. Most accidental ingestions involve children, so the responsibility for prevention rests with adults. A tour of one's surroundings on hands and knees (mentally, at least) usually reveals surprising poisoning opportunities that can be rectified. Prevention and treatment include the following two measures:

(1) When moving into new living quarters, obtain the number of the nearest Poison Information Center from the local medical society or telephone company and post it by the telephone.

(2) Keep handy a bottle of Syrup of Ipecac. A tablespoonful will usually induce vomiting and is the first treatment in *most* poisonings; *adults* should drink six 8-ounce glasses of water in addition to ipecac because it works best when the stomach is full. Syrup of Ipecac can be obtained without prescription and is often given free by drug stores. However, *always check with a Poison Information Center before actually giving Syrup of Ipecac.* Some substances—such as acids, lyes, petroleum products—should *not* be treated by induced vomiting.

Burns

The first aid of burns boils down to "the less the better"—which is a way of saying that butter, grease, or other creams are of no value. Cold compresses or actual immersion in cold water (until the pain is gone) will relieve the pain of a burn and may minimize the extent of injury. Any burn which involves more than first degree damage (that is, more than the redness of a sunburn) or that involves a critical area of function or appearance (such as face, hands, or joints) should be evaluated by a competent medical person.

There is, however, one type of burn which requires immediate action even before seeking medical advice—namely a *chemical burn* produced by corrosive substances. Such burns should be treated by *rinsing with as much water as possible as quickly as possible.* If clothing is involved, remove it *while rinsing with water.* If the eyes or mouth are involved, get water into these areas in any way possible. One should rinse with copious amounts of water for at least fifteen minutes before worrying about calling for help. And the answer is water—not other liquids which might counteract the corrosive.

Bleeding

The true first aid of bleeding is quite simple—direct pressure on the site of bleeding. Information concerning tourniquets or pressure points may be useful to the professional, but *direct pressure applied to the bleeding site with the cleanest material available* is adequate to stop all but the most massive kind of bleeding. Two points should be stressed:

(1) Sterile materials are not necessary, though the cleaner the material used to apply direct pressure, the better. In a true emergency, anything will do—clothing, towels, and so on.

(2) To be effective, pressure must be continuously applied for at least ten minutes *by the clock.* To be honest, the exact amount of time will vary in given situations, but ten minutes is a good minimum to remember. If bleeding starts when pressure is removed, quickly reapply for at least another ten minutes. Most nosebleeds can be stopped in the same way with continuous pinching of the nose for ten minutes by the clock.

Transportation to medical care should be undertaken after an attempt has been made to control bleeding. Obviously, pressure may be applied en route.

Cuts

There is probably no more common dilemma in the household inhabited by young active children than this: "Should I take Johnny to the doctor?" The ultimate answer has to be, "If in doubt, check it out." But short of that, there are some guidelines that suggest when medical attention might be needed:

(1) *If the cut results in skin edges that pull apart rather than fall easily together.* Such wounds, if left to heal by themselves, not only run a higher risk of infection—since the underlying tissue is no longer covered by nature's greatest barrier to infection, the skin—but they will "fill in" with scar tissue rather than normal skin.

(2) *If the cut is in a cosmetically sensitive area, such as the face.* Again, the purpose of stitches for even small cuts in such areas is to minimize scarring.

(3) *If the cut is in an area of movement*—such as over or near a

joint. The movement will continually pull open the skin edges and delay healing.

(4) If the cut is "dirty" or if it is caused by an animal (or human) bite. (Here stitches are usually not advisable.)

(5) If movement or sensation is lost—suggesting an underlying tendon or nerve injury.

If there is any chance that medical care might be necessary, evaluation should be sought as soon as possible. After 6–8 hours contamination might make it necessary to forgo stitches and keep the wound open for secondary healing by scar formation.

Sprains

The term "sprain" is used when the stretching (or tearing) of joint ligaments—the fibrous bands that hold bones together—is suspected. (The word "strain" is more appropriately used for the stretching or tearing of a muscle.) The usual response to a sprain is pain and swelling of the affected joint. And the best first aid—at least until the degree of sprain can be determined—is *ice, elevation, and no weight bearing.* The ice and elevation will help reduce swelling and pain; staying off the joint will prevent further damage. If, after twenty-four hours of conservative treatment, no swelling or distress is apparent, gradual return to weight bearing and use is usually safe. However, if distress persists, a medical evaluation should be sought.

In cases of severe ankle sprain accompanied by pain and marked swelling and bruising, the use of "stress" x-rays should be considered if routine x-rays are negative. Stress x-rays may require some form of anesthesia to eliminate pain and muscle spasm, to allow stretching of the joint in a manner simulating the actual injury. X-rays taken when the foot is held in this position may demonstrate abnormal movement between the bones of the ankle—indicating stretched or completely torn ligaments. Such damaged ligaments must be treated either by immobilization in a plaster cast or, in the presence of severe tears, by surgical repair to avoid permanent instability of the ankle joint. *The moral:* severe ankle injuries should be examined by stress films if fractures are not demonstrated on routine x-rays.

Hazards of Living

MYTH 2

*A bare head and wet feet increase
your chances of getting a cold.*

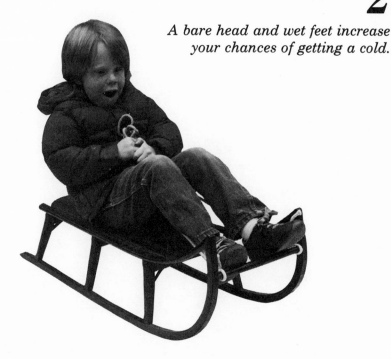

Smoking

It is an unequivocal fact that cigarette smoking is this nation's number one injurious personal habit. Smokers expose themselves to over 1,000 different chemicals each time they light up, increasing the risk of:

Lung cancer: Up to a 20 times greater chance that heavy smokers will develop this number one cancer killer, versus non-smokers—not to mention an increased chance of developing *mouth, lip, voicebox, pancreas, and urinary bladder cancer.*

Heart attack: A two to three times greater chance of dying from a heart attack than a non-smoker—and given the fact that more than 600,000 Americans die of a heart attack each year, doubling or tripling the risk is no small item. The exact reasons for this association are not clear but most experts agree that carbon monoxide (which decreases the amount of oxygen the blood can carry) is a major contributor.

Stillbirths and sick infants: A twofold increase in risk for spontaneous abortions (miscarriages) in smoking mothers. Children born to smoking mothers weigh 200 grams less on average than children born to non-smokers. And studies in Britain and Israel show that infants of mothers who smoke are more likely to be admitted to the hospital during the first year of life for bronchitis or pneumonia.

Wrinkles: Dermatologists are starting to report observations that women who smoke are more likely to develop facial wrinkles as they grow older; this may be the most convincing argument for those who tend to worry more about how they look than about how they feel.

Money up in smoke: The cost of a two-pack-a-day habit now approaches $600 a year—enough to buy two tailor-made suits or a week at a resort.

Etc.: Not to mention a decreased sense of smell and taste, a constant cough, an increased chance of dying in bed from a fire, a tell-tale odor on clothes and breath and in the home and car, etc., etc., etc.

DOES IT PAY TO QUIT?   That question is often asked by a smoker seeking motivation to fight the cigarette habit. And it is eloquently answered by Dr. Richard V. Ebert of the University of Minnesota in the November 10, 1978, issue of the *Journal of the American Medical Association*—in an article worth reading in its entirety. Dr. Ebert summarizes some of the pertinent findings of the now classic report of Doll and Peto who followed 34,000 British physicians for 20 years to determine the effects of smoking—and to measure the results in those who quit. Among the more pertinent findings:

(1) The annual death rate for cancer of the lung in physicians who continued to smoke cigarettes was 16 times that of lifetime non-smokers. The death rate for those who had successfully broken the habit for 5 to 9 years was only six times that for non-smokers. And those who had not smoked for more than 15 years had a death rate from lung cancer only twice that of non-smokers.

(2) Relatively few cancers occurred in those who had smoked cigarettes for less than 20 years; *after 20 years of smoking, cancer rates rose rapidly.*

(3) Persons who ceased smoking before 54 years of age had a lower death rate from coronary artery disease than those who continued. Quitting after age 54 did not affect the death rate from coronary artery disease.

Ebert concludes that "there is overwhelming evidence of the danger of smoking after the age of 40 years." He goes on to suggest that we should concentrate our efforts to help people stop smoking on the middle-aged smoker who has been smoking for less than 20 years. Do you qualify? If you would like information on how to stop smoking, contact your local American Cancer Society office or write to the Office on Smoking and Health, Room 158, Park Building, 5600 Fishers Lane, Rockville, Maryland 20857.

(Incidentally, the results from a 1975 survey of smoking habits, when compared to a similar survey in 1967, indicate that the proportion of physicians who smoke dropped from 30% to 21%; dentists, from 34% to 23%; and pharmacists from 35% to 28%.)

Cigarette Advertising

By now, most people have been exposed to the content of the Surgeon General's report on smoking—probably to the point of boredom. Our Advisory Board goes on record as supporting any reasonable effort—even the publication of a 1200-page government document—that might aid persons in stopping a habit so clearly injurious to their health. However, we would also seize this opportunity to point out that the most effective tactics in the war on smoking are those designed to prevent young people from starting in the first place—versus those addressed to a lifelong struggle against tobacco addiction. We have no quarrel with the "right" of a consenting adult to engage in hazardous living—as long as that choice does not infringe on the rights of others. (Some would argue, of course, that smoking does just that—in terms of both personal annoyance and health costs.) However, we would point out that the combination of seductive advertising and enormous peer pressure often makes the choice of a teenager less than truly informed. Therefore, we respectfully call upon appropriate government officials to move vigorously to accomplish the following:

(1) Programs that reduce the availability of tobacco to minors.
(2) Elimination of *all* advertising that presents smoking in an enticing manner and an intensification of educational programs to portray the often horrible results of smoking.

We are realistic enough to know that tobacco will not be eliminated from the face of the earth. However, we feel it *is* appropriate to protect those whose choices are not entirely informed. We think it proper to protect our young from fire, malnutrition, and alcohol. Why not tobacco?

WHO'S COME A LONG WAY?   Some alarming statistics have emerged from the Connecticut Cancer Epidemiology Unit. Between

1945 and 1949—when male smokers predominated—lung cancer in men was almost five times greater than in women in Connecticut. By 1974, the ratio had dropped to less than two to one. And in 1975, for the first time, there were more cases of lung cancer in women than in men in the age group 35–44.

What makes this report even more frightening is some evidence that women smokers are more susceptible to lung cancer than men smokers. The Third National Cancer Survey indicated that women who smoke heavily have a 16 times greater chance of getting lung cancer than women non-smokers—versus an increased risk of ten-fold between comparable male groups.

Surveys continue to show that while the proportion of male smokers is declining, more women are smoking. Unless this pattern changes, it seems that those who predict a new lung cancer epidemic secondary to increased numbers of women smokers are going to be tragically correct. This killer disease, which now strikes more than 100,000 new victims each year in this country, will claim even more—as women pay the price for lighting up.

A Safe Cigarette? Not a Safe Bet

Nearly half of American billboards advertise cigarettes—most of them low-tar, low-nicotine brands. The unstated implication of this enormous campaign is that lowering the tar and nicotine delivery of cigarettes makes them safer. The public appears to be buying this message and the cigarettes: Americans smoked 620 billion cigarettes in 1979 (up 5 billion from the year before) and 43% of these were low-tars.

The evidence that "old-time" cigarettes have been killing smokers is rock-solid. The average male smoker loses six to eight years of life from his habit. For women, the statistics are only slightly less alarming, and the picture is becoming worse as more women with a long-term, heavy habit reach the age at which they must pay its full price. But the question now being asked by scientists and smokers alike is this: Are the new cigarettes really safe—or at least safer than brands that are higher in tar and nicotine?

WE'D RATHER SWITCH THAN DIE   Several studies of people who switched to filter-tips from the high-tar brands smoked during the 1940s and 1950s have shown that filter smokers ran a slightly smaller risk of lung cancer (and probably heart disease) than those stubborn individuals who stayed with older smokes. However, the two groups of smokers are not strictly comparable; those who switched to filters were self-selected and they may have been puffing or inhaling less to begin with. Therefore, these studies cannot be taken as conclusive proof that switching to a filtered brand was what made the difference.

In theory, switching to low-tar, low-nicotine cigarettes should be protective because it has been pretty well established that the danger of smoking is proportional to the amount of inhaled tar and nicotine (plus carbon monoxide, a component that is harder to reduce). People who smoke ten cigarettes a day are at lower risk than those who smoke twenty and so forth. But there are some practical problems with the theoretical advantage:

(1) Tar and nicotine delivery is measured by machine. The method is not completely standardized, and different types of cigarettes may not be accurately compared. Smokers can easily get more than the official amount of tar and nicotine from a cigarette, and many of them undoubtedly do.

(2) There is good reason to believe that smokers who switch to cigarettes with less tar and nicotine compensate by smoking more cigarettes, inhaling more deeply, or puffing more often.

(3) The "tar" produced by newer brands is not necessarily the same as that from heavier types. It *could* contain higher amounts of the most dangerous components. Data on this point are hard to obtain and, once available, will probably be even harder to interpret.

HOOKED ON NICOTINE   Why do some smokers who switch to lower-tar brands defeat their own purpose by inhaling more smoke? For most of them, the reason appears to be addiction to nicotine. Whatever psychological reasons there may be for cigarette use, the fact is that as many as 95% of smokers are physiologically dependent to some degree on the nicotine they inhale. They suffer discomfort and craving when deprived of it.

Nicotine is most addicting when it is inhaled into the lungs, and less so when absorbed from the lining of the nose and mouth, as occurs with cigar or pipe smoke, chewing tobacco, or snuff. With each puff of cigarette smoke, blood in the lungs is loaded with a high concentration of the drug, which is then carried to the brain in seven seconds without further dilution (Heroin shot into a vein in the forearm takes fourteen seconds, and it is diluted along the way.) Cigar and pipe smokers, chewers, and snuffers do not get equally high doses of nicotine delivered with such rapidity.

After months to years, the addicted cigarette smoker has need for high levels of nicotine in portions of his or her brain. Inhaling is the most efficient way to get this effect. But nicotine also produces unpleasant symptoms, such as nausea and wooziness, when blood levels get too high. Smokers thus have a difficult balancing act to perform. They want the pleasant sensation that a rush of nicotine provides them and they want to prevent withdrawal, but they don't want to overdose and get sick. With experience, the majority of smokers can tolerate high levels of nicotine in the blood, but all of them have their limits. Most smokers take 200 to 300 puffs a day, and with all that practice they become adept at regulating their nicotine intake.

The most powerful incentive to smoke, for someone who has been smoking a few years, is preventing withdrawal. Indeed, smokers find a cigarette "relaxing" largely because it reverses the irritability of beginning withdrawal. When they go without their cigarettes for very long, they begin to complain of jumpiness and craving followed by nausea, headache, constipation or diarrhea, and other physical symptoms. Many of them gain weight. At the same time, brain wave patterns change, levels of certain hormones fall, heart rate slows, and blood pressure goes down. Inability to concentrate is a very common subjective complaint and it may persist for weeks or months. When smokers who are abstaining are given tasks that require vigilance or tracking, they perform less well than when they are smoking—objective evidence that the difficulty in concentrating is real.

Although these symptoms often abate during the first ten days of not smoking, some of them (such as drowsiness, difficulty with concentration, and craving) may become worse about two weeks after quitting. According to one study, craving continues for as *long as five to nine years* in about one-fifth of reformed smokers. This means that smokers who quit are extremely vulnerable to relapse.

THE ROLE OF LOW-TARS   Do low-nicotine, low-tar cigarettes help people quit by "tapering off"? There is little evidence on this point to date, but one group of investigators has recently reported that quitting cold-turkey (perhaps after a bit of psychological preparation) is more effective than tapering the habit, presumably because exposure to a little nicotine from time to time makes withdrawal worse. In other words, it is *possible* that using low-nicotine cigarettes to help "cut down" actually prevents some people from quitting altogether.

Worse yet, the new cigarettes are undoubtedly helping a whole new group of people to get hooked. It is well known that the number of adolescent girls and young women who smoke has been increasing in the past ten years. A major reason for this trend appears to be the availability of low-tar cigarettes. Females, according to a recent study, are more sensitive than males to the unpleasant side-effects of nicotine. Given access to low-nicotine cigarettes it is easy for them to begin smoking in response to social pressure, the desire to look grown-up, and so forth. In time as they become tolerant to nicotine they may well switch to the heavier brands, which are still available.

This turn of events is particularly tragic when the young woman becomes pregnant. Infants of smoking mothers are born smaller and run a higher risk of death before or at birth. Their deliveries are sometimes more complicated. Children of mothers who smoked during pregnancy *may* have impaired growth and development. As children exposed to a smoking parent, they may also suffer more respiratory disease than children of non-smokers, as well as subtle but measurable damage to their lungs. Finally, when they approach adulthood, they are at a higher risk of becoming smokers themselves.

In short, *the overall value of the new low-tar, low-nicotine cigarettes to health is highly questionable.* Using them may prevent some people who would otherwise quit from doing so. We can expect that many people who are addicted to nicotine will either find the new cigarettes unsatisfying or will smoke them more heavily than their old brands—with results that cannot be foreseen.

Smokers who are concerned about their health should make every attempt to quit. A period of tapering (to cut out the day's "extra" or "unnecessary" cigarettes) may help, but sooner or later a cold-turkey decision has to be made. The real difficulty though is not quitting. Just as for the alcoholic, the challenge comes weeks to months later, when the temptation to try "just one" arises. About 75 percent of the people who manage to quit eventually fail to stay off cigarettes, largely because of the temptation to smoke "just one" some time later.

Smokers who believe they are incapable of quitting might, in theory, benefit from smoking cigarettes that are relatively *high* in nicotine (to satisfy craving) and low in tar (to reduce risk). As a rule, the two components rise and fall together, but a few low-tar brands are higher in nicotine than their competitors. However, there is simply no guarantee that these are the "safest" brands, especially as the role of nicotine in causing disease has not been determined.

IN CONCLUSION   Inhaled nicotine is powerfully addicting. Almost all smokers begin their habit during adolescence and unfortunately the earlier they start, the heavier the habit. For this reason, the greatest effort of any anti-smoking campaign should be to prevent teenagers from starting. Education is important. More stringent legal restrictions, such as banning cigarette machines and increasing the penalties for selling cigarettes to minors should be considered. The value of low-tar, low-nicotine cigarettes is questionable, especially in view of their role in helping girls to become addicted; policies encouraging their use should therefore be re-examined.

Is the Smoke of Others Dangerous?

That question is among the more emotional issues faced by our society. And to date, the scientific answers have been scanty and frustratingly difficult to come by. There is no evidence that exposure to the smoke of others actually *causes* serious diseases of the lungs or heart. However, the March 27, 1980, issue of the *New England Journal of Medicine* carries a study of 2,100 workers demonstrating that healthy non-smokers chronically exposed to the smoke of others had a measurable change in two lung function tests similar to that of those who inhale between one and ten cigarettes per day. In an accompanying editorial, two scientists from the National Institutes of Health praise this study as providing for the first time a quantitative measurement of a physical change in healthy non-smokers exposed to the smoke of others. They conclude that the study "constitutes a foundation to be used by health planners and legislative bodies to stimulate the search for a public policy that is not only equitable but based on irrefutable scientific evidence."

PASSIVE SMOKING AND ANGINA   In a study at the Long Beach VA Hospital in California, ten males with known exertional angina (the development of chest pain during exercise) were tested to see how long it would take to develop pain during measured exercise *before* and *after* exposure to the cigarette smoke of others. The "after" testing took place after sitting in a room (11.5 by 10.5 feet) for two hours, during which time 15 cigarettes were smoked by three other persons (five each). The results were clearly significant: it took an average of 22% less time to develop chest pain after exposure if the room was ventilated and 38% less time after exposure in an unventilated room. In other words, chest pain developed considerably sooner during exercise after being in the smoke-filled room. (Resting heart rates and blood pressure were also increased after exposure.)

These results do not indicate that passive smoking *causes* heart disease, but they do suggest that persons with known exertional angina are adversely affected by exposure to the smoke exhaled by others.

Alcoholism

Consider that half of all deaths in automobile accidents, half of all homicides, and a fourth of all suicides are related to alcohol abuse; that persons with a "drinking problem" are seven times more likely to be separated or divorced than those in the general population; that the total annual cost of alcohol abuse in this country may approach 5 *billion* dollars; that an alcoholic's life span is shortened (on average) by 10–12 years; and that *at least* ten million persons in this country abuse alcohol. No wonder some have labeled alcoholism the most devastating socio-medical problem faced by human society short of war and malnutrition. It is obviously worth asking these questions: Why do so many in our society become alcoholics? How can one identify or even predict a "drinking problem"? What are the biological effects of alcohol? What are the best methods of solving a drinking problem?

DEFINITIONS   When experts attempt to define "alcoholism," as many definitions as experts usually emerge. Some argue the relative merits of biological ("it is a disease") versus social or psychological ("it is a behavior disorder") theories, but most settle for descriptive definitions—such as this one from the Rutgers University Center of Alcohol Studies: "An alcoholic is one who is unable consistently to choose whether he shall stop or not." Ultimately, all will agree to descriptive definitions which point out that for the person with a serious drinking problem, tremendous disruptions occur in health, interpersonal relationships, and the basic activities of life—eating, sleeping, and working.

THE EFFECTS   Whatever the root causes of excessive alcohol intake, the effects on the human body are well documented and potentially devastating. The following list is only partial—but clear enough to establish that large amounts of alcohol are not good for the biological machine that must receive, distribute, and eliminate this chemical known as ethyl alcohol (ethanol):

(1) Liver damage: Four to five drinks daily for several weeks result in increased accumulation of fat in liver cells. This early stage of liver change is not harmful and is completely reversible with abstinence. A more serious type of liver disease is known as *alcoholic hepatitis*—an inflammation of liver tissue with actual destruction of its cells. While there is some debate about the continued progression to the irreversible stage of liver disease known as *cirrhosis,* there is no question that cirrhosis will develop in about 15% of heavy drinkers. Cirrhosis, in turn, leads to severe complications (intestinal bleeding, kidney failure, fluid accumulations, and so on) and eventual death if drinking is not stopped in time.

(2) Other gastrointestinal disorders: Alcoholics have a much higher incidence of *peptic ulcers* and *pancreatitis* (inflammation of the pancreas) than non-alcoholics. In addition, many suffer from repeated episodes of nausea, vomiting, and abdominal distress—most often due to superficial *gastritis* (inflammation of the lining of the stomach).

(3) Nervous system damage: Well-known are the acute problems of *intoxication* and (in the physically addicted person) *withdrawal*—including the DTs (delirium tremens) which leads to death in about 10% of cases. Alcoholism also contributes to permanent damage to the brain and peripheral nerves. Among such chronic effects are *Wernicke's disease* (rapid mental deterioration, paralysis of eye movements, stumbling gait); *polyneuropathy* (loss of sensation and strength due to nerve damage); and *cerebellar degeneration* (degeneration of the part of the brain controlling stance and balance). A recent report from Denmark (*Lancet,* October 13, 1979) suggests that intellectual impairment may be a serious problem for the younger alcoholic. The Danish study involved measurements of intellectual functions and liver damage in 37 alcoholic men under age 35 in whom no other explanation for possible brain damage could be found. Nineteen percent of the group turned out to have cirrhosis, but 59% showed signs of intellectual impairment on standard testing (memory, concentration, comprehension) with 11 of the

37 showing enough impairment to be described as "occupationally disabled." The researchers concluded their report with this chilling statement: "Disabling intellectual impairment may be the earliest complication of chronic alcoholism and may arise early in the alcoholic career."

(4) *Heart disease:* Despite recent information suggesting a possible beneficial effect of small amounts of alcohol on coronary artery circulation, there is little doubt that large amounts of alcohol can damage heart muscle directly—a disease described as *alcoholic cardiomyopathy.*

(5) *Sugar and fat metabolism:* When liver supplies of glycogen (a storage form of sugar) are depleted—as occurs in malnourished alcoholics—alcohol ingestion can lead to hypoglycemia (low blood sugar). Alcohol also produces elevated levels of blood fats—especially triglycerides and very low density lipoproteins. These elevated fats contribute to the "fatty liver" described earlier.

(6) *Other metabolic changes:* The oxidation of excessive alcohol (90% of which occurs in the liver) can lead to severe *metabolic acidosis* due to the accumulation of excessive acids in the body. Chronic alcohol ingestion causes proliferation of liver enzymes that inactivate drugs and other substances which may result in disordered drug metabolism, and it also reduces the amount of circulating testosterone. This may be responsible for the feminization observable in many male alcoholics. Alcohol also affects both red and white blood cells, contributing, respectively, to problems of anemia and infection.

(7) *Drug interactions:* The Food and Drug Administration estimates that 2,500 deaths (most *not* intentional) occur each year in this country because of interaction between alcohol and other drugs—not surprising, given the fact that half of the one hundred most frequently prescribed medicines in this country have at least one ingredient known to interact adversely with alcohol. For example, alcohol enhances the effect of many drugs taken for high blood pressure, with the potential danger of a sudden drop in pressure that might cause loss of consciousness. Many antihistamines and tranquilizers combine with alcohol to produce a potentially serious loss of judgment and alertness; a strong sleep medicine, when mixed with alcohol, can produce coma.

(8) *Fetal alcohol syndrome:* The April 5, 1976, issue of the

Journal of the American Medical Association described 41 infants born to mothers who had abused alcohol during their pregnancies; the label "fetal alcohol syndrome" was used to describe the many physical and mental defects noted in these infants—and the syndrome has since become well known and widely recognized. No one knows for sure just how much alcohol consumption during pregnancy can increase the risk for birth defects, but some experts suggest that more than two drinks per day (of *any* kind of alcoholic beverage) can lead to an increased chance for this syndrome. Obviously, the safest choice is not to drink at all during pregnancy.

The list could go on, but the above is enough to indicate that excessive consumption of alcohol eventually demands payment—sometimes permanent—from our bodies.

CAUSES   As with many of the complex "abuse" problems of modern times (whether the object of abuse be food, heroin, or alcohol), the search for causes generally leads in three directions:

(1) Biological: While a great deal has been learned about the metabolism of ethanol (the type of alcohol found in alcoholic beverages), there is still no good evidence that persons with a drinking problem consistently demonstrate biological differences that separate them from others. It is known that alcoholics metabolize alcohol a little faster than persons not addicted to alcohol. There are also some identifiable physiological effects of excessive consumption—such as the development of physical dependence which leads to withdrawal symptoms on abstinence. Some intriguing studies of adopted children indicate an inherited tendency toward alcohol abuse. For example, one survey of 133 Scandinavian men raised by foster parents showed that sons with biological fathers who were alcoholics were four times as likely to become alcoholics themselves as were sons of non-alcoholic biological fathers. But despite these pieces of evidence, few are prepared to state that alcoholics are biologically destined to become so.

(2) Behavioral: Though it is tempting to judge alcoholics as "weaker" and "without will power," the evidence argues otherwise. Many alcoholics function remarkably well during periods of abstinence. Only about 5% of all persons with a drinking problem fit the

skid-row stereotype. It is true that alcoholics in general have a higher rate of other psychological disorders (particularly manic-depressive illness) and that their drinking problem may eventually lead to tragic disorder in their emotional lives. But it would be a great oversimplification to blame alcoholism on personality deficiencies.

(3) Social: Some feel that the serving of liquor has become the event itself in much of our social life. Sociologists have long been intrigued by national differences in the handling of liquor. For example, both Italy and Israel have low rates of alcoholism; in these societies, drinking is culturally accepted as a companion to socializing—rather than as the occasion itself.

TREATMENT   If an alcoholic does not stop drinking, he or she too often ends up in one of three places—prison, an institution for emotional disorders, or the morgue. Therefore, urgent attempts to cure the problem are understandable. However, given the complexity of the root causes of alcoholism, it is probably misleading to talk about "treatment" in the traditional medical sense of that word—a pill or procedure that will predictably cure the disease. Indeed, it is not surprising that many different approaches to problem drinking have been and are being used. Whatever the approach, all experts agree that *the chance for success is directly proportional to the degree to which a person is willing to acknowledge that he or she has a drinking problem—in short, to be able to admit to being an alcoholic.* Once this plateau of self-honesty has been reached, any or all of the following approaches may have a useful role:

(1) Aversion therapy: This approach is based on associating miserable physical reactions with alcohol by the supervised injection of emetine (which causes severe nausea and vomiting) and the ingestion of alcohol over a period of days; the goal is to induce a long-term aversion to alcohol. While still employed, aversion therapy has never become widely popular—in part because of cost and in part because of the "aversion" of many to this approach.

(2) Antabuse: Many are often surprised to hear that there is a pill available for the treatment of alcoholism. Disulfiram is the generic name for a drug (often better known by one of its trade names, Antabuse) that has been available for over thirty years. It acts by interrupting the body's metabolism of alcohol, leading to the build-

up of another chemical, acetaldehyde. This, in turn, makes the person who consumed the alcohol wish he or she had never taken a drink. The nature of the reaction varies, but usually includes headache, nausea, and vomiting; in more severe cases, breathing difficulty, chest pain, and dizziness are experienced. Therefore, the treatment involves taking a daily oral dose of Antabuse. Some alcoholics have done this for over twenty years, knowing that any subsequent drinking will cause them to feel very ill.

Not all alcoholics are candidates for this treatment method. A commitment to stop drinking is required; daily Antabuse is most useful in the person who does not plan to drink but is susceptible to impulse or spree drinking. Some people—such as those with serious heart or liver disease—cannot tolerate the potential reaction to the drug. But Antabuse should be strongly considered as one of many possible methods of helping an alcoholic return to a normal life.

(3) Psychotherapy: Classical "talking-it-out" may be helpful for some, but most experts minimize the practical role of this time-consuming and expensive approach for the majority of alcoholics.

(4) Industrial programs: Many private and public clinics for alcoholics claim excellent success rates. One of the most exciting developments in the last decade has been the increasing involvement of industry in treatment programs for employees. There is solid evidence to suggest that the threat of losing one's job is an excellent inducement to solving a drinking problem—as is the threat of any significant loss, such as divorce or institutionalization.

(5) Alcoholics Anonymous: Although it is not the answer for all who are in need, this remarkable organization has supplied more help and "caring curing" to alcoholics than any other method or treatment available; in part, this can be attributed to its sheer pervasiveness—over a million members organized into more than 28,000 groups which meet throughout the week in convenient locations at no cost. No one pretends to understand the full genius of this movement, but most suggest that the example and involvement of persons who are themselves alcoholics—and willing to admit it—brings a degree of unique authenticity and understanding to the person wanting help. As the Big Book, the "bible" of A.A., puts it: "Most of us sense that it is a real tolerance of other people's shortcomings and viewpoints (and) a respect for their opinions and attitudes which make us more useful to others. Our very lives, as ex-problem drinkers, depend upon our constant thought of others and how we may help meet

their needs." Members of A.A. are immediately available on a 24-hour basis to those seeking help. Persons of all backgrounds are welcome and many meeting groups are set up for those with common interests.

SUMMARY   The key to recovery from alcoholism is a willingness to acknowledge the problem. Once this stage of awareness is reached, many approaches to the prevention of further drinking are available. The vast majority of people with extensive experience in treating alcoholism agree that those afflicted can never resume drinking even small amounts of alcohol without great risk of again drinking out of control.

Could You Be in Danger?

The key to a successful solution for a drinking problem is a willingness to admit to being an alcoholic. The following questions (reprinted with permission from Ayerst Laboratories) are recommended as a means of self-testing for a drinking problem:

EARLY SYMPTOMS   (the first stage of alcoholism)

Yes   *No*

____ ____   Are you beginning to lie or feel guilty about your drinking?

____ ____   Do you gulp your drinks?

____ ____   Must you drink at certain times—for example, before lunch or a special event; after a disappointment or a quarrel?

____ ____   Do you drink because you feel tired, depressed, or worried?

____ ____   Are you annoyed when family or friends talk about your drinking?

____ ____   Are you beginning to have memory blackouts and occasional passouts?

MIDDLE SYMPTOMS   (an extension of early symptoms)

Yes   *No*

____ ____   Are you making more promises and telling more lies about your drinking?

____ ____   Are there more times when you need a drink?

____ ____ When sober do you regret what you have said or done while drinking?

____ ____ Are you drinking more often alone, avoiding family or close friends?

____ ____ Do you have weekend bouts and Monday hangovers?

____ ____ Have you been going "on the wagon" to control your drinking?

____ ____ Are memory blackouts and passouts becoming more frequent?

LATE SYMPTOMS   (the advanced stage of alcoholism)

Yes No

____ ____ Do you drink to live and live to drink?

____ ____ Are you obviously drunk on important occasions—for example, a special dinner or meeting?

____ ____ Do your drinking bouts last for several days at a time?

____ ____ Do you sometimes get the "shakes" in the morning and think it helps to take a "quick one"?

____ ____ Do blackouts and passouts now happen very often?

____ ____ Have you lost concern for your family and others around you?

Marijuana

After several years of being more or less ignored, marijuana is again attracting attention as a potential health problem. The current concern does not arise because there are any major new findings about the health effects of marijuana, but rather because marijuana is being consumed in larger amounts and by younger people.

Only in the past fifteen years has marijuana become a truly common recreational drug in the United States. By 1977, some 43 million Americans had tried marijuana and over 16 million used the drug regularly. Use has been increasing most rapidly among young teenagers; in 1977, at least 4 million youngsters between the ages of 12 and 17 (about one-sixth of the total population of this age) reported that they were using marijuana. In 1979, 10% of high school seniors claimed to be *daily* users.

How will this change in the nation's habits affect the physical and mental health of Americans? Unfortunately, there is no conclusive evidence on the subject. Tobacco and alcohol are still our major problem drugs—the most frequently used and the most costly to health. On the basis of information assembled so far, marijuana appears to be relatively safe—but the same thing could have been said about tobacco in 1920. After experimenting on themselves for a half century, during which the amount of cigarette smoking increased dramatically, Americans (and many others) proved that inhaling tobacco smoke is a deadly habit. Now marijuana is the substance being tested and once again people must be their own guinea pigs. Animal experiments can give us some clue as to possible risks, but they cannot be trusted to predict the actual outcome in human users. Experiments with people are possible, but ethical considerations and time limitations restrict their utility. Even observations made on heavy marijuana smokers elsewhere (Jamaica, Costa Rica, Egypt,

Greece) have limited applicability to Americans because of differences in environment and pattern of use.

HIGHS AND LOWS   People using marijuana for the first time are commonly motivated by curiosity about its effects or by the urging of friends. Those who return to it usually want the "high"—a mild euphoria, a loosening of inhibitions, and possible alterations in the quality of perceptions and sensations without true hallucinations. Other aspects of the marijuana high are extremely variable. The drug's subjective effects usually last for two or three hours.

Objective changes also occur. While high, marijuana users may become somewhat clumsy (though they may feel graceful); they react more slowly than normal, perceive the passage of time less accurately, pay attention less well, and do arithmetic less well; they also show defects in short-term memory during the high. Impaired driving can pose a serious threat to health; even in low doses, marijuana clearly interferes with driving (or piloting) skills although it does not appear to stimulate aggressiveness behind the wheel the way alcohol does. Moreover, the effect on driving skills lasts several hours beyond the period when a person feels high; even someone who feels "normal" drives worse than usual. *It is foolish and dangerous to drive while under the influence of marijuana.*

A few individuals may react to the marijuana high by becoming extremely anxious; they have a minor "bad trip." As a rule, this problem is best handled by reassuring them and helping them wait out the period of intoxication. There is no solid evidence that other, more serious or lasting psychological effects are likely to result from marijuana use. A marijuana high may trigger prolonged symptoms in unstable people, but does not itself appear to be responsible for mental illness.

Some heavy users of marijuana can become tolerant to its effects—meaning that they have to smoke larger amounts than before to get the high. A few may become dependent on marijuana—and there are a few reports of people showing physical symptoms when they stop using it. True addiction of the sort produced by nicotine or heroin seems to be rare or nonexistent.

Marijuana has been blamed for leading to apathy, loss of motivation, and narrowing of interests in people who use it heavily. There is no evidence that the drug does indeed produce such an "amotivational syndrome." On the contrary, young people who are depressed and have low expectations for themselves—and whose parents expect little of them—are more likely than others to make heavy use of marijuana. In other words, heavy use may be a *symptom* of depression and low self-esteem, *rather than a cause.*

PHYSICAL CONSEQUENCES No convincing report has yet been published to show that marijuana permanently damages the brain. It would not be particularly surprising if there were some effect from heavy, prolonged use, but the weight of the evidence, at the moment, suggests that there is none.

THC (tetrahydrocannabinol, the "active ingredient" of marijuana) opens the air passages of the lungs, and for this reason smoking marijuana during an asthma attack was sometimes recommended in the last century, when medicinal use of the drug was still legal. But *heavy* smoking, it now appears, has the opposite effect: a narrowing of the air passages and inflammation of their lining. Sufficiently heavy, long-term marijuana smoking probably leads to chronic bronchitis, just as tobacco smoking does. Marijuana smoke contains more than 400 chemicals besides THC, and some of them are quite similar to tobacco "tars," including those that contribute to lung cancer. It is likely that smoking marijuana can lead to cancer of the lung, but, even if the risk is fairly high, another 15 to 20 years must pass before enough evidence accumulates in this country to show how much marijuana smoking is necessary to create a significant risk.

During the high, marijuana causes the heart to beat faster and work harder. Although this effect is insignificant in healthy people, it may be a hazard for anyone with heart disease.

Production of the male hormone testosterone and of sperm can be reduced by marijuana, although the effects appear to be temporary and reversible; the significance of these changes is unclear. Effects on females are even less well studied, but it appears that marijuana is capable of disturbing the menstrual cycle. During pregnancy, THC can pass into the placenta (where it tends to be stored) and the fetus. A nursing mother almost certainly would pass the substance in her milk. Milk production itself can be reduced by exposure to THC. Whether typical marijuana use causes genetic damage is simply not known. The subject has been controversial for more than a decade, and it remains so. Marijuana may, however, be capable of causing miscarriages or birth defects. *Women who are pregnant should avoid all drugs except those that are medically necessary;* the list of substances to avoid includes alcohol, tobacco, and marijuana. Both men and women who are planning to conceive a child should avoid drugs whenever possible.

Because THC can lower pressure within the eyeball, it has seemed promising as a treatment for glaucoma. However, its effects on the heart make the drug inappropriate for use in many older people, the group most likely to need glaucoma treatment. THC clearly can relieve the nausea and vomiting that sometimes accompany chemotherapy for cancer. Patients for whom other treatments have been ineffective have benefited from THC, though not all of them respond, and it is said that older patients are more likely to be distressed by the "high" than to find it enjoyable.

PLAYING IN THE GRASS   Little is known about marijuana's long-term effects on the children and adolescents who use it. Thus, their widespread use of the drug is a form of mass self-experimentation. These young "volunteers" can hardly be thought to have given their "informed consent." Even if marijuana proves to have few or no adverse effects on the health of young people, the time they spend "high" is time that could be spent in normal learning and physical activity. *Growing up should be as drug-free as possible.* It seems appropriate to take measures that will diminish marijuana use by young boys and girls, but how to do so is not very clear. Research conducted in the past ten years has some tentative implications for parents who wish to discourage their children's use of marijuana:

(1) Limiting access to the drug is one way. If a school or other area becomes identified as a source of supply, parents can take action to change matters.

(2) Peers are the major influence on youngsters' use of drugs; encouraging friendships with non-using companions may help to reduce the incentives and opportunities to indulge.

(3) Attempting to delay a child's experience with marijuana is probably worthwhile. The later someone begins to use the drug, the less likely he or she is to become heavily involved, according to some

studies. (Most often, use tapers off spontaneously after the age of twenty-five.)

(4) It is always good policy for parents to reconsider their own approach to drink and drugs. The children of parents with a relatively casual attitude are more likely than others to become involved with all drugs.

Parents protect their children from drug use by being close to them, remaining actively involved with them and their friends, supporting their self-esteem, and expressing high expectations for achievement in school. However, once heavy drug involvement has begun, as it may even in close and supportive families, parents are often not able to help their children give up the habit, which in the case of marijuana is likely to taper off of its own accord in a few years.

It probably is not productive to let marijuana become ammunition in the war between the generations or to treat experimentation as a catastrophe. And some perspective about drugs should be kept. Just because tobacco and alcohol are more familiar does not mean that they are safer than marijuana. They are a very real threat to health at every age. Marijuana is still a somewhat uncertain factor, and it may have serious drawbacks, but it does not threaten lifelong severe addiction in the way that cigarettes do. Nor is it as toxic as alcohol. However, these comparisons should not lead to the conclusion that marijuana is safe.

Stress

"Stress" is one of those words we all think we understand—until we are forced to become precise about its meaning and implications. It is, therefore, a word around which all kinds of myths and misunderstandings have gathered. The goal of this essay is to sort out some of the fact from the fiction concerning stress.

THE DEFINITIONAL DILEMMA   It *is* possible to define stress rather precisely in *physiological* terms as a collection of predictable body responses—increased heart rate, soaring blood pressure, rapid breathing, and increased muscle tension. Indeed, the famous description (by the Harvard physiologist Dr. Walter B. Cannon in 1914) of this arousal as the "fight or flight" response points to the exquisite ability of a living organism to prepare itself almost instantaneously for an appropriate response to physical threat. Years later (1946), Dr. Hans Selye of Montreal first popularized the word "stress" while describing this adaptational response of the human body.

Since then, of course, the word has become widely used to cover not only predictable physical responses but a whole spectrum of social and psychological stimuli that might provoke such reactions. Indeed, we now use the word as a synonym for less precise terms—such as anxiety or tension—to indicate our feeling that stress, far from being constructive, is potentially damaging to a person who is "under stress."

In short, the word stress in current usage no longer refers to an appropriate body response—as experienced by a runner at the starting block—but to a wide range of modern psychological devils that prod our bodies into a state of arousal for which no appropriate release can be found. It is not often acceptable to fight against or flee from the enemies of our time; the nasty office memo, instead, arouses a state of smoldering frustration that we instinctively sense does us no good. What happens next may be a translation of mental suffering into physical expression, but we still face a great deal of uncertainty as to how and when this happens.

THE DISEASE CONNECTION   It is not too hard for us to imagine that such temporary conditions as a tension headache or an upset stomach might be rather directly related to stressful situations. But what about the more chronic and serious states of "disease"—especially the two major killers of modern time, cardiovascular disease and cancer? Here the waters become muddy—or at least less clear:

(1) Heart disease: Many laboratory studies using animals have demonstrated clear and direct lines of connection between isolated stimuli (such as electric shocks or separation from mates) and the development of heart disease. It is, however, much more difficult to study and isolate all of the potentially stressful variables in the human environment. Two California cardiologists (Drs. Friedman and Rosenman) have popularized the concept of the "Type A" personality—competitive and time-conscious—as being prone to coronary artery disease. However, others have not been able to duplicate their correlations consistently. Also, some studies of large companies have suggested that persons typically described as "fast-paced" or "hard-driven" may have fewer heart attacks than those with less obvious stress at lower levels of the company hierarchy. In short, while many case reports seem to point directly to the role of stress (from a change in jobs, divorce, and so on) in the development of heart disease, it is hard to generalize from this to the point where we can say that specific persons are certain to have heart attacks—and others are certain to escape.

(2) High blood pressure: In recent years, the work of behavioral scientists showing that various meditation techniques can lower blood pressure moderately has pointed to a connection between emotions and elevated blood pressure levels; indeed, meditation has become a useful part of the treatment program for some persons with relatively mild hypertension. Again, however, it would be misleading to automatically equate "high-strung" with "high blood

pressure"—or to suggest that an apparently placid person is immune to high blood pressure.

(3) Cancer: The fear surrounding this most dreaded of all diseases has been heightened for some by recent reports suggesting that destructive emotions can contribute to or cause cancer. One popular theory suggests that such emotions can weaken the surveillance mechanisms of our body which are constantly destroying abnormal cells that might otherwise cause cancerous growths. There is also increasing research interest in the possibility that healthy emotions might be harnessed by a cancer patient to "fight" his or her disease. And while these theories deserve further study, it is currently unwarranted to suggest that any cancer is caused by faulty emotions; there is no hard evidence to date to support this position.

(4) Other diseases: The list of diseases thought to be related to if not caused by stress is almost endless—and includes asthma, allergies, ulcers, ulcerative colitis, and migraine headaches. Indeed, physicians have the instinctive impression that stress is a very important contributing factor in making any medical problem worse in terms of symptoms and total impact upon a patient's life. *Again, however, it is very difficult to isolate stress as the critical event in the natural history of these diseases,* in spite of its evident role in "making things worse."

In short, the straight-line connection between stress and disease is often difficult to establish. But most health professionals are increasingly aware of the role of emotions in arousing physical responses that might be damaging to the body.

AN APPROACH TO STRESS   Given the above uncertainties, what should we do about the concern we tend to have about the damaging role that stress might play in our lives? The following may be no more useful than all of the other easy words of advice offered by so-called "experts," but we suggest them in the hope they may be helpful to some:

(1) Avoid equating "pace" with "damaging stress": It is possible that inappropriate anxiety is aroused by the simplistic labeling of an apparently "hectic" pace as dangerous. As emphasized by many stress researchers, the person who works long hours and leads a busy

life may be far less frustrated than the person trapped in a limited position with no sense of release or accomplishment. Furthermore, we all differ in our needs; for some, the fast pace is indeed too fast but for others it may be just right.

(2) Consider the role of regular exercise in reducing stress: For years we have emphasized the potential physical benefits of regular exercise while largely ignoring its possible emotional benefits—a sense of control over one's body, a feeling of accomplishment, a release for pent-up frustration, and so on. More recently, however, there has been increasing emphasis on the role of regular exercise as an effective treatment for emotional problems. And some intriguing biochemical research suggests that regular exercise may increase the levels of brain chemicals (endorphins) that result in good feelings. (In fact, some have proposed that persons who seemingly become addicted to exercise might literally have become addicted to an increase of such body chemicals.)

(3) Periodically re-evaluate priorities: This bit of advice may indeed be trite—given the fact that many are trapped by circumstances over which they have little control. But given that obvious restriction, most of us can still identify areas of our lives that we could change *if* we periodically took the time to identify what it is we do well and enjoy.

IN SUMMARY   Stress should be recognized as a legitimate concern, but one which is potentially manageable and not necessarily the dominant predicament of our lives.

Sleep Disorders

Most people spend a third of their lives sleeping. It's no wonder that complaints about difficulty getting to sleep, staying asleep, or getting enough rest from sleep are very common. The following questions about sleep and insomnia are answered by Dr. Quentin R. Regestein, Associate Professor of Psychiatry, Harvard Medical School, and Director of the Sleep Clinic of Brigham and Women's Hospital.

What is "normal" sleep and what is insomnia?

"Normal" sleep leaves one refreshed the next day. Continuous laboratory measurement of brain waves, eye movements, and muscle activity discloses that different stages of sleep (for example, light, dreaming, or deep sleep) appear in predictable sequence each night. People who sleep with satisfaction sleep about the same total number of hours from week to week. Some people get along on six hours a night, while others need nine hours, although both may sleep "normally." The elderly, in particular, are sometimes preoccupied by their apparent lack of sleep. The normal 85-year-old spends about one fifth of the night in wakefulness. This normal lessening in the soundness of sleep, however, does not correlate much with the complaint of insomnia.

Some doctors define insomnia as sleeping less than six hours a night or taking more than 45 minutes to fall asleep. Others insist that only a record of sleep obtained in a laboratory can conclusively diagnose inadequate sleep. There are people who sleep more than they think they do when studied in a laboratory that records sleep stages with electrical equipment. However, I feel that if a person complains that he sleeps too little, he deserves to be helped, regardless of the recordings. It does one little good to be told that his laboratory tests are normal if he nevertheless feels he sleeps poorly all the time.

What are the common causes of insomnia?

The list of possible causes is long (see table). However, most cases of insomnia can be traced to one of several common problems, including irregular bedtimes, irregular arising times, night work, overuse of caffeine or other stimulants, or chronic abuse of drugs affecting the nervous system—especially tranquilizers, sleeping pills, and alcohol. Other "culprits" are daytime naps (especially by unemployed or older people) and a completely sedentary daytime routine.

Common Causes of Chronic Insomnia

Irregular sleep schedules
   (night work, irregular rising times, or irregular bedtimes)
Hyperarousal
"Endogenous" depression
Daytime naps
Boredom, purposelessness, and inactivity
   Old age
   Unemployment
Drugs
   Sleeping-pill tolerance
   Side effects of:
      Anti-arrhythmia drugs
      Anti-hypertensive medication
      Steroids
      Hormonal preparations
      Alcohol
      Asthma medications
Stimulants
      Caffeine
      Diet pills
Various disease conditions, for instance:
      Those involving pain, itching, or breathlessness
      Endocrine gland disorders
      Neurological disorders

There are some people who are constantly more alert than others. They tend to be sensitive individuals, often perfectionists who ruminate about details long after the event. Some of them take a long time to "wind down" each night. They often take a while to fall asleep, but usually sleep soundly once they do. They manifest particular electrical properties of the nervous system, and their condition is known as "hyperarousal."

A sudden crisis (a financial reversal, divorce, court case, and so on) can obviously interfere with sleep; such "insomnia" should disappear when the crisis is over. More commonly, chronic depression underlies disordered sleep, especially when early morning awakening occurs. Often these depressions are unrecognized because the patient does not feel "sad." But early morning awakening combined with the inability to enjoy customary pleasures, the appearance of irrational fears, or even temperamental outbursts may indeed signify depression. The types of depression associated with insomnia are often readily relieved once the depression is recognized and treated.

Finally, one should always think of physical problems (pain, fever, breathlessness), underlying diseases (such as thyroid, kidney, heart), and medications (hormonal preparations or drugs for cardiac rhythm disturbances) as possible causes of disordered sleep. Many blame environmental discomforts for their chronic insomnia, but these rarely underlie insomnia, since most people can sleep well in a noisy city on a lumpy mattress.

How do you approach treatment for insomnia?

Since most cases of insomnia are related to the common "life-style" problems described above, initial treatment efforts are directed toward changing these patterns, with emphasis on regular bedtimes, regular arisings, and the avoidance of naps and caffeine beverages. For such people, a uniform time for "hitting the sack" should be observed, and sleeping late in the morning should not be permitted even when they feel tired. This is true for weekends as well as weekdays. It is amazing how many sleep problems will evaporate when caffeine drinks are avoided; some people are so exquisitely sensitive to caffeine that even a single morning cup of coffee will disturb nighttime sleep. I am also convinced that regular exercise and the time-honored glass of warm milk before bed can be helpful. Relaxation exercises and meditation procedures can be especially valuable for those "alert" individuals I described earlier. Of course, these relatively simple measures (not so simple in terms of breaking habits) will not work for everyone. But the majority of people with sleeping problems can be helped in this manner—and this is where we usually start.

What is the role, if any, of medications in treating sleep problems?

Obviously, if sleep problems can be traced to underlying physical problems that require medications, they should be used. It is also important to stress the value of antidepressant medications in people with a true depression underlying their sleep problems. Too often, these medications are not used in sufficient dosage for long enough periods of time.

Having said that, I would like to stress the terrible dangers involved in using sleeping pills indiscriminately. Particularly dangerous are the barbiturate drugs—so widely used in the past as sleeping pills. Apart from the dangers of suicide and addiction, there is no good evidence that they improve sleep over the long run. Indeed, the evidence is to the contrary; they tend to disrupt normal sleeping patterns. A person who has become addicted to these drugs must be withdrawn slowly under the careful direction of a physician.

The drug most commonly used as a "sleeping pill" today is flurazepam (Dalmane), a tranquilizer similar to the familiar drugs Valium and Librium. These drugs are less dangerous in overdose than the barbiturates—but they, too, must be used with caution. Regular use of Dalmane causes daytime sedation, which is detected by performance tests but unrecognized by the user (see below). Also, there is little evidence to support effectiveness of these—or any— drugs when used for more than 20 days at a time. Despite a current interest in the amino acid tryptophan, there is no evidence at present that this agent relieves chronic insomnia.

What do frequent nightmares mean?

Nightmares can occur because of recent horrible experiences; however, chronic psychological troubles may also cause nightmares.

Surprisingly, nightmares may also come as side effects of withdrawal from various medications, including sedatives. In a few people, nightmares appear as a problem without any obvious cause, occasionally associated with sleep walking. Sometimes drugs which suppress "deep sleep" (when nightmares usually occur) can be helpful in alleviating them.

Where should people with sleep problems go for help?

There are clinics which specialize in the treatment of sleep problems. If a patient cannot find adequate help locally, he can obtain a list of such clinics by writing to: Dr. William Dement, Association of Sleep Disorders Centers, Stanford University School of Medicine, Stanford, California 94305, or the Brigham and Women's Hospital Sleep Clinic, 75 Francis Street, Boston, Massachusetts 02115.

Dalmane and Sleep

Dalmane (the trade name of flurazepam) is now the most frequently prescribed sleeping pill in the United States. A member of the benzodiazepine family of drugs, which includes Valium, Librium, and Serax, Dalmane is generally effective and considerably safer than the barbiturates. However, as stressed in a report from the Institute of Medicine of the National Academy of Sciences (*New England Journal of Medicine,* April 5, 1979), there are potential problems with this and the other benzodiazepines when they are used for sleep. With regard to Dalmane, the report emphasizes the following points:

(1) Dalmane is converted by the body to active products that can remain in the blood for up to eight days. Therefore, its effects can last far beyond the night when they are taken and may, in fact, become cumulative with repeated use.

(2) Dalmane combined with alcohol makes people very drowsy. People who have taken Dalmane in the last several days and plan to drive should not drink alcohol.

(3) The report also urges the use of a 15-milligram dose—not the typically prescribed 30 milligrams—because the smaller amount is adequate to induce sleep and has fewer side effects.

Nevertheless, Dalmane is an improvement over the barbiturates for people who truly need medication, temporarily, to aid with sleep. What is important is that Dalmane be prescribed cautiously and for limited periods—no more than two to four weeks in people who are not already dependent on pills as a result of chronically using them.

Leg Cramps

Leg cramps during the night afflict some people to the point where an uninterrupted night of sleep is rare. All kinds of remedies (including magnets under the mattress) have been tried without much success. Therefore, a recent letter to the *New England Journal of Medicine* (July 26, 1979) from Dr. Harry Daniell of Redding, California, describing a stretching technique that was successful in 44 people with recurring night cramps, is of interest.

He writes: "Patients were instructed to stand with their shoes off, face a wall two to three feet away and then lean forward, using the hands and arms to regulate their forward tilt and keeping the heels in contact with the floor, until a moderately intense, but not painful, 'pulling sensation' developed in their calf muscles. The stretching position was held for 10 seconds, then repeated after a five-second period of relaxation. This sequence was repeated three times daily until all leg cramps were gone, then used with whatever frequency was necessary to maintain a cramp-free state." As Dr. Daniell points out, the above technique (similar to what runners often use as a warm-up exercise) has not been subjected to controlled studies. But since it is without cost or danger, it may be worth a try for those of you who scramble from the bed at night because of (eerie music, soft voice) "cramps in the night."

Mental and
Emotional Illness

More than 2 million people in the United States are currently under formal treatment for emotional illness. Psychiatrists outnumber pediatricians and obstetricians. Despite the evident need, controversy concerning the treatment of mental disorders is widespread. Diagnosis often lacks precision. Careful evaluation of effectiveness is lacking for some treatments. Drug therapy for mental disorders can be abused; the very possibility of abuse leads some critics to regard drugs with suspicion, even when there is evidence that they are effective. Such uncertainties place the "consumer" of treatment for mental illness in a difficult situation. We cannot provide final answers to these concerns, but we will attempt to offer information about two commonly asked questions: How can one recognize serious mental disturbance? What kinds of treatment have been shown to be reasonably effective?

While it is theoretically helpful to categorize emotional illnesses, most classification schemes turn out to be artificial. Nonetheless, we will begin with brief discussions of "neuroses" and schizophrenia, followed by a more extensive review of the most common of all emotional disorders, depression. Finally, we will turn to three potentially controversial areas relating to emotional illness: evaluating therapy, using minor tranquilizers, and treating agoraphobia.

THE NEUROSES   This term includes a wide range of psychological and behavioral responses whose common denominator is anxiety. Neurotic responses are generally less disruptive than psychoses, but some, such as severe phobias or compulsions, can markedly impair both work and social adjustment. The following information is important to understanding what we know about neuroses:

(1) Some neurotic behavior is clearly abnormal—such as washing one's hands every five minutes because of the fear of germs. More often, neuroses are expressed in more indirect ways, such as fatigue or irritability or even depression. Complaints about body functions—or actual symptoms such as numbness or heart palpitations—may be an expression of anxiety. Since neurotic reactions are extensions of common behaviors, it is often difficult to decide exactly when help is needed. While no rule covers all situations, it is useful to evaluate the individual's ability to function in basic ways—working, sleeping and eating, making and keeping friends, and enjoying recreational activities. When these are impaired by anxiety, evaluation should be sought.

(2) The range of psychotherapeutic and behavioral treatments that have been proposed for neuroses is almost endless. That in itself suggests that no single form of treatment works all the time. However, there are *some* effective approaches to troublesome neuroses—such as desensitization treatment for phobias. To be avoided are treatment fads which "guarantee" success.

(3) The use of "anti-anxiety" drugs (commonly known as "minor tranquilizers" to distinguish them from the drugs used for psychoses) has become one of the more controversial practices in our society (see below). The benzodiazepines (Valium, Librium, and so on) are *quite safe when used in short-term recommended doses and when not mixed with other drugs or alcohol.* Other sedative drugs—especially barbiturates—are potentially dangerous and should seldom be used, if at all, in the treatment of anxiety or insomnia. Over-the-counter drugs are rarely effective and can cause serious reactions if taken in excessive amounts.

SCHIZOPHRENIA Schizophrenia is a psychosis marked by progressive withdrawal from reality, grossly inappropriate behavior, abnormalities of thought, and a discrepancy between thought content and mood (for example, the patient may smile while stating that he is about to die). Disturbances of mental function include delusions ("I am Jesus Christ") or hallucinations ("hearing" or "seeing" things that are not audible or visible to other people). Full-blown schizophrenia is easy to diagnose; less severe forms are more difficult to recognize.

Drug treatment for schizophrenia was revolutionized in the

1950s with the introduction of a category of drugs referred to as "anti-psychotics" or "major tranquilizers." Before the introduction of these drugs, conventional treatments consisted of shock therapy (of limited usefulness in schizophrenia) and heavy sedation. The great benefit of the newer anti-psychotic drugs is their ability to diminish or eliminate disturbance in thought and behavior while allowing the person to function at work and with friends. Indeed, the introduction of these drugs has been the single most important factor in the dramatic reduction of state mental hospital beds, a reduction of over 50% since 1955. Unfortunately, anti-psychotic drugs have serious side effects in some cases and their administration *must be closely monitored by a competent physician.* Of particular concern is the development of uncontrollable muscle spasms; such side effects usually occur after prolonged use at large doses.

There is strong evidence for genetic predisposition to many psychoses, including schizophrenia. For example, schizophrenia is more common in identical twin pairs (who have exactly the same genetic composition) than in fraternal twin pairs (who are no more similar than siblings). This and other evidence strongly point to a biochemical factor underlying schizophrenia. The precise chemical abnormality (or abnormalities) have not yet been clearly identified.

DEPRESSION   This word is used to identify normal reactions to the sorrows of life as well as serious mood disturbances. There are three major reasons why understanding serious depression is important: *(1) Recognition of serious depression is sometimes difficult;* many studies indicate that both physicians and non-medical observers often fail to perceive major depressive illness. *(2) Effective treatment for depression is often possible*—especially when therapy is prompt and vigorous. *(3) Suicide is a common and tragic result of serious depression.* Conservative estimates put the number of suicide attempts at over a quarter of a million per year in this country, with at least 25,000 ending in death. It is the second leading cause of death in the 15–24 age group.

(1) Recognition: Classic and full-blown depression is usually described in terms of the loss of the capacity to enjoy life combined with a poverty of thought and movement. Typical symptoms include *weight loss, decreased sexual desire, difficulty in sleeping, and fa-*

tigue. Serious depression may sometimes be disguised by anxiety or excessive complaints about body function or chronic pain—especially headaches. *Early morning awakening* in a person who generally sleeps later may herald depression. Some diseases, such as hypothyroidism (underactive thyroid gland), may produce depression while others, such as heart disease or arthritis, commonly bring on a depressive reaction. Certain drugs may cause depression—especially steroids (cortisone-like drugs), rauwolfia drugs (such as reserpine), and, less commonly, oral contraceptives (birth control pills). Since the range of manifestation of depression is almost endless, there is *no easy "rule of thumb" for recognition other than the interference with ability to function in basic ways, such as eating, sleeping, working, and relating to other people.* When in doubt, professional advice should be sought.

(2) Treatment: Fortunately, most people with severe depression can be helped. In the early and acute stages of depression, the goal is to reduce symptoms and prevent suicide. The following medical approaches are useful:

> *Anti-depressant drugs* most commonly used today are known as "tricyclics" and are marketed under trade names such as Tofranil, Elavil, and Sinequan. The many tricyclics are thought to be equally effective and to differ only in dosage forms. (Another category of drugs known as MAO inhibitors have potentially more dangerous side effects and are therefore less often used.) While tricyclics have not proved effective in all studies, most experts strongly advocate these drugs when used in *proper amounts* for *appropriately selected cases.* Specifically, tricyclics must be used in amounts sufficient to produce detectable side effects (such as a dry mouth) for at least three weeks before they can be considered to be ineffective. Tricyclic drugs should be administered only under the supervision of a physician since side effects—such as markedly altered blood pressure or heart rhythm abnormalities—are possible. These drugs should be used with caution in persons with certain forms of heart disease—including conduction blocks and recent heart attacks. Elderly people are generally more sensitive to the adverse effects of tricyclics.
>
> *Lithium carbonate* has been used since 1949 and is the drug

of choice for controlling the variant of depressive disease known as "manic-depressive" disease. (In manic-depressive disease, there are swings of mood which include episodes of "mania"— exuberance of thought and movement during which the person might be very volatile and grandiose and do things that are embarrassing and very much out of character.) Lithium is most effective in *preventing* attacks of mania and, to a lesser degree, depression. Lithium may require several weeks to exert its effect and must be *very carefully monitored with blood tests* to avoid excessive levels, which can cause serious side effects.

Electroconvulsive therapy (also known as ECT or shock treatment) has received a "bad press" in recent years—much of it justified as a response to past misuse. However, ECT still has an important role in the treatment of severe depression not responsive to drug therapy—particularly the severe depression of middle life known as "involutional melancholia." Present techniques, which include pre-medication with muscle relaxants and short-acting anesthesia, are less unpleasant than the techniques used earlier. The major side effect of ECT is short-term memory loss—a deficit which increases in proportion to the number of treatments given. While the idea of ECT is unpleasant, it should be remembered that there are times when it is a life-saving measure in the face of severe suicidal preoccupation. Most experts would agree that there is little use for ECT for conditions other than severe depressive illnesses.

When depression has been brought under control by one of the above measures, psychotherapy may be important in helping to remedy underlying interpersonal and social problems.

(3) Suicide prevention: Depression of any kind—as well as other emotional and physical disturbances—may lead to suicide. *Most suicides are not impulsive, but are well-planned.* In the process of planning, many persons will communicate their intent—either indirectly (such as by revising a will) or in direct statements. *Any threat of suicide—even if made in apparent jest—should be taken very seriously.*

Statistically, suicide is more likely in men, older persons, and in those who have recently experienced a significant loss, such as that of a mate or a job. A family history of suicide also adds to the risk, as does a previous attempt. Persistent worries about the development of serious disease raise the possibility of suicide.

When a person discusses suicide, you owe him the favor of seeking protection for him, even over protests to the contrary. At the very least, you should arrange for a person who speaks openly of suicide to be taken to a mental health facility or nearby emergency room. *Any suggestion of suicidal intent constitutes a psychiatric emergency.*

(4) Reactive depression: The discussion thus far has concerned mood disorders for which no obvious cause can be found. Much more common are mood changes which are provoked by external events—such as the death of a loved one, marital discord, or serious disease. Grieving is a normal response to loss. The failure to grieve may lead to psychosomatic symptoms months or even years later. When grief reactions continue beyond 3 months, or interfere seriously with the capacity for work, they are a cause for concern.

Seeking Help for Emotional Problems

People experiencing emotional distress often feel helpless, so that the challenge of finding competent professional help can seem all the more overwhelming to them. We have asked Dr. Leon Eisenberg, Professor of Psychiatry at Harvard Medical School, to answer some questions concerning this dilemma.

What is the first step for someone with an emotional problem to take?

It is important to make sure that the symptoms of distress are not due to a primarily physical disorder. Although most episodes of anxiety and shakiness, for example, are psychological in nature, they can result from an overactive thyroid gland, low blood sugar, or other medical conditions. Most headaches result from tension, but some can be caused by a tumor, high blood pressure, or other causes for which psychiatric care by itself would be ineffective. A thorough medical evaluation should be the first step in assessing the need for treatment of emotional difficulties.

If it appears that psychiatric or psychological intervention is warranted, your family physician or internist may be in a good position to make the appropriate referral. Besides knowing you, a family doctor is likely to know the professional reputation of other practitioners and may have had some experience with successful referral of other patients to a particular specialist. If you are not able to use the family doctor in this way, or don't have one, you can, instead, call a mental health clinic; many general hospitals and psychiatric hospitals provide outpatient services.

As with any medical specialist, it is worth learning whether the person you are going to consult has been appropriately certified and/or is on the staff of a hospital or the faculty of a university. To be sure, gifted people may lack such credentials and mediocre ones may have them; neither certification nor a faculty appointment guarantees competence, but they do improve the odds.

Does it matter whether the therapist is a psychiatrist, psychologist, or other mental health worker?

Psychiatrists are medical doctors who have special training in emotional and mental illness. They are generally better equipped than psychologists to manage *severe* mental disorders; they are the only mental health professionals who can prescribe medications, which are often required in addition to psychological treatment for such conditions as schizophrenia and severe depression.

Psychologists with the most advanced training have received doctorates from graduate programs devoted to the study and treatment of abnormal thoughts, feelings, and behaviors. For "problems of living" that are best managed by psychological methods, a psychologist may be as well equipped as a psychiatrist, may be less expensive (but not necessarily), and may, depending on his or her training and experience, be more skilled. Other kinds of mental health professionals, such as psychiatric social workers and psychiatric nurses, also practice as therapists. Depending on their training and experience these professionals may be helpful with emotional problems. It is important to make certain that the individual professing to be competent has the requisite qualifications; affiliation with a university or teaching hospital is a useful criterion where there is no state certifying mechanism.

How should a patient settle on a particular therapist?

Even after the patient (or "client," as the person receiving non-medical help is often called) has gotten as far as the first appointment, his or her judgment is crucial in making the final decision to enter treatment with the therapist. There are several important questions to ask: Can I work with this psychotherapist? Do I trust him or her? Does the method make sense, at least provisionally? The patient has the right to ask the prospective therapist for an explanation of the method to be used, for a guess about the length of treatment and its cost, and for an opinion about goals and results that can be expected. Bear in mind that these matters can be difficult to assess at the beginning of treatment. Patients should be wary of anyone who promises certain "cure," but they have a right to approximate estimates and a firm agreement to reassess progress and remaining needs after a reasonable trial of treatment.

The patient and the therapist should be specific about the broad goals of treatment. Is the main purpose to obtain relief from certain symptoms, such as a phobia, sexual dysfunction, or poor performance at school? Is it to discover the cause of a problem, such as marital tension or a persistent sense of sadness? Is it a desire to increase one's self-understanding, perhaps to enhance one's creativity? When the purposes of treatment have been spelled out, it will be useful for the patient and therapist to agree on criteria for assessing whether these goals are being attained.

If, after a few sessions, the patient is in doubt about continuing with a particular therapist, it is perfectly appropriate to look further. Some people may prefer to visit a few therapists before making a final decision.

How does one choose among the many varieties of psychotherapy?

The most common kinds of psychological treatment today are psychotherapy conducted with individuals or groups; family therapy; behavior modification; relaxation training; and biofeedback. No one method is ideal for all problems, and a therapist skilled in more than one is desirable. Sometimes patients are best served by seeing a diagnostician at the outset who can give advice on the best method to use.

Psychoanalysis is the most intensive form of individual psychotherapy; sessions take place four or five days a week for periods of several years. This approach is appropriate for those seeking to change long-standing personality problems, but not for acute treatment of disabling psychiatric disorders. Psychoanalysis is based on a meticulous exploration of the past and of the relationship between patient and analyst as a corrective for distorted developmental experiences. Other forms of individual psychotherapy may use similar principles; some are more oriented to current problems. They vary in intensity (one to several times a week), duration (limited to 10 or 15 sessions, or continuing indefinitely), and method.

There is no solid evidence, as yet, that the school of therapy makes a difference in the results; the skill and personality of the therapist and the fit between therapist and patient appear to be more decisive. Thus, it is important for the patient to decide within a few sessions whether he or she feels enough confidence to continue.

Group therapy offers the advantage of sharing experiences with others. It is likely to be particularly useful to people who are uncomfortable in social situations, and it involves a lot of learning from peers. People who have difficulty talking about their feelings—even to one person—may not be able to profit from a group. Family therapy is based on the belief that problems exist more *between* members of a family than *within* the individual. It is most often used to treat children and adolescents, or as "couple" therapy to help people with marital difficulties.

Behavior modification applies learning theory to the elimination of troublesome symptoms. It disdains the past and focuses exclusively on existing situations that help maintain the symptoms. Phobias and the habit disturbances of children are particularly responsive to this approach; with other emotional problems behavior modification is not clearly any more or less effective than other forms of therapy.

Relaxation training is a form of behavior therapy often useful in modifying physical symptoms, such as headache or back pain, resulting from tension. Biofeedback employs mechanical devices to make the patient aware of bodily functions (such as heart rate, blood pressure). Despite early enthusiasm for this method of treating psychosomatic problems, recent evidence suggests that biofeedback is no more effective than relaxation training, and it can be much more cumbersome.

Psychotherapy can be—and most of the time *is*—effective in diminishing emotional distress. There is by now a substantial scientific literature which demonstrates significantly better outcomes for patients who have received psychological treatment in contrast to comparable "control" patients in the untreated condition. Moreover, there is evidence of better results from combined psychotherapy and drug therapy in the treatment of depression than from the use of either alone. The major challenge in psychotherapy research is to identify which types of therapy are best for which kinds of patients. This is currently a major area of investigation. Until those findings are in, the point to remember is that psychotherapy does help to relieve mental distress as well as the physical symptoms which express it.

Anti-Anxiety Drugs

The human race has long sought substances that would ease the pain of anxiety; herbs and alcohol have probably been the ones used most widely. In more recent times—described by the poet Auden as the "Age of Anxiety"—this search has intensified. Barbiturates were the chief drugs used earlier in this century, both to relieve anxiety and induce sleep; subsequent attention to their serious side effects has greatly reduced their use for these purposes.

In the mid-50s, the discovery of a compound known as meprobamate (sold as Miltown and Equanil) led to an intensive search for others that could provide relief of anxiety without heavy sedation. In 1957, a chemist at the Hoffman-LaRoche company submitted a new kind of compound—a benzodiazepine—for testing. This first member of the benzodiazepine family—subsequently named Librium—led to the discovery of many others, including Valium (approved by the FDA in 1964), Serax, and Tranxene. These drugs are commonly called minor tranquilizers.

Each year, doctors in the United States write more than 50 million prescriptions for Valium alone—which translates into about 3 billion tablets and retail sales valued at more than half a billion dollars. Approximately 10–15% of American adults take Valium with some regularity, and women exceed men by a sizable margin. Such widespread use has led to understandable concern on the part of health authorities and government agencies—and to some sensational charges in the public press of "abuse," "national tranquilization," and portrayals of a nation of housewives who couldn't make it through the day without "mother's little helper." The following remarks are intended to provide a balanced perspective on Valium and related anti-anxiety drugs in the benzodiazepine family.

The benzodiazepines are remarkably effective in alleviating the misery of severe anxiety which almost all persons have experienced at one time or another in their lives. When such anxiety relates to an isolated event—the unexpected illness of a loved one or a major crisis at work—few would quibble with the short-term use of these drugs to reduce the anguish. The real problems arise from people who resort to them as a first response to *any* degree of tension, and from doctors who use them as a ready prescription for "minor symptoms" of anxiety (such as headaches and bowel upset). Such inappropriate use has the potential to cause both physical and psychological addiction, particularly in those prone to such problems with other drugs and with alcohol. In recognition of this fact, the producers of benzodiazepines have acceded to a 1980 FDA request to caution physicians that these drugs are not generally required for the tension associated with the stress of everyday life.

Clearly addiction is less common with the benzodiazepines than with barbiturates, their predecessors for anxiety relief a generation ago. And life-threatening problems owing to overdose (accidental or intentional) are really quite rare in contrast to barbiturates. Some people who are very sensitive to minor tranquilizers will note the lightheadedness and a feeling of being "spaced out" on even small doses; it is an uncomfortable sensation that often curtails further use. Everyone receiving benzodiazepines should recognize that these drugs depress the central nervous system—which means that even activity such as automobile driving can be affected by blunted reflexes and reduced alertness. It also means that when alcohol and benzodiazepines are combined, their effects are additive; the "calming" effect of either can be transformed into grogginess when they are used together.

In summary, the benzodiazepines are effective anti-anxiety drugs that are generally safe—which is probably the reason why overuse is common. As with any drug which affects the psyche, dependency and addiction can occur in people who are predisposed to drug abuse.

Agoraphobia

Hundreds of thousands of persons are victims of sudden attacks of panic that seem to defy rational explanation. Embarrassment and despair over these attacks are natural. We have asked Dr. David V. Sheehan, Assistant Professor of Psychiatry at the Massachusetts General Hospital, Harvard Medical School, to provide some insights into this common problem.

What is agoraphobia?

Agoraphobia has sailed through medical history under a wide variety of aliases. The term derives from the Greek word "agora" meaning "a place of assembly" or "crowded place." Although a fear of crowds is the most frequent and disabling problem, a great diversity of other symptoms typically accompany agoraphobia. For this reason, it is one of the great imposters in medical practice. Patients with this condition have usually visited many physicians over several years for relief. The cardiologist may be consulted to investigate a rapid pulse, pounding heart, and chest pain; the neurologist for light-headedness and headaches; the ear, nose, and throat specialist for a lump in the throat and dizziness; the gynecologist for hot flashes; the endocrinologist for possible thyroid disease or low blood sugar; and the pulmonary specialist because of difficulty breathing or hyperventilation. Often the cancer specialist is consulted because of a preoccupation concerning malignant disease.

When no underlying disease can be found, the person with agoraphobia attracts such diagnostic labels as "hysteria," "anxiety neurosis," "hyperventilation syndrome," "cardiac neurosis," "hypochondriasis," "depression," and even "autonomic epilepsy." In a large series (over 100 patients) seen at Massachusetts General Hospital, 70% had consulted more than 10 physicians during their 12 years of symptoms and had received an average of 3.8 years each of psychiatric treatment. Ninety-eight percent were on tranquilizers.

Yet without exception they remained severely disabled by their symptoms.

What is the "natural history" of agoraphobia?

The disorder usually starts with attacks of anxiety that strike suddenly, without warning and for no apparent reason. These attacks usually begin in later adolescence or early adulthood. Eighty percent of patients are women. There is often a family history of similar symptoms among close female relatives. Patients describe these spontaneous panic attacks as a special brand of anxiety never before experienced, even under stress. Many report feeling disoriented, a sense of complete loss of control, and fears of impending death or insanity. A pounding heart, lightheadedness and dizziness, rubbery legs, a lump in the throat, difficulty breathing, hot or cold sensations, and a sinking, nauseated feeling in the abdomen usually accompany the feeling of panic. Strange sensations may follow, such as the feeling that the ground is moving underfoot or the visual impression that objects are becoming more distant or shrinking. A "flight response" follows ("I've got to get out of here in a hurry"), although the person is at a loss to say what he or she is fleeing from. These episodes last from minutes to several hours. As time progresses, symptoms may occur in small clusters and need not even be accompanied by much anxiety. They leave the victim wondering when the next attack will strike.

Over the next few months, morbid fears (phobias) develop. The type of phobia is usually dictated by the circumstances in which the spontaneous panic attacks occur. For example, if a severe panic occurs whenever the patient is in a crowded store, the store by association becomes capable of triggering anxiety. Later, if the patient even approaches the store, the anticipation of panic actually provokes it. Within a few years, many phobias are conditioned (learned) in this way. The victim, in an attempt to avoid these attacks, begins to avoid situations associated with such panic attacks in the past. Finally, the person may become so disabled by phobic anxiety that he or she becomes housebound.

Thus, what started as unexplained medical problems or anxiety attacks matures into its full-blown form and the patient is now said to suffer from "agoraphobic syndrome." The condition typically fluctuates in severity over the course of years.

How is agoraphobia treated?

The physician is faced with two major problems in dealing with these patients. First, the basic anxiety must be controlled. Then the patient must overcome patterns of avoiding specific situations (the agoraphobia and other phobias) that complicate the original anxiety.

Effective control of the anxiety can be accomplished with drugs. However, the value of minor tranquilizers such as diazepam (Valium) has been greatly exaggerated. In our study, 57 patients had consumed approximately 2/3 of a million minor tranquilizer tablets, yet all continued to have spontaneous panic attacks. No reliable evidence supports the use of anti-psychotic drugs (so-called major tranquilizers), although they are prescribed for nearly half of all persons afflicted with agoraphobia. However, recent studies indicate that two classes of drugs are uniquely effective for relieving spontaneous panic attacks—the MAO inhibitors (notably phenelzine) and the tricyclic anti-depressants (imipramine and desipramine). In our study of agoraphobics disabled for an average of 13 years, both were superior to placebo, with phenelzine showing superiority over imipramine. Doses less than 45 mg/day of phenelzine or 150 mg/day of imipramine are rarely effective; in practice, 40% of patients require higher doses than these. The dose at which some mild "postural hypotension" (lightheadedness when assuming an upright position) occurs is usually the dose at which phenelzine will be effective. It is unusual to observe a positive effect from either drug in less than 3–4 weeks.

Although these drugs are traditionally regarded as anti-depressants, their effectiveness is independent of the presence of depression. Physicians are often surprised to learn how useful these drugs may be when all other measures have failed, and how well the patients tolerate them *after* the initial side effects of the first 3 weeks. It is important to understand that many persons will require drug treatment for extended periods.

When the spontaneous panic attacks are controlled, the learned avoidance behaviors (phobias) can be more easily overcome with a variety of behavior therapy techniques, such as desensitization. However, behavioral therapy in the absence of drug treatment does not appear to be nearly as effective. For example, Zitrin and Klein at the New York Psychiatric Institute demonstrated that behavior therapy plus imipramine was significantly superior to behavior therapy used *alone* for the relief of these symptoms. The evidence now available suggests that psychotherapy, behavior therapy, and group therapy when used alone are not as effective as once believed and alone offer little lasting or significant benefit. Consequently, the thrust of psychological treatment is now addressed to the proper use of drugs and to encouraging the patient to approach and re-enter the long avoided phobic situations.

The usefulness of specific drugs supports the hypothesis that agoraphobia is linked to an underlying biochemical imbalance. This is also suggested by the fact that agoraphobia clusters in families and tends to appear within a specific age range. However, final understanding of this condition is still elusive.

Headaches and Painkillers

Each year approximately 20 million Americans seek medical help for headaches, the most common of all the problems that are brought to physicians. However, despite being so common, headaches are still often difficult to sort out in terms of a specific diagnosis and treatment program. Even a careful search of current medical wisdom on the topic leaves one bewildered by the complexity, confusion, and missing links in our knowledge. (It's enough to cause a headache.) Nonetheless, some general principles and enough specifics can be garnered to serve as a beginning guide for those who suffer from headaches.

INITIAL EVALUATION   One of the first questions that arises when a headache problem begins is this: Is this serious enough to merit medical attention? Indeed, the question is often more blunt: Do I have a serious disease—like a brain tumor? Fortunately, the vast majority of headaches are not ominous in the sense of signaling life-threatening disease—though they may raise havoc with daily living. The following types of headaches are more likely to be serious:

(1) Headaches that come on "like a bolt out of the blue" with shattering severity should receive *immediate* medical attention since bleeding inside the skull may be the cause.

(2) Headaches accompanied by specific neurological abnormalities—visual blurring, seizures, mental confusion, loss of alertness or consciousness, loss of body function or sensation—also demand immediate evaluation.

(3) Headaches accompanied by fever *and* neck stiffness may mean meningitis and should be promptly evaluated; obviously, the

124

line between such headaches and those caused by cold and flu viruses may be blurred initially, but when there is doubt, a physician should bear the responsibility of making decisions.

(4) Headaches that become recurrent or that increase in frequency or intensity should be checked out—though it must be stated that the initial severity of headaches usually bears no direct relationship to any potential danger.

(5) Headaches that are localized to a specific area (ear, eye, one side of the head) should also be reviewed by a doctor.

The fact remains that the overwhelming majority of headaches do not mean a serious underlying disease; some ultimately become labeled as "chronic, non-specific"—a term that sounds intelligent but really means that there's a continuing problem that we don't know much about. Attempts at classification will probably never be fully satisfactory because of the many variations that occur in real life. Nonetheless, it is useful to consider headaches in terms of the following types, with special reference to a somewhat broader definition of migraine.

MIGRAINE   The word "migraine" comes from the Greek word meaning "half of the skull"—a logical designation, since this type of headache is often confined to one side of the head. The *classic migraine* consists of "prodromal" (early) symptoms—for example, flashing lights or flickering vision—followed by an initially throbbing or pulsating headache which later becomes steady or dull. However, most migraines do not occur in the classic form, and experts increasingly use the phrase *migraine variants* to cover other kinds of headaches (and other associated symptoms such as nausea and vomiting) that do not fit this classic description. For example, *cluster headaches*—so-called because they tend to occur in clusters over a period of days, weeks, or months—are probably part of the migraine family. It should also be stressed that some headaches formerly labeled as sinus headaches, because they were accompanied by nasal stuffiness and pain in the sinus area, are now being recognized as migraine headaches accompanied by tear formation and nasal discharge. *The common underlying bond for all the headaches labeled "migraine" is a role played by the blood vessels of the neck and head.* There is solid evidence that the early symptoms are usually related to constriction of these vessels and that the actual headache occurs when the vessels subsequently expand. The exact reasons for these blood vessel changes are not certain, though current interest is focused on the role of platelets and chemicals (like serotonin) which act on blood vessels. Whatever the exact cause, the following two areas of prevention and treatment are effective in many patients:

(1) Identifying and minimizing trigger factors: Many headache experts emphasize the importance of carefully trying to determine factors that seem to trigger headache attacks rather than jumping in immediately with drug therapy. As might be expected, the list of potential "triggers" is almost as long as the list of those who suffer from migraines, but the following seem to be most common:

Dietary factors: Changes in eating pattern (fasting or missing meals), specific foods (such as cheese, chocolate), alcohol, excessive caffeine (or sudden withdrawal from caffeine drinks), food preservatives (the nitrates and nitrites of cured meats such as cold cuts and hot dogs), and flavorers (MSG or even salt) can produce headaches in some people.

Hormone and drug factors: Hormones (as in birth control pills) and the change in hormones at the time of menstruation are clearly implicated in many women; reserpine (used in treating high blood pressure) is a drug known to produce headaches.

Emotional factors: While the stereotype of the migraine personality as rigid and compulsive is far from true for many migraine sufferers, there is general agreement that when perfectionists are subjected to stress, they are more likely to have headaches. Biofeedback techniques are being widely employed for such persons and for many others with no readily identifiable emotional factor.

Environmental factors: Temperature extremes, cigarette smoke, perfume, glaring light, and sudden changes in barometric pressure can trigger migraines.

(2) Careful drug therapy: The word "careful" is used to emphasize the need for attention to both proper use (timing and dosage) and potential side effects. Indeed, one of the hallmarks of the modern headache expert is the individualized manner in which he or she

prescribes drugs for a given patient. In addition to the usual pain relievers such as aspirin, Tylenol, Darvon, and codeine, the following drugs are in common use for the treatment of migraine and other headaches:

Ergot alkaloids: Long the mainstay of migraine treatment, these drugs act to prevent blood vessels from expanding; therefore, they are most effective in the early stages of a migraine before the throbbing phase of the headache becomes established. Because of the critical importance of dosage and timing with these drugs—and the danger of habituation and other physical side effects—they must be used only under the careful guidance of a knowledgeable physician.

Anti-depressants: Studies have demonstrated the effectiveness of these drugs (particularly amitriptyline)—even in persons without apparent depression. Obviously, long-term use is less than ideal, but judicious therapy with anti-depressants may be helpful in some people.

Propranolol: Recently approved by the Food and Drug Administration for the treatment of migraine, this drug is being widely used in headache treatment programs. It has the apparent advantage of minimal side effects when compared to other standard migraine drugs—and reports thus far support its effectiveness in many migraine sufferers.

Diuretics: Women who suffer from menstrual headaches may benefit by taking diuretic pills to promote fluid loss at the time of their period.

OTHER HEADACHES   *Tension headaches* refer to those that are primarily caused by contractions of the muscles of the scalp and neck; as suggested earlier, there is often an overlap between muscle and blood vessel contributions to a given headache. Treatment for this type of headache usually involves heat and massage for the involved muscles and simple pain medicines or muscle relaxants. However, in persistent cases, attention to underlying emotional factors becomes important in treating "up-tight" muscles. *Post-injury headaches* are common following head and neck injuries; sometimes these headaches do not begin until weeks or even months after an injury but they invariably clear with time—and the assurance that they are not serious. *Sinus headaches,* as indicated earlier, should as a rule be accompanied by signs of infection—local tenderness, fever, discharge of pus, and so on—in order to qualify as headaches not in the migraine family. Headaches associated with *high blood pressure* are uncommon (and more often associated with treatment for high blood pressure) but when they do occur, they are typically located in the back of the head, are worse upon arising, and improve as the day progresses. Significant *eye problems* are seldom the cause of headaches, though acute glaucoma should always be thought of as a possible cause, particularly in older persons who have accompanying visual changes.

Chronic headaches usually get labeled with one or more of the terms discussed above. Far more important than finding a quick label, however, is finding a physician who will take the time to evaluate thoroughly and patiently any headache problem that interferes with one's life. The National Migraine Foundation (4214 North Western Avenue, Chicago, Illinois 60625) can provide a list of specialists in headache problems.

The Painkiller War

The above title comes from a *Newsweek* article on the battle between manufacturers for the $720,000,000 that Americans spend for painkillers each year; significantly, the article was in the Advertising rather than the Medicine section of the magazine. The lines are drawn between *aspirin* (*salicylate*) and *acetaminophen,* which is marketed under many brand names, including Datril, Liquiprin, Lyteca, Nebs, Tempra, Tylenol, and Valadol. Some of the manufacturers have taken advantage of the fact that aspirin is seldom referred to by a specific brand name: a Tylenol ad says that doctors suggest their brand (of acetaminophen) more than all *brands* of aspirin combined. But the more revealing statement is that aspirin is still much more recommended than acetaminophen—largely on the basis of cost. For those of you "torn apart" by the advertising wars between aspirin and acetaminophen, the following facts may be useful:

(1) The two agents appear to be equally effective for the relief of mild to moderate pain or fever. *Only aspirin, however, has addi-*

tional anti-inflammatory effects—useful in the treatment of certain forms of arthritis, in which case the aspirin must be taken in higher (and potentially more dangerous) doses than are required for pain or fever. Both aspirin and acetaminophen are available generically (by asking for the compound itself, not the brand name given to it by the manufacturer), and they are generally cheaper when purchased in this manner.

(2) Side effects of aspirin include gastrointestinal irritation (aspirin may worsen symptoms in patients with ulcers and distress), prolongation of bleeding (aspirin should not be used by people with certain bleeding disorders), and a true allergic reaction (very rare, but potentially dangerous). Acetaminophen does not cause these problems and is an excellent substitute for persons who develop reactions to aspirin.

(3) Both aspirin and acetaminophen can cause serious toxicity and death in *large* overdose, as might be taken by children or those intent upon suicide.

For most people the choice between aspirin and acetaminophen would seem to boil down to cost. For those relative few who cannot tolerate aspirin, acetaminophen is an excellent substitute. When *anti-inflammatory* properties are specifically needed, aspirin should be selected.

ANALGESICS AND KIDNEY DISEASE   Kidney disease has been clearly associated with chronic, excessive use of the common pain medicines aspirin and phenacetin when taken in combination over a period of years. While it is not certain if either of these drugs is alone responsible for kidney damage, it has been known for some time that when they are taken routinely for persistent headaches, backaches, or even as stimulants, their cumulative impact can be the subtle development of serious kidney injury.

The problem occurs mainly in women (about 4 times as often as men). Typically, anywhere from 5 to 10 pain tablets containing both aspirin and phenacetin are taken each day for relief of headaches. Often, there is poor awareness of the number of such pills that are consumed. Until the right questions are asked, doctors may scratch their heads as to why the person's kidneys are failing. Recent estimates suggest that about 5% of all cases of "end-stage" kidney disease in this country can be traced to excessive analgesic (pain medicine) use. Unfortunately, some victims will pay the price of severely damaged kidneys and may even require dialysis treatment or a kidney transplant. Fortunately, many who develop kidney problems will improve—or at least stabilize—if the pain medicines are stopped.

Backaches

It is not surprising that the only persistently upright mammal on the face of the earth often reacts to general trouble with the woeful lament, "Oh, my aching back." Indeed, for millions of Americans, this cry is more than figurative, as it aptly describes either new or recurring pain in the lower part of the back. Each year, over 200,000 Americans submit to the surgeon's knife in the hope of curing—or at least lessening—such pain. Many anatomists and philosophers trace the back problems of *Homo sapiens* to the evolutionary accomplishment of traveling on twos rather than fours—thereby putting apparently unintended stress on the bones and supporting structures of the back. All experts agree that the ability to handle such stress has been lessened by the increasing trend to a sedentary life—which weakens the support muscles that aid the back in maintaining the upright position. This essay, however, is not concerned with the past—but with the present possibilities in the prevention, diagnosis, and treatment of lower back pain.

SPECIFIC CAUSES   The list of possible causes of lower back pain is seemingly endless and includes diseases of abdominal organs, cancer, arthritis, osteoporosis (weakening of bone due to hormonal changes or aging), and infections. However, the majority of back problems are due to strain or disc herniation.

(1) Strain: This all-purpose word is most often used for lower back troubles that are believed to be due to stresses on muscles and ligaments that surround the vertebral column. Often, localized areas of muscle spasm can be felt. At other times, deeper structures (muscles, joints, or ligaments) are assumed to be the site of the strain even though specific areas of tenderness or other abnormalities are not evident. Some feel that degenerative and traumatic changes in

the discs are the underlying reasons for susceptibility to back strains. Most back strains are relieved by adequate rest—often with the aid of pain-relieving and muscle relaxing medicines. In fact, it is generally accepted that no matter what is done, roughly 70% of back sufferers get well and are left with no symptoms or only intermittent problems that are not truly disabling.

(2) Disc problems: The spinal column (see diagram) is composed of 24 bones (vertebrae) which are surrounded by muscles and ligaments, all of which combine to provide both flexible support for the upright body and protection for the spinal cord and its nerve roots. Between the vertebrae are cushions known as "discs." These discs, which have a soft jelly-like center contained within a fibrous casing, make the spine flexible; they tend to degenerate (become less jelly-like and more compressible) with age. These changes account in part for the actual loss in height that occurs in many individuals as they grow older. Such degeneration usually causes no more than mild, intermittent backache and stiffness.

The more significant cause of disc pain results from relatively rapid protrusion (herniation) of the softer center through its outer casing, often due to stressful back movements. When this protruding material presses on the adjacent nerve root emerging from the spinal cord, classic "sciatica" occurs—pain that follows the distribution of the sciatic nerve to the back of the thigh, the outer part of the lower leg, and the foot. Sensory changes such as tingling and numbness in the leg and muscle spasms with eventual wasting of leg muscles may also occur with herniated discs.

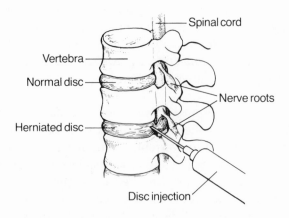

If these symptoms do not subside with rest (presumed to cause shrinkage of the protruded tissue), the logical treatment for such an anatomical derangement would seem to be removal of the protruding disc material—and thousands of such operations are done in this country each year. However, before disc surgery is considered, careful diagnostic studies must be done to prove with reasonable certainty that a particular disc is the culprit. Even then, physicians advise treatment with conservative measures (bed rest, pain medicines, some form of back support, and gradually increasing exercises to strengthen muscles) *since the majority of persons affected with apparent disc problems respond partially or completely to non-surgical treatment.* More recently, disc injection treatments have been used—but great controversy surrounds this technique (see p. 135). In short, the treatment of many disc problems is controversial—and often as much a matter of judgment as of scientific certainty. Second opinions are often appropriate—especially when one is confronted with a recommendation for early surgical treatment.

EVALUATION   Quite frankly, many physicians are "turned off" by back problems, especially those of people who have been to many doctors without getting relief. Nonetheless, physicians who specialize in back problems usually arrive at an accurate diagnosis using the following techniques:

(1) Careful history and physical examination: A complex back problem requires that the physician listen carefully to the patient's story (when does the pain occur? where is it felt?) and examine the patient thoroughly—observing him sitting, walking, and bending; touching and probing for sensitive areas; putting the legs in various positions to elicit symptoms; checking reflexes (ankle and knee), muscle strength, and sensation in the legs; and doing rectal, pelvic, and abdominal exams (as needed) for sources of "referred pain."

(2) Routine tests: At the very least, a blood count, urinalysis, and sedimentation rate should be done. Other tests may be used to check for malignancy or metabolic abnormalities. Structural changes in bones and joints, as well as "collapsed" discs, can be demonstrated by standard back x-rays.

(3) Special studies: These may be required to locate the offending disc(s)—and are considered mandatory before surgery by most

experts. *Myelography* involves fluoroscopy done after the injection of dye into the space surrounding the spinal cord and nerve roots; a protruding disc (or tumor) distorts or blocks the flow of dye as seen on x-rays. While this procedure is not routine, modern technique has minimized the discomfort and decreased the associated risk. *Discography,* another x-ray study done after injection of dye directly into the discs, is controversial. Measuring the speed of nerve impulses to muscles is sometimes useful in assessing nerve damage.

PREVENTION   Throughout this essay, we have hinted at conservative treatment measures—which can be used to aid in recovery from back pain. Of more importance, many of these same measures can help to *prevent* further attacks. We would like to emphasize some of them:

(1) Exercising: Any exercise that strengthens body muscles in general also helps the back. Most specific back exercises emphasize strengthening the abdominal muscles to aid the "front line" of defense against a sagging back. Many different exercise programs have been recommended and most will work if habitually performed; when tolerated, sit-ups with the knees bent are among the best.

(2) Learning proper lifting and bending: By now, most of us have gotten the message that bending and lifting from the waist are bad for the back. Instead, the knees should be used for bending—and heavy objects should be kept as close to the body as possible.

(3) Maintaining proper posture: While mother's strictures against slumping may have been excessive, most experts agree she had a point. Sleeping posture is also important—meaning that it is best to avoid sleeping on one's stomach and instead adopt the side or back positions. A firm—not hard—mattress is also helpful. Finally, high heels may be fine for fashion, but they are bad for the back.

(4) Losing excess weight: This seems to be the answer to everything—but logic clearly points to excessive weight (especially abdominal overhang) as extra strain on the back.

The above measures will not prevent all back troubles, but they will help many persons avoid surgery (not a bad trade-off) and prevent further attacks of back pain.

Disc Injection

Surgery for a herniated disc has long been a difficult and controversial decision. A recent development has added another reason for this controversy—the possibility of an alternative form of therapy, known scientifically as chemonucleolysis and popularly as "injecting the disc." Since such therapy was first tried in 1963, it has become enmeshed (in the U.S.) in a tangle of federal regulations that eventually resulted in temporary withdrawal of approval for further investigational use in this country. We have asked Dr. Thornton Brown, Associate Professor of Orthopedic Surgery at the Massachusetts General Hospital, Harvard Medical School, and Editor Emeritus of the *Journal of Bone and Joint Surgery,* to answer some questions about disc injections. (See diagram, p. 132.)

What is chemonucleolysis?

Chemonucleolysis is the procedure in which chymopapain (the enzyme present in meat tenderizers) is injected into the soft or jelly-like central portion of an intervertebral disc in order to dissolve this portion of the disc structure. If one visualized the intervertebral disc as a water bed, the injection of chymopapain would "let the water out of the mattress." Chemonucleolysis is a highly technical procedure performed under anesthesia (local or general); x-rays must be used to guide the insertion of the needle. When placement is correct, the surgeon injects Discase—a solution of chymopapain in a fluid composed of chemicals that in themselves may have some deflating effect on the disc. In successful injections, sciatica is relieved very promptly due to reduced pressure on nerve roots, but back pain may be severe for 12 to 48 hours. Once pain has subsided to a tolerable level, the patient can get up and leave the hospital—usually in a day or two. Return to light work is possible after one to six weeks and to heavy work in about three months. Gradual narrowing of the "disc space" between the vertebral bones, when seen on x-ray, is a favorable sign.

What is the success rate?

In general, chemonucleolysis will relieve symptoms in about 70% of patients with disc herniation causing sciatica, but the injection is relatively ineffective in (1) patients who have had a previous unsuccessful operation for back and leg symptoms; (2) patients with symptoms due to spinal stenosis (a narrowed spinal canal causing nerve pressure); (3) patients with spinal instability due to disc degeneration; and (4) patients whose back symptoms are inextricably intermeshed with emotional and personality problems.

What are the risks?

Although there were a few early cases of paralysis after injection, which have been cited frequently by those who disapprove of chemonucleolysis, it is now well established that if the injection is done properly, the risk of nerve damage is almost nonexistent (no signs of damage after approximately 15,000 injections of Discase). Life-threatening allergic reactions have been reported in less than 1% of patients injected; although these pose a real danger, their treatment is usually very effective when preparations have been made in advance. Other complications include infection or non-bacterial inflammation of the injected disc space, as well as the usual risks involved in any surgical procedure with anesthesia. Overall, the risks of injection are less than those of surgical removal of a disc. Also in favor of injection treatment are a shorter hospital stay and an easier convalescence.

If chemonucleolysis fails, is surgery still possible?

Yes. Surgical removal of the disc protrusion or removal of bone to decompress a nerve root can still be done, usually about six weeks after an unsuccessful injection. Opinions vary as to whether a prior injection may make surgical treatment more difficult.

Why is the procedure not done in the United States?

The answer to this question is complicated. The Food and Drug Administration initially approved the use of chymopapain on an experimental basis and the enzyme was used extensively by some 1,600 physicians. By 1975, the FDA appeared to be ready to approve the drug for general use, subject to certain restrictions. However, in July of that year investigators were instructed to discontinue chemonucleolysis and return all enzyme in their possession to the manufacturer. Subsequently, a double-blind study (neither doctor nor patient knew what was injected until the code was broken at a later date) was described at a conference—but not reported in print until 1976. In this study, approved by the FDA, the results of the injection of Discase were compared with those after injection of the diluent alone. After rather short follow-up, the data showed that the results after the two injections were not statistically different. Although the validity of this study was criticized for a variety of reasons, the FDA refused to release chymopapain without further evidence, and the manufacturer withdrew its application for approval of a new drug. In addition, for a considerable time the manufacturer declined to proceed with the development of the product. Finally, after much negotiation, a new FDA-approved double-blind study was developed and begun in late 1979. In this study, either the enzyme chymopapain, the diluent solution, or plain salt solution is injected without the patient's or doctor's knowing which agent was injected until the code is subsequently broken. This study is currently in progress, but because patients are being selected for inclusion in the study according to very strict criteria designed to insure that the results are scientifically valid, it is anticipated that it will take several years before any conclusions as to the true value of chymopapain can be drawn.

In the meantime, in a study of 114 patients treated between 1972 and 1975 and re-evaluated 3 to 6 years later (*Journal of the American Medical Association,* May 23/30, 1980), nearly 73% continued to have marked improvement. In addition, reports from Canada, Australia, Yugoslavia, and elsewhere have shown success with the procedure in properly selected patients.

Assuming chemonucleolysis becomes available in the United States, when should it be used?

The exact role of chymopapain in the treatment of the "back-pain problem" has not been established. One opinion expressed by a Canadian orthopedic surgeon with extensive experience is that chemonucleolysis is the last step in the conservative (non-operative) treatment of lumbar disc herniations, the step before operation when all else has failed. Certainly, time-proven conservative measures, including rest in bed and anti-inflammatory medications, should be tried for two weeks at the very least (and preferably much longer) before chemonucleolysis is considered. The word "injection" may imply a minor procedure, but this is not so. Chemonucleolysis should only be done in hospitals equipped and staffed to deal with any complications. It should also be done only after a complete diagnostic work-up, including x-rays, myelogram (in the opinion of some authorities), and other studies—among them psychological tests—have established that the patient is a candidate for the procedure. People who have been considered unsuitable for chemonucleolysis include those with a history of allergy to the enzyme in meat tenderizers, those with myelograms showing a complete block to the flow of the dye or a possible tumor, those with rapidly developing loss of muscle power or sensation, or any disturbance of function of the urinary bladder or bowel attributed to the disc protrusion, and women who are pregnant. Previous treatment with chymopapain is also probably a reason not to have further treatment by this method.

Disc injection is no cure-all for an aching back, but it might save time and expense if the problem is a herniated disc that has not improved after adequate non-operative treatment. The final answer awaits further carefully controlled studies for which the stage has now been set.

Temporomandibular
Joint Syndrome

In recent years, the temporomandibular joint (TMJ) has become the object of both intense scientific interest and popular folklore. This joint (where the lower jaw attaches to the skull near the ear) has been blamed for many problems—some of which really relate to the muscles that activate it. Several years ago, an article in the Sunday supplement *Parade*—entitled "The Great Imposter"—kindled even more interest in the TMJ. We have asked Dr. Walter Guralnick, Professor of Oral Surgery at the Massachusetts General Hospital, Harvard School of Dental Medicine, to answer the following questions:

In simple terms, how does this joint work?

The TMJ can be portrayed as a hinging of the lower jaw (mandible) onto the upper part of the skull in a manner analogous to a ball and socket (see diagram). The top of the mandible is ball-shaped and fits into a hollow area in the temporal bone of the skull—giving rise to the name of the two bones involved, temporomandibular joint. As in several other joints, there is a small disc (meniscus) which separates the two bony parts and the entire joint is sheathed by a capsule of supporting ligaments.

When the mouth is opened or closed, only the mandible moves. It is controlled by several large muscles that can move it up and down and, to a lesser degree, sideways. However, TMJ movement is unique in two ways. Any movement on one side depends on appropriate "cooperation" from the paired TMJ on the other side. Also, tooth problems can significantly influence TMJ function.

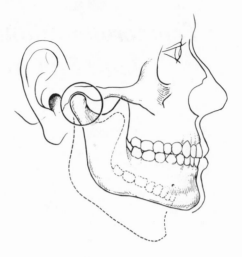

Finally, it's worth noting that the TMJ is within two or three millimeters of the inner ear canal, which explains why an "earache" is a common symptom of TMJ trouble.

What kinds of problems can be traced to the TMJ?

Our understanding of the TMJ stems from some remarkable studies during the past thirty years which indicate that the majority of TMJ problems are unaccompanied by pathological changes and only a small proportion (5 to 10%) are caused by identifiable anatomic disturbances in the structure of the joint. Such changes include ankylosis (fusion) of the joint, a serious problem usually arising from an injury at an early age. Arthritic destruction of the joint may also occur; while some damage to the TMJ is seen in some persons with rheumatoid arthritis, severe deformity of the joint is relatively rare. Tumors of the TMJ are very rare.

Far more common are "functional" problems—restricted motion, facial pain, noisy or clicking joints—in which no structural changes can be found. The research of the past thirty years has indicated that the majority of these complaints can be attributed to what is now generally termed the myofascial pain-dysfunction (MPD) syndrome—a fancy phrase which means that the trouble lies in the muscles that control the lower jaw.

In order to understand this phenomenon better, we should consider how often we all use our jaw muscles to express emotion. Such phrases as "grimacing in pain" or "gnashing his teeth" or "clenching his jaw" stem from real life. Tension habits such as grinding the teeth during sleep (bruxism) or clenching teeth when concentrating are common. These habits can understandably lead to fatigue and spasm of the jaw muscles which, in turn, can produce many of the typical symptoms associated with the TMJ. The other major contributing factor to the MPD syndrome is malocclusion—the improper meeting of teeth when jaws are in the closed position. Something as simple as a "high" filling or as complex as a bite "thrown off" by missing teeth can lead to continued discomfort in the region of the TMJ.

What are typical TMJ symptoms?

The most common symptom is a one-sided "ear" pain which is often dull and constant, typically worse in the morning and often increased by chewing; the pain may radiate to the temple, neck, or angle of the jaw. The TMJ may be tender to touch and there may be some restriction of jaw motion; the jaw often deviates to the painful side on opening. Occasionally, with severe muscle spasms, the jaw will "lock" and have to be forcibly opened.

How do you treat TMJ problems?

Structural problems can often be treated by surgery, and many ingenious procedures are available today. Fusion, for example, can be treated by removing the fused area of bone and replacing it with a piece of silicone rubber. Sometimes an artificial joint is the answer.

It is essential to stress, however, that surgery is recommended for only a very small percentage of persons with TMJ troubles. As already discussed, the vast majority of TMJ pains are caused by undue muscle tension and do not require surgical intervention—unless secondary structural problems have resulted. It is, of course, necessary to correct any dental disturbances that might contribute to myofascial pain-dysfunction.

When the MPD syndrome is diagnosed, it is important to approach it as a psychosomatic problem and deal with the underlying psychological components. Counseling is often required to ease the tension underlying such habits as grinding or clenching teeth; a sympathetic and thorough explanation of the problem can be of great help. Application of heat along with muscle-relaxing or pain-relieving medicines can also be useful. A soft diet to decrease chewing is often recommended. Finally, "midline opening exercises" to retrain the jaw muscles in normal function are sometimes advised. With these simple measures, more than 75% of persons with TMJ symptoms can be cured eventually.

What kind of doctor should someone with TMJ problems consult?

Many persons do not suspect TMJ problems as the cause of their symptoms and thus go to doctors appropriate for their complaints—ear specialists (otolaryngologists) for ear pain, as well as arthritis or orthopedic specialists for bone pain. However, almost all people with TMJ problems will benefit from seeing a dentist or dental specialist who has a specific interest in TMJ problems. Usually such specialists can be identified by calling a nearby dental school or hospital dental department. However, if there is any question that pain in the TMJ region may be due to other causes, full evaluation by others—such as ear-nose-and-throat specialists—is in order.

Colds and Flu

During each winter season, much of the country turns its medical attention to those annoying afflictions of the human race we label as colds or flu—not surprisingly since these diseases account for over 50% of all acute illness, up to 50% of time lost from work in adults, and up to 80% of time out of school in children. And while they seldom cause death (except in the very young and very old or in persons seriously ill with other disease), these afflictions are surrounded by considerable misunderstandings that can lead to unnecessary anxiety and poor medical practice.

THE "BUGS" Basic to an understanding of any infectious disease is the fact that there are two major kinds of germs in this world— bacteria and viruses. In the case of colds and flu, this distinction becomes critical because most of these "winter blahs" are caused by viruses. And since viruses are not affected by antibiotics, the obvious conclusion is this: *the vast majority of colds and flu should not be treated with antibiotics.*

THE TERMINOLOGY Generally, infections are named for their location followed by the suffix "-itis." Thus an infection in the major breathing tubes to each lung—the bronchi—becomes "bronchitis." (Other examples are laryngitis, pharyngitis, and tonsillitis.) The following terms are often not clearly used or understood:

(1) URI (upper respiratory infection): This phrase is used for infections located in the upper part of the breathing system—that is, above the lungs. This is what the term "cold" generally refers to— the infamous collection of symptoms such as runny nose, sore throat, weepy eyes, and so on. URIs may be caused by many differ-

143

ent families of viruses. Some of these families are themselves very large. For instance, there are over 100 types of rhinoviruses, the viruses most commonly associated with fall and spring colds.

(2) Flu (influenza): Generally these infections are distinguished from URIs by the suddenness and severity of symptoms and the more generalized ill feeling ("ache all over") and prostration (being "pooped out") that usually accompanies the flu. Unlike URIs, flu often is accompanied by fever greater than 101 °F. When flu occurs in large epidemics, it usually is caused by influenza type A viruses.

(3) Croup and bronchiolitis: These common infections in young children are apt to produce obstruction to air flow that *results in considerable breathing difficulty.* Signs of such difficulty—such as stridor (a harsh, shrill noise) or retraction (pulling in) of chest muscles during breathing—signal the need for immediate medical attention.

(4) Bronchitis: As mentioned above, this term refers to infection in the major breathing tubes leading to the lungs from the windpipe. This diagnosis is often invoked when no evidence of infection in the lungs can be found but chest findings such as deep cough and wheezing are present.

(5) Pneumonia: This word should be used only for infection in the lungs. (The word "lungitis" might be more logical—but the term pneumonia, stemming from the Greek word for lung, has long been used.) Such infections are more likely to be treated with antibiotics. Viral pneumonias are common, however, and may be difficult to distinguish from bacterial pneumonias.

TREATMENT IN GENERAL   It is important to *distinguish between viral and bacterial infections since viruses should not be treated with antibiotics.* Sometimes this distinction is not easy even after careful examination and many tests (such as blood count, chest x-ray, microscopic examination and cultures of sputum). And sometimes it is legitimate to treat with antibiotics, even though the infecting organism is not certain. *But as a general rule, the doctor who takes time to examine you and then indicates that antibiotics are not necessary is doing you a favor by avoiding unnecessary expense and possibly severe reactions to antibiotics. Instead of requesting antibiotics, you should be asking if they are really necessary.* Obviously, self-medication with antibiotics is totally inappropriate; in addition to the danger involved, antibiotics can confuse culture tests that might be needed.

TREATMENT FOR COLDS   Given the above, a section on treatment for a condition caused by viruses may seem unnecessary. There is, however, a "cure" agreed to by all experts, including Mother Nature: Large doses of "tincture of time." Many remember the old maxim: "If you do nothing, you will get better in a week, but if you treat the symptoms of a cold vigorously, you will get better in seven days." In some cases, bacterial complications that require antibiotics—such as sinusitis, ear infections, even pneumonia—may occur subsequent to viral infections of the upper respiratory tract. But a pure cold is the kind of problem medically described as "self-limited"—meaning that it will run its course and get better without specific treatment. Given this fact, it is amazing that Americans spend over 500 million dollars each year for over-the-counter (OTC) non-prescription cold remedies—*not* including aspirin. While almost anything can be found in some cold remedies (including antacids and laxatives), most OTC cold products contain one or more of the following categories of medications:

(1) *Decongestants:* Decongestants used in cold remedies are usually members of a class of drugs known as "sympathomimetic amines"—meaning that they constrict blood vessels (among other actions). When used *topically* (sprays, drops), they may produce a "rebound" in which the nose later becomes even more congested; prolonged use of nasal sprays or drops can therefore *produce* problems. When taken *orally,* doses of decongestant required to constrict nasal vessels will also constrict vessels elsewhere in the body and therefore cause potential dangers, especially for persons with high blood pressure.

(2) *Antihistamines:* There are about twenty different kinds of antihistamines available in the United States. When used in cold remedies, the theory is to take advantage of "anticholinergic" properties (see below) which may dry up nasal secretions in the early stages of a cold. However, these same properties can also cause blurred vision and urinary retention, and may pose problems for those taking medication for glaucoma. A major side effect of antihistamines is sedation, and persons who are especially sensitive to this

reaction should avoid driving or other potentially hazardous activities. There is no scientific rationale for combining different antihistamines in a single product. Some specific antihistamines—such as chlorpheniramine—are available generically, at much lower cost than when sold in combination trade-name products.

(3) Anticholinergics: These drugs are sometimes placed in cold remedies in the hope that they might contribute to a drying out of the nasal passages. In doses commonly used, it is unlikely that they alone will have such an effect, but when combined with antihistamines, some nasal drying *may* result. However, such a combination increases the danger of sedative effects from the antihistamines.

(4) Antipyretics (anti-fever) and analgesics (anti-pain): This category of medication—including aspirin and acetaminophen—is used to suppress the aches and pain often associated with viral infections, colds or otherwise. Most colds are not accompanied by actual fever, even though the patient may feel warm. Almost all OTC cold remedies contain either aspirin or acetaminophen—or both. In fact, claims made for "the ingredient most often prescribed by doctors" usually refer to nothing more than simple aspirin. And the reason for including more than one of these agents may be nothing more than to provide a backing for the claim of "more than one active ingredient." People who might be sensitive to aspirin may be surprised to learn that it's in their favorite cold remedy.

(5) Antitussives: These cough medicines are designed either to promote the raising of sputum (expectorants) or to decrease coughing (suppressants). It is important to raise excessive sputum that is filled with pus. Many experts argue that humidifiers and vaporizers are better than any expectorant for liquefying secretions and thus raising sputum. Cough suppressants can be useful for persons whose "dry" or "hacking" coughs interfere with sleep, but should not be employed when excessive sputum exists.

(6) Vitamin C: Despite several studies of the issues, there is *no good evidence to date that high doses of vitamin C are effective in preventing or treating the common cold.* Although the dangers of vitamin C have probably been exaggerated as well, *proof of safety* should be required from those who introduce new treatment, and that has not been established for large doses of vitamin C.

(7) Etc.: Almost anything can be found in some so-called cold

remedies—vitamins, tranquilizers, quinine, and even laxatives. Some remedies contain caffeine to attempt to counter the sedative effects of their antihistamines.

Given the incredible number of OTC remedies, the average consumer is understandably bewildered by the array of products confronting him when he staggers into the drug store to find something that might help the miseries of the common cold. In fact, OTC remedies are generally overrated. Often single-ingredient medications will meet a specific need. For example, simple aches and pains of a cold are best met with a plain aspirin, or acetaminophen for those not able to tolerate aspirin. And, as pointed out initially, the essential fact is that persons with nothing more than a cold, however miserable they may feel, will get better in a few days. And, believe it or not, there is some evidence to support the benefit of chicken soup; supposedly it helps the flow of mucus in congested nasal passages.

PREVENTION   It is impossible to avoid the viruses of colds and flu, and there is no evidence that bare heads and wet feet increase the chances of getting a cold. (The increased incidence during winter is caused by many factors, including greater exposure to viruses due to indoor gathering of people.) The only two preventive measures available are the flu shot and amantadine. We have asked Advisory Board member Dr. Stephen Schoenbaum, a specialist in infectious diseases and a member of the Public Health Service Advisory Committee on Immunization Practices, to comment on the controversies surrounding the influenza vaccines and the use of amantadine in preventing influenza.

What are flu shots?

The flu shots currently used consist of large quantities of influenza viruses which have been grown in eggs, killed, and purified. Being dead, they cannot reproduce within the body to cause disease. But they will stimulate the body to produce antibodies which will protect against similar live viruses. A full-blown infection should then be prevented—or at least curtailed.

Why are flu shots controversial?

First, the influenza vaccine is only 60–70% effective in preventing illness, while vaccines for polio, measles, and some other viruses are over 90% effective. Also, influenza viruses are notorious for constantly changing their surface coat which antibodies attack. Major changes often result in large epidemics, while minor changes are associated with smaller epidemics. The antibodies produced by older vaccines will be less effective, and sometimes totally ineffective, against the newer strains of virus, so the vaccine's protective value is reduced. In other words, influenza viruses tend to keep "fooling" older vaccines, and the vaccines need frequent updating which involves some scientific guesswork.

Second, influenza vaccines seem to lose their effectiveness after one year—though the exact duration of their effectiveness is unknown. For this reason, annual immunization is advised.

Third, there is a high reaction rate associated with influenza vaccines. Sore arms are common after a shot, and some people will have a fever for a day or two. Although the surveillance program for vaccine reactions resulting from swine flu shots uncovered a previously unknown problem—the occurrence of the Guillain-Barré syndrome of paralysis in about one out of every 100,000 recipients of this particular vaccine—there has fortunately been no evidence of such increased risk with the usual flu vaccines used each year, even though it has been in the years since the swine flu program.

Who should get flu shots?

Current evidence still suggests that it is important for selected individuals to receive the vaccine—those in the so-called "high-risk" groups (people with chronic diseases, those over 65, and people in high-risk occupations, such as hospital employees). Each time there is a large epidemic caused by an influenza virus, an excess number of hospitalizations and deaths beyond that normally expected occurs. These flu-related deaths are most common among high-risk groups. Since 1968, influenza epidemics have been rather small compared with those seen in the past, and they have changed in pattern as well, occurring annually in a limited geographic area, rather than nation-wide every two or three years. Nevertheless, deaths are still occurring that are attributable to the influenza virus and an annual flu shot could *partly* prevent this problem. The question is whether the benefits from vaccination outweigh the risks and the costs involved. That question has been examined on several occasions, and each time it appears that the most sensible policy is yearly immunization of high-risk groups with vaccine made from viruses similar to the strains expected to be prevalent during the winter season. Vaccination of the entire population is recommended only in years when very large epidemics are expected—years in which a major change in the influenza virus has been detected.

What is the difference between the flu shot and the pneumonia vaccine?

Some people confuse the annual flu shot (changed each year to combat the specific influenza viruses expected) with the pneumonia vaccine—a vaccine designed to protect against 14 strains of the pneumococcus bacterium, one of the most common causes of pneumonia. These two shots are very different in composition and preventive effect—though they are both typically recommended for the same people, namely, the elderly and those with serious chronic diseases. They can be taken at the same time, but it is important to remember that while the flu shot is designed to offer protection only for the coming flu season, the protective effect of the pneumonia vaccine is expected to last from three to five years.

Of what value is amantadine in preventing influenza?

Though vaccination must be considered the principal approach to prevention of influenza on the basis of proven efficacy over a long period of time, safety for use in very large populations, and relatively low cost, a second approach is available and merits consideration for special patients or groups. The drug amantadine (used in Parkinson's disease) is about 60–70% effective at preventing influenza, *if it is being taken at the time of exposure*. Since the drug must be taken at least once daily, and a course of the drug is considerably more expensive and less convenient than the flu shot, it has not come into widespread use for prevention of influenza. Amantadine also can be used to treat persons with influenza, and can lead to shortening of the illness; but to be an effective treatment, amantadine must be given within 48 hours of the appearance of the first symptoms. This means that amantadine must be given before the complications of influenza, such as pneumonia, set in. Thus, by the time a physician is seen for persistent illness or increased severity of symptoms, it is usually too late to use the drug.

Like all drugs, amantadine has potential side effects. Among the most troublesome are mental problems such as depression, anxiety, and difficulty concentrating. Generally, however, fewer than 10% of persons who have been started on the drug in clinical trials have had to stop taking it because of side effects.

Amantadine works only in preventing or treating illness caused by influenza A viruses. It does not even work for the very similar influenza B viruses; and it is, of course, totally ineffective for all the other viruses which cause URIs and even flu-like illnesses.

Nevertheless, there is a place for amantadine. Sometimes there are vaccine shortages at times of major influenza A epidemics. Unvaccinated persons in the high-risk group might be protected with amantadine. Regrettably, only a fraction of the high-risk populations—about 20%—receives vaccine in the fall before the onset of the influenza season. And, once a flu epidemic starts, it has been considered too late to give vaccine because the protective effect takes about two weeks to develop. However, by receiving amantadine for those two weeks, a person could be protected until the vaccine is itself effective. Furthermore, vaccine and amantadine can work in concert, so that both might be used for people with severe respiratory diseases who are at very high risk from influenza infections. Finally, by instructing patients in advance, physicians should be able to start high-risk persons on amantadine during known influenza epidemics within 48 hours of onset of symptoms, thus taking advantage of the therapeutic effect of amantadine.

Allergies

Sneezing. Itching. Weeping. Wheezing. As many as a fifth of our readers experience these miserable symptoms of allergy. Probably the most common form of allergy is "hay fever," which is a classic misnomer since it is not caused by hay and there is no fever. The more accurate term is *allergic rhinitis* ("rhin-" meaning *nose,* as in "rhinoceros"). Related conditions that are less common but can be more debilitating include *asthma*; "eczema," also known as *atopic dermatitis;* "hives," or *urticaria,* most commonly from foods or drugs; and a life-threatening reaction known as *acute anaphylaxis.*

In a rather casual way people often say they are allergic to this or that substance when they are not truly allergic at all. For example, many so-called food allergies result from the inability to digest a particular food in a normal way. In other cases, an irritant may produce discomfort which is not based on an allergic response.

BASICS   Allergies all result from a characteristic defect in the immune system, which normally serves to protect our bodies from microscopic foreign invaders. The defect in question is a tendency to overreact to foreign substances, such as pollens, that otherwise would be utterly harmless.

Here's an outline of what happens when an allergic reaction to pollen takes place. Other allergic reactions are similar in principle, but the details can be quite different.

(1) A pollen grain, coated with its distinctive molecules, lands on the membranes of the nose or lungs.

(2) If a person is allergic, antibodies that recognize these particular foreign molecules are in the neighborhood. They are capable of attaching themselves to a particular type of defense cell known as a

151

mast cell—or some of them may already be on the mast cells' surfaces.

(3) The antibodies become stuck to the foreign molecules. In the case of pollen, many identical molecules are carried on the surface of a single granule, so they consequently can become stuck to more than one antibody. In turn, each antibody can hitch up with two molecules on the pollen surface. Thus, antibodies and granules easily form a lattice or network.

(4) The lattice, as it forms, acts as a switch to turn on the mast cell. The cell then releases *histamine* and a variety of other substances which go on to produce the symptoms of allergy.

(5) Histamine causes the itching; it also makes tiny blood vessels dilate and become leaky—hence the swelling and redness associated with allergy. The itchy, runny nose and sneezing of hay fever are mainly produced by histamine. Another substance released by mast cells makes trouble for asthmatics. It causes the air passages in their lungs to constrict, and the narrowed air passages produce the characteristic wheezing of asthma.

This basic course of events and its variants are responsible for all allergic reactions. Why one person gets hay fever from ragweed, another gets hives from seafood, and yet another gets eczema from exposure to various substances—these differences in reaction pattern simply are not understood.

As a rule, the first time someone is exposed to an allergen (the foreign molecule that sets off an allergy) nothing very obvious happens because antibodies are not yet present to start the chain reaction. But exposure, which may occur only once or may have to be repeated many times, stimulates production of the "allergic" type of antibody (known in the business as immunoglobulin E, or IgE for short). And then symptoms develop. Any kind of allergy can appear at any time in life, and often an allergy will go away or become milder after a few years. Eczema and asthma are often at their worst in early childhood and get better after that. Hay fever, on the other hand, may begin in adulthood or even old age. Whenever an allergy develops, a combination of factors must be present to bring it on: (1) an inherited (genetic) tendency, (2) exposure to a molecule that acts as an allergen, and sometimes (3) yet another triggering event—some kind of stress—that helps to get the ball rolling.

DIAGNOSIS   Often it's fairly obvious that someone has an allergy. Yet hay fever can resemble a cold, and it may be recognized for what it is only after the patient notices that he or she gets the "cold" at precisely the same time every year and that it also goes away on schedule. Year-round allergies (for example, a dust allergy) may be harder to spot. Hives are usually easy to identify, though allergy may cause subtler rashes. Asthmatic attacks may or may not have an obvious allergic trigger.

The hallmark of allergy is a recurrent association of symptoms with a change in the environment. If a change of seasons, location, job, diet, or habits brings on the condition or makes it go away, patient and doctor have a clue to its cause, and painstaking review of the events leading to an episode can serve to pinpoint the culprit.

Skin tests: For certain kinds of allergy—mostly the variants of "hay fever"—skin testing is an invaluable method of identifying the allergens that affect a particular patient. A very small quantity of the suspected allergen, in highly purified form, is injected into the skin. The allergic person responds in short order by developing a patch of red, itchy skin around the injection site. This type of testing, although it is associated with some discomfort, is the cheapest, most convenient, and most reliable way of identifying allergens. Yet skin tests have only been proved valid for a limited range of substances: the pollens, drugs, certain foods, and perhaps (in asthmatics) animal dander. There is little or no support for the notion that other substances can be tested in this way.

The RAST: It would be nice if the minor discomfort of skin testing could be avoided and a sample of blood used for a laboratory evaluation of allergy. The most successful test of this sort, so far, is the RAST (radioallergosorbent test), which, unfortunately, does not appear to be as sensitive or as accurate as skin testing. At present, the RAST is used mainly to test for food allergies. It is also helpful when a skin disorder such as eczema makes skin testing too difficult.

TREATMENT   Avoiding the offending agent would be the ideal approach if it were only possible all the time. But people who are allergic to oak pollen usually can't leave town every spring for a desert vacation. And people who are allergic to bee stings can't stay indoors their whole lives. Fortunately for people with various kinds of allergic disease, real progress is being made in treatment methods.

Hay fever: The sneezing, itching, and weeping that come from allergy to pollens, dusts, animal dander, and so forth are caused by the action of histamine that has been released from mast cells. Antihistamines, of which there are very many (see below), are drugs that prevent the released histamine from causing symptoms. They are the mainstay of treatment for hay fever and help two-thirds or more of the people who try them. For the best effect, antihistamines should be taken around the clock (usually four times a day). Sometimes, a very slight increase over the starting dose will improve a person's response; some trial-and-error may be needed.

The main problem with antihistamines is their common side effect: sleepiness (which is made much worse when alcohol is also taken). Fortunately, the wide variety of antihistamines makes it possible to experiment with various types to see which produce the best protection with the least drowsiness. In the following list of common antihistamines, those marked * are reported to produce relatively little drowsiness; but you have to find out for yourself which works best for you:

tripelennamine*	brompheniramine*
pyrilamine*	pyrrobutamine
thonzylamine*	triprolidine
diphenhydramine	promethazine
phenyltoloxamine	trimeprazine
dimenhydrinate	cyproheptadine*
chlorpheniramine*	phenindamine*

Decongestants, on the other hand, may actually favor the release of histamine; they probably should not be routinely used but rather reserved for times when nasal stuffiness interferes with sleep or creates discomfort. (One decongestant, ephedrine, doesn't release histamine, but it has other side effects that limit its usefulness.) Three commonly used decongestants are pseudoephedrine, phenylpropanolamine, and phenylephrine.

Immunotherapy (previously called "desensitization shots") was at one time regarded as a questionable treatment for allergies. It has by now proved its worth: in a few cases it cures allergies, in many more it markedly reduces the severity. In immunotherapy gradually increasing doses of an allergen—beginning with very small amounts—are injected into a patient's skin. The injections must be given at weekly intervals over a period of three to five years, and if the sequence is interrupted it has to be started all over again. At the end of this period, the patient should show improvement; there is no point to continuing for years on end with no clear sign of progress.

However, immunotherapy still has many limitations. Its value has been conclusively demonstrated only for pollen allergies—mainly those to ragweed, which is the most common cause of hay fever in the United States, and certain of the grasses and trees. The procedure may also help with allergy to house dust. No conclusive studies have demonstrated the value of immunotherapy for allergies to food or animal dander.

Some good news has recently appeared. It is possible to modify the ragweed allergen in a way that makes it much more effective for immunotherapy than the purified substance itself. Treatment with the new material is often effective after only a season. In time, it may be possible to modify other allergens to produce similar results.

Nevertheless, the cost, inconvenience, and (modest) risk of immunotherapy make it appropriate only for patients who are disabled by their symptoms but cannot take antihistamines without drowsiness or other adverse effects.

Anaphylaxis: Some people have a violent allergic reaction to insect stings or to drugs such as penicillin. At its worst, this reaction—known as anaphylactic shock—leads to collapse and rapid death. Immunotherapy has been developed for insect allergies and has been shown to work very well if a purified preparation of the insect's venom is used. People who are allergic to the sting of bees, wasps, or fire ants should consider protecting themselves with a course of venom immunotherapy. In any case, susceptible individuals should keep "sting kits" at hand so that epinephrine can be injected promptly in the event of a sting reaction.

Allergy to penicillin, it now appears, can be rapidly overcome by a few hours of immunotherapy. In this case, the patient is given a tiny *oral* dose of the antibiotic and then the dose is doubled every fifteen minutes until it reaches moderately high levels. If further studies confirm the initial report, this procedure may benefit many patients.

Asthma: Asthma cannot be cured as yet, but in the past few years improvements in drug therapy have made treatment much more effective, and still better drugs appear to be on their way. Whereas treatment for hay fever is mainly directed at blocking the effects of histamine once it is released, drugs for asthma work to prevent the release of substances that produce symptoms. All the drugs traditionally given to prevent or relieve an attack appear to have this effect, and all of them have been improved in ways that reduce their side effects. There is reason to believe that optimal control is achieved when the drugs are used in combination.

PREVENTION   Adults subject to allergic reactions can only prevent them by avoiding the cause of their symptoms. Staying inside as much as possible during the pollen season may help those with hay fever. Air conditioning or filtration may be necessary, but the systems that really work to reduce indoor pollen counts are likely to be expensive. Synthetic fabrics used for blankets, pillows, and rugs are less likely to cause reactions than natural fibers. Certain foods—such as eggs, shellfish, nuts, tomatoes, and chocolate—are notorious allergens and may have to be avoided. Venom reactions, as we've said, can be prevented by immunotherapy. The chance of stings can be minimized by commonsense measures—avoiding bright colors and smells which attract insects, wearing protective clothing, etc.

New parents with a history of allergies in their families may want to take certain measures to reduce the child's risk. Although the following recommendations are not based on rock-solid evidence, they seem warranted: breast feed the infant as long as possible; avoid cow's milk and cow's milk products for at least six months; also delay giving eggs, fish, and citrus juices, as well as solid foods in general; don't keep pets; don't have wool fabrics or feathers around the house; take measures to minimize dust and mold; don't smoke. And good luck!

Diseases from Pets

Thirty-eight percent of American households have a dog, twenty percent have a cat, and another fourteen percent have other pets. This translates into the startling fact that approximately sixty million dogs and cats share living quarters with families in this country. Given this common mingling between Americans and pets, we have asked Dr. Ann Sullivan Baker, Assistant Professor of Medicine at the Massachusetts General Hospital, Harvard Medical School, to answer the following questions concerning health hazards presented by pets.

**What are the most common dangers posed
by household pets?**

The problems caused by pets include bites, infections, and allergic reactions. An *allergic reaction* (such as asthma or sneezing) is generally rather easy to spot and, unfortunately, treatment usually is removal of the pet from the household. It is estimated that more than one-half million animal *bites* occur in the United States every year, and the dog is the most common offender. The biting dog is usually young and often caged or tethered. Dogs that have been trained to attack may turn on children, and serious mutilating injuries have occurred in this circumstance. The major problems posed by bites are wound infections caused by bacteria from the mouth of the animal or on the skin of the victim. Careful washing of a wound and leaving it open after a bite are important measures in preventing an infection from developing. In the view of the general public, the most worrisome problem posed by household pets is that they might transmit *infections*. Although a number of such diseases can be listed, the most important point is that most of them are rare.

What are the important infections that cat and dog owners should know about?

Perhaps it would be best to begin by mentioning a few problems that have been overblown, so that fears can be allayed. *Rabies,* for example, is almost unheard of in the urban, domestic, immunized dog. In fact, several places, such as New York City, have been declared rabies-free, meaning that a person bitten by a local dog ought not to receive rabies immunization. (However, dog bites in rural areas are more likely to involve rabies. Anyone bitten by a bat, raccoon, skunk, or fox should receive a full course of rabies prophylaxis.) The considerable concern that cats spread *leukemia* should also be allayed because there is *no evidence* that "cat leukemia virus" can grow in humans or that it plays a role in human cancer. Finally, there is *no proof* that exposure to small animals causes *multiple sclerosis.*

There are some transmitted diseases, though, that cat and dog owners should be aware of. Some involve persons at special risk. Young children (ages 1–3), for example, may ingest material contaminated by cat or dog excreta as might be present in sand boxes, and thus be vulnerable to *visceral larva migrans.* This illness is caused by a round worm (a parasite that is present in most young puppies). If the eggs of the parasite (present in the feces) are swallowed by the child, they may cause intestinal symptoms, or their hatched larvae may migrate to other organs. Infestation of the lungs, for example, can lead to symptoms of pneumonia or bronchitis. Puppies' feces should be examined for round-worm eggs; if present, repeated worming is recommended. *Leptospirosis* is a bacterial infection that can be transmitted to young children playing in water contaminated by infected dog urine. A relatively rare disease, it can have a variety of clinical appearances and is usually not serious. *Toxoplasmosis* is another parasitic disease that humans can acquire by contact with feces (in litterpans and soil) from infected cats. When contracted during pregnancy, transmission to the fetus can produce blindness, mental retardation, and other serious birth defects. *Pregnant women should wash their hands after handling cats and should avoid handling litter boxes.*

Cat owners should be aware of *cat scratch fever,* a mild, self-limited disease in which fever and swollen lymph nodes occur after (usually young) cats scratch (usually young) people. No specific treatment is required, although lymph nodes may need to be drained if they become filled with pus. Rarely, a deep cat scratch (or bite) can result in a wound infection with *Pasturella multocida.* This infection is easily treated with penicillin, which is recommended after a *deep* cat scratch or bite.

Several skin problems should also be mentioned. *Ringworm* is a fungus found in both cats and dogs—causing them to suffer hair loss and skin redness at the infected site. Humans can contract the fungus from animals (as well as the soil), resulting in a characteristic raised, itchy, red, circular rash. *Mites* that cause "mange" in animals can survive for only a few days on human skin, but during this time may cause severe itching. On the other hand, *fleas* are transmitted freely from animals to man and tend to cause skin problems in young children. *Ticks,* which can be transported by dogs to humans, can spread several generalized diseases including *Rocky Mountain spotted fever* and *tularemia.*

What about other pets?

Because hamsters may carry a virus that can cause neurological infection *(lymphocytic choriomeningitis)* in humans, they should be obtained from colonies that have been screened for this virus.

Birds such as parakeets, chickens, pigeons, and parrots are a source of lung infection known as *psittacosis.* Pigeon droppings may also be the source of fungal infections in humans *(cryptococcosis* and *histoplasmosis)* which involve the lungs as well as other organs.

Pet turtles have been reported to spread *salmonella.* Monkeys, in particular, may carry tuberculosis or viruses which may cause hepatitis or encephalitis in humans.

What preventive measures are helpful?

Wild animals such as raccoons, foxes, monkeys, and skunks make dangerous pets; this practice should be discouraged.

Immunizations, usually started around six weeks of age, are imperative for both cats and dogs. Dogs are immunized against rabies, distemper, hepatitis, and leptospirosis. Immunizations for cats include feline panleukopenia, respiratory viruses, and rabies.

For humans, general hygiene is of foremost importance. Children should be taught to wash hands after fondling animals. Utensils used for an animal's food should be separate from household crockery. Beds should not be shared with animals. Since toxoplasmosis is mainly a threat to the unborn fetus, litter boxes should be emptied daily by someone other than a pregnant woman.

Humans should be immunized with tetanus toxoid and all bite wounds must be carefully cleaned. Deep bites from cats should be treated with penicillin. Those living or vacationing in tick areas should carry out "search and remove" operations nightly.

In summary, commonsense hygiene, avoidance of wild or sick animals, and attention to recommended immunizations will make pet ownership a "healthy" experience for most people.

Radiation

Those undergoing x-ray examinations (over 130 million people per year in this country) often wonder how harmful the radiation they receive might be. We have asked Dr. Reginald Greene, Associate Professor of Radiology at the Massachusetts General Hospital, Harvard Medical School, to answer some questions about the sources and effects of radiation in order to provide an informed perspective on the real and imagined hazards of medical x-rays.

What are x-rays and where do they come from?

X-rays are high-energy electromagnetic impulses that comprise part of a spectrum that includes radio, light, and heat waves. They were discovered by Wilhelm Konrad Roentgen in 1895, and in his honor, the term "roentgen" has been chosen as the unit to express amounts of radiation. Large doses, in the order of thousands of roentgens (for example, 5,000R), may be necessary in radiation treatment of cancer. On the other hand, diagnostic x-ray examinations require rather small amounts of radiation, usually described in milliroentgen (1/1,000 of a roentgen) units. For example, exposure to the skin of the chest from a chest x-ray (20mr) is only 20/1,000 of one roentgen.

There are three major sources of radiation to which people are exposed:

(1) Natural background radiation contributes an average exposure of about 100mr per year. This radiation originates from two sources: (1) cosmic rays from our solar system and outer space and (2) radioisotopes (such as uranium 238) in the earth's crust. Background radiation varies, depending on altitude and on local concentrations of earth's isotopes. At sea level, the average exposure to

cosmic radiation is only 28mr per year, but in Denver, Colorado (one mile high), it is 50mr. The importance of the protective layer of the atmosphere is further illustrated by the fact that cosmic ray exposure from a single five-hour transcontinental flight at 39,000 feet altitude is 2.5mr. The annual background radiation from earth's isotopes averages 15mr along the coastal plains where isotopes are not plentiful, as compared to 57mr on the Colorado plateau, where there are significant uranium deposits.

(2) Non-medical man-made radiation accounts for a small amount of exposure (7mr per year), as compared to the 100mr exposure caused by natural background sources. Most of this exposure is the result of above-ground nuclear weapons testing that took place prior to 1962. There are also a number of less important man-made sources of radiation, including television receivers, electron microscopes, airport inspection systems, and radio-luminous watch-face materials. The Environmental Protection Agency estimates that by the year 2000, exposure from all the planned nuclear power and fuel reprocessing plants will be about 0.4mr per yer. It is unlikely that the maximum allowable annual exposure (500mr) for non-medical man-made radiation, recommended by the National Council on Radiation Protection, will ever be exceeded—barring nuclear disasters.

(3) Medical x-ray studies produce greatly varying amounts of radiation exposure. The chest x-ray, which accounts for 50% of all x-ray studies, is the most common source of medical radiation. The average exposure to the gonads (the sex organs—where genetic mutations are of concern) from a chest x-ray is 0.04mr in adult men and 0.2mr in adult women. By way of comparison, it would take 2,500 chest x-rays in a man or 500 in a woman to produce the same gonadal exposure as occurs each year from natural background sources. For another comparison, the gonadal dose from a single transcontinental air flight is equivalent to 60 chest x-rays in men and 12 chest x-rays in women.

X-rays of the skull and extremities also result in very low radiation exposures. However, x-rays of thicker parts of the body, especially the abdomen and lower back, directly expose the gonads and result in higher skin and gonadal doses. The gonadal dose from a single x-ray of the abdomen is 12mr in men (equivalent to 300 chest x-rays) and 125mr in women (equivalent to 600 chest x-rays).

Other types of medical x-rays which can result in similar radiation levels include fluoroscopy, tomography, magnification radiography, computerized tomography, and special examinations which require repeated exposures (such as angiography). Because radiation from each of these procedures is apt to approximate or exceed the annual exposure from background radiation, a potentially important medical benefit should be apparent before any is carried out. However, patients should not refuse x-ray examination solely to avoid radiation exposure because the health risk from omitting the study may far exceed any potential radiation hazard.

What are effects of radiation on the body?

Although a massive amount of radiation (such as 5,000R) can be given to *small areas* of the body in divided doses to destroy malignant tumors, a lesser amount (such as 500R) given as a single dose to the *whole* body can be lethal. The effects of large radiation doses given over short time spans are fairly well understood, but much less is known about the effects of very low-dose radiation received over a prolonged period. Our limited knowledge is based on animal studies and projections from high-dose human exposures, such as the Japanese atomic bomb victims. The two most important radiation effects relate to genetic changes (mutations) and cancer.

Animal studies indicate that relatively high doses are required to cause genetic mutation. About 1,000mr (1R) of gonadal exposure is required to raise the natural mutation rate by one per cent. The real risk of cancer from low-dose radiation is much less certain. Low-dose radiation appears to result in less injury than estimates from high-dose exposures would predict, probably because the low doses cause few cell injuries and enough time is available for cell repair to occur. The best evidence indicates that there is not a threshold (or particular accumulated dose of radiation) below which there is no added theoretical risk of induced cancer. However, the added cancer risk from low-level radiation appears to be very low. A committee from the National Academy of Sciences in 1972 roughly estimated that if the entire population were exposed to an additional 100mr (equivalent to doubling the natural background for one year), the added cancer deaths for each of the 25 years after that exposure would be one per two million persons.

What guidelines would you suggest for the wise use of medical x-rays?

(1) If you do not understand why x-rays are being ordered, do not hesitate to ask your physician.

(2) If you are concerned about the radiation you may receive from any x-ray study, your radiologist or technician ought to be able to provide you with information. They may compare the dose to that received from a chest x-ray, for instance.

(3) Elective (not urgent) abdominal examinations in females of childbearing age should be restricted to the first 14 days of the menstrual cycle to avoid the possibility of an early pregnancy.

(4) Pregnant females should avoid all non-essential medical radiation, especially of the abdomen.

(5) Young adults should avoid repetitive x-ray exposures of the gonads unless medical indications are clear.

(6) Keep track of the dates and locations of previous x-rays. They may be useful to you in the future and reduce the need for additional x-rays.

(7) No diagnostic x-ray study gives "too much" radiation *when* there are important medical reasons for it.

Asbestos

An asbestos curtain was once the very symbol of safety and security. When primitive stage lighting made the risk of theater fires a constant worry, the presence of a fireproof curtain reassured audiences that a blaze could be contained long enough for them to escape it. Now the tables are turned; disease caused by asbestos has become a matter of serious concern.

Since antiquity, asbestos had been made into such items as permanent lamp wicks or novelty fabrics that would not burn. But early in this century, the use of asbestos grew like wildfire (so to speak). A potential health hazard was suspected very early, but it wasn't until the 1960s that its full magnitude became evident.

THE MATERIAL   Asbestos is a family of similar minerals that all occur naturally as a kind of soft rock made up of compressed fibers. One of the best insulators known, it protects what it covers from heat, corrosion, or electrical damage. It is also strong and durable. The mineral fibers can be handled in ways similar to vegetable fibers; they can be spun, made into felt, or bonded with other substances to form durable materials.

By now there are 3,000 uses of asbestos. Insulation for buildings is made from the material; huge amounts have also been used to insulate boilers and pipes in ships; automobile brake linings and clutch plates have been made of asbestos since the early 1900s. Asbestos has been incorporated into cement to strengthen it for use in pipes and other formed objects. Asbestos filters are used in the manufacture of some imported wines. For many years, hair dryers were insulated with the material. Until recently, asbestos was commonly incorporated into the spackling and taping compounds used for drywall construction. From 1946 to 1973, asbestos was added to coatings that could be sprayed onto walls or other structures in lieu of plastering them.

In all, some 30 million tons have been used in the United States since the beginning of this century, and by its end, according to one estimate, some half a million people will have died as a result of their exposure to asbestos.

THE PROBLEM   Asbestos produces disease only when it is inhaled (or possibly swallowed). Minuscule fibers of the material (some too small to be seen with a standard microscope) are drawn into the lungs. There the fibers are taken up by cells responsible for cleaning the air passages, but these fibers cannot easily be broken down for removal. Instead, the fibers remain in place or migrate slowly toward the periphery of the lungs. Some may even travel across the diaphragm into the abdominal cavity (peritoneum), whereas others probably arrive there after being swallowed.

It appears that asbestos creates problems solely because of its physical properties, not because of its chemical nature. The tiny size of asbestos particles is important; if they were larger, the fragments would settle out in the large airways, which are better equipped to remove foreign substances than the very small ones. The shape also matters; needle-like dimensions, which are typical of the asbestos crystal, appear to increase its ability to cause disease. Unfortunately, many of the possible substitutes for asbestos, such as certain newer types of fiberglass, acquire these characteristics in the process of being developed into better insulators. In other words, the desirable properties of asbestos as an insulating material are also the ones that make it dangerous. Even so, it appears so far that asbestos is more potent in causing disease than other effective insulating substances, such as fiberglass and rockwall.

Thirty or so years after asbestos dust is inhaled, but sometimes much sooner (depending on dose), it begins to cause several types of detectable disease:

(1) Asbestosis is a sometimes fatal condition that results from significant, but not necessarily heavy, exposure. It hardly ever occurs except in people who have worked with asbestos or with products containing it. This is, however, the most common disease produced

by exposure to the material, though not the most common cause of death, which is lung cancer. Asbestosis is a kind of scarring process, one that takes place within the lung tissue itself or on its outer surface. Asbestosis causes the air spaces to become smaller or obstructed, and the lung itself to become more rigid. There is no effective treatment to prevent or reverse the scarring. As a result, breathing is difficult, oxygen and carbon dioxide are poorly exchanged, and lung infections are easily acquired. This disease or its complications can progress, even without further exposure to asbestos.

Lung infections, such as pneumonia or bronchitis, are extremely threatening to people with asbestosis. They should be vigorously treated, usually with antibiotics, at the first sign of a respiratory infection. Stopping smoking is critical: cigarette smoke not only makes asbestosis more dangerous, difficult to live with, and hard to treat, but it markedly increases the risk of lung cancer in anybody who has been exposed to asbestos.

(2) *Lung cancer* is extremely common among people who have worked with asbestos, many of whom smoke. For some unknown reason, the combination of cigarette smoke and asbestos is much worse than would be predicted by adding together the risks from each. Anyone who has been exposed to even small quantities of asbestos dust should do everything he or she can to stop smoking. The outlook for those who stop is much better than for those who continue. As is the case with all lung cancer, by the time symptoms occur, it is usually too late for curative treatment, and no good tests for earlier detection are available.

(3) *Mesothelioma,* another type of cancer, occurs mainly in people exposed to asbestos dust. These tumors arise from the membrane that lines the chest or abdominal cavity, and they are highly malignant. Although they are rare, mesotheliomas can occur even after a limited exposure to asbestos dust and may affect people who were not directly involved in handling the material, such as relatives of asbestos workers. A very long time—forty years or more—can elapse between exposure and the appearance of mesothelioma, although many cases appear earlier.

Some other types of cancer, occurring outside the lungs, also appear to be somewhat more common in people exposed to asbestos dust. A few other diseases may also be more common, and it appears that the suicide rate in former asbestos workers is as much as two to three times higher than in the general population.

WHAT TO DO?   The asbestos situation raises two questions: What can individuals do to protect themselves and their families? What should we do as a nation to prevent further injury from exposure to asbestos?

The answer to the first question is reasonably straightforward for people who do not work with the material. Asbestos is only dangerous when it produces dust. Left undisturbed or bonded into durable slates, tiles, or other materials, it presents virtually no risk. But asbestos-containing insulation around pipes or boilers and in walls, wall coverings, or spackling compounds that are sawed, cut, sanded, or are exposed to damage from routine use may give off considerable quantities of asbestos dust. Nobody should work with such materials unless he or she is adequately trained and is fully protected from inhaling the dust. Deteriorating asbestos materials should be removed, covered with an effective sealant, or enclosed under another covering. Expert advice is needed both to determine whether there is an asbestos problem in a given area and to choose the proper method for dealing with the hazard.

Spray-on wall coverings that contain asbestos present a special problem. This inexpensive technique was rarely used in homes but quite frequently in school construction. Water damage, heavy use, and occasionally vandalism have caused the coatings to start disintegrating in some schools, and several states have begun programs to detect and correct the problem. Unfortunately such efforts are expensive and, all too often, underfunded.

People who work with asbestos and its products, including those who repair existing objects that contain the material or are covered with it—such as plumbers, shipyard workers, brake and clutch workers, construction workers—are entitled to protection from asbestos and the diseases it causes. They should be fully aware of the amount of asbestos dust that they breathe while they earn a living. Unfortunately, employers—both private industries and the government—have often been negligent, failing to inform employees about asbestos exposure or to protect them from it. Workers at risk of exposure should insist that the air they breathe be frequently sampled and analyzed by an appropriate method. Employers and workers should cooperate in bringing fiber counts in the air well below the current legal standard (2 million fibers per cubic meter), which is probably at least twenty times too high. Face masks and respirators are not as effective as ventilation control or improved handling methods, such as "wet processing."

The second question—what national action should be taken—is much more difficult to answer. There is no doubt that asbestos represents a major public health problem, one that extends beyond the large group of people who suffer from occupational exposure. Every possible way should be found to remove it from the human environment. But eliminating the substance from existing structures or from industrial applications may not be feasible for technical, economic, or political reasons. Meanwhile, there is controversy about the amount of asbestos exposure that is compatible with good health. Enforcing existing regulations, let alone more stringent ones, is difficult.

To date there has been no coherent, effective government program for dealing with the asbestos problem. Responsibility has fallen partly on the states and partly on several federal agencies. At a minimum, the federal government should be expected to take the initiative in developing a unified program to conduct research on asbestos diseases, measures to control exposures, and substitute materials. Technical advice and support should be offered to local control programs, and a policy should be developed for the future. Asbestos diseases become a medical problem only when it is too late to make them go away. Preventing these diseases is a political challenge, not a medical one.

Food Additives

The topic of food additives too often generates more heat than light. In the first section of this chapter, Dr. Judith Wurtman, a member of the Department of Nutrition at the Massachusetts Institute of Technology, answers the most commonly asked questions about these additives.

Why are additives put in food?

The major function of additives is to preserve food from the destructive effects of their own enzymes, as well as bacteria, fungi, and the environment. Enzymes in foods cause them to discolor or to become overripe too quickly; bacteria and fungi cause food to spoil and become dangerous to eat; heat, humidity, or oxygen can cause foods to become dry, soggy, or rancid. In short, additives are put in foods to keep them safe and edible.

Additives are also involved in the technical processes of industrial food preparation. *Leavening agents* (yeasts, baking powder) cause baked goods to rise; *glazing agents* make food surfaces shiny; *anti-foaming agents* allow containers to be filled completely with liquids; *foaming agents* put bubbles on drinks such as instant chocolate mix; *emulsifiers* keep oil or fat-containing ingredients mixed with the water base and give baked goods a light texture; *firming agents* maintain the firmness of fruits and vegetables during canning; *humectants* prevent foods like marshmallows or shredded coconut from absorbing water; *thickeners* give foods a smooth, thick texture and prevent ice crystal formation in frozen foods such as ice cream; *sequestrants* bind metals to prevent discoloration and to inhibit reactions which cause them to turn rancid; *artificial flavors and colors* enhance or impart flavor and color to foods (margarine is

170

colored yellow to resemble butter, for example); added *nutrients* increase the vitamin, mineral, and protein content of foods; and *imitation ingredients* replace the natural ones to reduce the calorie or cholesterol content of foods or to decrease the cost.

Some say that additives are dangerous; others say that they are safe. How do we know what to believe?

Additives are ingredients added to foods in which they are not *naturally* present. Thus, vitamin A is a natural ingredient in butter, but is an additive when put in margarine. Additives are chemicals, but so are *all* food constituents. Although some people feel that eating chemicals is dangerous, they would starve to death if they eliminated chemicals from their diets.

All additives that have entered our food supply since 1958 have undergone rigorous testing for their safety. Permission to use a new additive comes only after it has been shown to be safe for consumption by pregnant women, infants, children, and adults. Additives which were in common use before 1958 and which had passed certain safety standards are now being reevaluated under more stringent conditions of use. These additives (known as GRAS or "generally recognized as safe") include commonly used ingredients such as salt and nutmeg.

In order to remain in food, these additives must be proven (1) harmless to fetal development, (2) non-carcinogenic, (3) non-toxic to any organ system, and (4) uninvolved in behavioral abnormalities.

Some GRAS substances have had the decision regarding their safety deferred until further research is carried out. The use of such additives ("BHT" and "BHA" are examples) is restricted to their present function in food processing. No new uses are allowed until a final decision is made. Some consumer groups have interpreted the postponement of the decision regarding safety of an additive as proof that the additive is dangerous. This is not true. It simply means that insufficient information is available with which to make a decision.

However, no additive or food can ever be consumed without *any* risk. Most foods, even water, are toxic if they are ingested in sufficiently large amounts. Moreover, there may be people with intolerances to certain food additives, just as there are those who cannot tolerate certain foods like chocolate or strawberries or eggs. Moderation in the consumption of foods and additives is the safest way to eat.

Nitrates, nitrites, and saccharin have been shown to cause cancer. Why are they still in food?

Nitrites and nitrates are still added to food because they perform a critical function. They prevent the growth of the deadly bacterium that causes botulism. These bacteria grow in oxygen-free environments and can flourish in improperly processed vacuum-packed meats or in the interior of cured or smoked meats and fishes (bacon, smoked fish). The concentrations of nitrates and nitrites in processed meats have been reduced considerably in the last few years (and will be soon reduced in beer, where they have also been found).

However, most of our exposure to nitrates and nitrites comes not from those additives in salami or ham but from natural sources such as green leafy vegetables and from the production of these compounds in our bodies. Considerably more nitrite than we ingest is actually formed within our bodies.

Nitrites combine with a by-product of amino acids (called amines) to form a group of carcinogenic compounds, *nitrosamines*. Small amounts of nitrosamines are formed in foods containing nitrates and nitrites; however, most nitrosamines are made in our intestines. Much research is focusing now on the question of how nitrosamine formation might be prevented. Some current theories suggest that the proteins, ascorbic acid (vitamin C), and tocopherol (vitamin E) we tend to ingest in foods that contain nitrates or nitrites may prevent these compounds from turning into nitrosamines.

Many processed meats contain little or no nitrates or nitrites. This makes them very susceptible to the growth of the botulism-causing organism. Be sure to follow the instructions on the package of such foods for proper storage; otherwise you may be exposed to a hazard much more deadly than cancer.

Saccharin remains in our food supply despite evidence that it causes cancer in laboratory animals because its perceived benefit in making certain foods available to diabetics and dieters is judged to be greater than its risk. Congress overruled a Food and Drug Administration decision to ban saccharin and allowed it to remain in foods for at least 18 months. As any consumer of diet beverages or foods knows by now, a food which contains saccharin must display a prominent warning attesting to its carcinogenic properties in laboratory animals. As soon as another non-nutritive sweetener becomes available, saccharin will be replaced. One likely candidate, aspartame, is undergoing a final round of testing.

Is saccharin safe? Yes, for adults. We don't know whether it is safe for the unborn child, children, or older persons. Several federally supported studies have detected little or no additional risk of contracting bladder cancer among people who use saccharin. In one National Cancer Institute study, no overall increase in cancer risk was found among saccharin users as compared to non-saccharin users. The study surveyed more than 9,000 people. Two cautions are needed, though. Saccharin may act as a "weak" carcinogen in heavy smokers: people who drink saccharin-sweetened beverages and smoke heavily may be at greater risk than heavy smokers who do not use this sweetener. In addition, we have no good information yet on the long-range effects of ingesting saccharin from early childhood through old age. It is probably prudent for children and pregnant women to consume saccharin in small amounts. (Remember, an alternative to diet soft drinks is the calorie-free, sugar-free, and relatively inexpensive beverage, water.)

Sorbitol and Diarrhea

A letter from two physicians in the *Journal of the American Medical Association* describes the experience of one of them following the consumption of twelve diet mints during a two-hour meeting—namely the development of severe abdominal distress (cramps, gas, diarrhea) about 30 minutes after swallowing the last mint. When a further episode requiring hospitalization occurred, the package label on the mints was read, and it was then discovered that sorbitol had been used as an artificial sweetener.

Sorbitol is described chemically as a non-digestible sugar alcohol—which means that it sits in the intestines and gets fermented by bacteria. The products of such fermentation set the stage for cramping and diarrhea. Unlike the more potent artificial sweetener saccharin, sorbitol must be added in large amounts to achieve a desirable taste effect. And if sorbitol-sweetened foods are consumed in quantity (12 mints in two hours), they can cause explosive diarrhea. Even in smaller amounts, lesser degrees of upset can occur—particularly in children. So if abdominal symptoms occur in conjunction with eating diet foods or candy, check for sorbitol as a possible culprit.

Sugar

The average American consumes an astounding 128 pounds of sugar per year, accounting for almost one quarter of this country's total caloric intake. Indeed, since much of that sugar comes from sweeteners added to the food we make and buy, it is not misleading to describe sugar as this country's number one food additive.

DEFINITIONS   The word "sugar" actually applies to more than a hundred substances that qualify as "sweet"—including honey, corn syrup, and molasses. The most basic of all sugars are *fructose* and *glucose*—the so-called "simple" sugar molecules (meaning only six carbon atoms) made by the green leaves of plants using energy from sunlight with water and carbon dioxide as raw materials. (Remember that photosynthesis equation we all had to learn in school?) From these basic building blocks, more complex sugars and carbohydrates are made—and consumed by both animals and man.

When most people speak of sugar, they are referring to sucrose, a 12-carbon molecule resulting from the linkage of glucose to fructose; sucrose is the sugar that is ultimately obtained from sugarcane or beets and refined to the white granules on our tables. The consumption of sucrose has remained stable for many years—just under 100 pounds per year per person in this country. However, the use of sugars derived from corn starch (corn syrup, corn sugar, corn sweetener) has jumped dramatically in the past twenty years from an estimated 13 pounds per person in 1960 to over 30 pounds last year. In other words, most of the increase in sugar consumption in this country in recent times has come in the form of sugars not usually identified as "sugar" but, in terms of sweetness and calories, very much the same as table sugar (sucrose).

Indeed, this lack of precision in defining "sugar" on labels makes it difficult for the average consumer to know how much sugar he is getting in the food he buys. For example, as pointed out in a *Con-*

sumer Reports article on sugar (March 1978), 29% of Heinz tomato ketchup is composed of sugar; most ice cream is 21% sugar; Wishbone Russian dressing is 30%; Coffeemate, 65.4%; Ritz crackers, 11.8%. In reading labels, it is important to remember that all carbohydrate sweeteners qualify as sugar, even though they may be called by other names.

DIFFERENCES AMONG THE VARIOUS COMMERCIAL SUGARS   Ordinary *table sugar* (sucrose) is, as mentioned, derived from sugarcane or beet plants. In initial stages of processing, the juice obtained from the cane is separated into *raw sugar* (crystals) and *molasses* (syrup). Raw sugar is banned in this country because of impurities such as insect parts and bacteria; white refined sugar, which results from several additional stages of raw sugar processing, is "safer" if not more "healthy." *Brown sugar* consists of sugar crystals coated with molasses syrup; in the United States, most of it is made by spraying refined white sugar with molasses syrup. *Honey* varies in composition depending on its nectar source, but it is essentially a mixture of simple sugars, mostly fructose. *Maple sugar and syrup* are, of course, derived from the sap of the maple tree and consist largely of sucrose. The various *corn sweeteners* are derived from corn starch and are composed mainly of dextrose, maltose, and more complex sugars.

The important point to be made is that all these sugars are essentially the same in that they consist largely of calories with very little else of nutritional value. There may be minor differences between various sugars in terms of minimal nutrients or sweetening power per calorie, but these differences are indeed minor.

IS SUGAR BAD FOR US?   Given the discussion thus far, you might be surprised to be reminded that blood sugar (glucose) is absolutely essential to the body's cells as an energy source. Indeed, almost all of the sugars and more complex carbohydrates we eat are processed, at least in part, into glucose by our bodies. A metabolic system of elegant precision maintains the amount of glucose in the blood within a relatively narrow normal range; excess amounts are stored in the liver as glycogen—or (the bad news) converted into fats to be stored you-know-where.

Although some sugar in our blood is essential to life, that "blood sugar" can be obtained from almost any source—including fruits and vegetables. So we might as well pick up some other useful nutrients (minerals, vitamins) along with the calories. It isn't even necessary to rely on commercial sugar products for so-called "quick energy," for unless we have been on a prolonged fast, our body stores of glycogen can be quickly converted to blood sugar to meet any sudden demand. Also, the inherent sweetness of sugar tempts us to eat more calories than we otherwise would.

In addition to this basic "empty-calorie" problem, sugar products *may* be associated with other health problems. There *is* a firm link between sugar exposure and tooth decay—though individual resistance and manner of exposure (constant caramels versus sugar with meals quickly brushed away) can make an enormous difference. Any causative role of sugar in diabetes is far from certain—though it may contribute indirectly via obesity. The same can be said of heart disease—no proven direct links, possible indirect contributions.

IN SUMMARY   Most of us need some sweets in our lives. The question, as always, is one of balance—in our diet and on the scale.

Cholesterol

The Food and Nutrition Board of the National Research Council created an enormous hubbub in the nation's kitchens in the summer of 1980 when it announced that the dangers of *dietary cholesterol* may have been overstated. Experts challenged the Board's conclusions, as did many organizations, including the American Heart Association. The general public was left to wonder whether the standard advice of some twenty years—to eat less fat and cholesterol—should be tossed out the window. As a guide for the perplexed, we offer the following information:

(1) Everyone still agrees that high levels of cholesterol in the blood signal an increased risk of heart attack. For example, the famous Framingham Heart Study has found that a man with 260 milligrams of cholesterol in 100 milliliters of his blood serum has three times the risk of a heart attack as a man whose count comes in under 195. At a cholesterol of 310, the risk is five times higher.

(2) Recently, it has been established that some of the cholesterol measured in the standard blood test isn't bad; it may even be good because it is in a form that leads to elimination from the body. So, even though total cholesterol is usually a reliable indication of increased risk, a better indicator is the proportion of bad versus good cholesterol (more of that in a moment).

(3) The big question, though, is one that has been debated for years: whether it pays to cut down on fat or cholesterol in the *diet* as a method of lowering cholesterol in the blood. Although there is some evidence that low-fat diets do not *always* improve the blood cholesterol, almost all experts still agree that such diets benefit some people, especially those with a strong family history of premature heart disease, those with established heart disease, and those who

are obese. These groups may be a majority of Americans, but it must be admitted that there are others who do not need to restrict dietary fats or cholesterol.

In short, the argument boils down—as is so often the case—to seeking a sensible recommendation based on incomplete information. Most experts agree that we *don't need* to eat a diet rich in fat and cholesterol, and there is a strong enough indication that dietary intake contributes to heart disease in the general population. Therefore, the prudent course is to hedge our bets and lower the amount of fat and cholesterol that we eat.

HDL-CHOLESTEROL   One form of cholesterol, commonly abbreviated as HDL because it is attached to high-density lipoproteins, is now attracting a lot of attention. HDL-cholesterol is a complex of fat and protein found in everybody's blood, and within the past five years, accumulated evidence has shown that people with relatively high levels of HDL in their blood have fewer heart attacks than others. Perhaps, then, HDL is protecting them from heart disease.

Lipoproteins exist for a reason. Because fat and water don't mix, the body needs a system for carrying fats (including cholesterol, which has many good uses) through the watery medium of the bloodstream. Proteins, in the main, serve this purpose for cholesterol; the two major classes are known as low-density and high-density lipoproteins (LDL and HDL). Produced by the intestine and liver, these proteins are secreted into the bloodstream, where they become attached to cholesterol. But there is an important difference between the two. LDL seems to serve as a delivery truck; it picks up cholesterol and deposits it in cells, including—under abnormal conditions—those of our blood vessels. HDL, on the other hand, is the garbage truck; it collects excess cholesterol—perhaps even removing it from cells—and (probably) carries the material back to the liver for elimination.

According to this scenario, a person's susceptibility to heart disease depends on the relative balance of the delivery and removal systems. Raise the proportion of HDL relative to LDL and potentially damaging excesses of cholesterol can be diminished. The theory is suggestive, and many people take it seriously, but it has not yet been proven.

According to Dr. William Castelli, director of the Framingham study, measuring the ratio of total cholesterol (which is mostly LDL-cholesterol) to HDL-cholesterol is worth doing once early in life—around the age of two—to find individuals with a genetic disorder called "type 2 hyperlipidemia," which predisposes to early, severe coronary artery disease. Such children should be started on a strict program to lower their blood-fat levels, and family members should likewise be checked to see whether they have the same disorder.

A second check is recommended sometime in early adulthood, in the twenties. If the value is acceptable, he advises subsequent checks at ten-year intervals. A high ratio, signaling the risk of heart disease, should lead to a program that attempts to lower it, and values should then be checked more frequently.

RECOMMENDATIONS   Because the HDL story is quite new, the medical profession is far from reaching total agreement on the implications of HDL levels or the proper approach to an abnormal value. Although a high ratio of total cholesterol to HDL-cholesterol clearly indicates a higher than normal risk of heart disease, purposely lowering the ratio has not yet been proven to protect against heart attacks.

However, certain measures seem prudent, and it should come as no surprise that most ways of lowering the ratio are already standard recommendations for reducing the risk of heart disease:

(1) Giving up cigarettes raises HDL, and it certainly reduces heart disease.

(2) Vigorous exercise appears to have a powerful influence on HDL. By comparison with their sedentary contemporaries, middle-aged runners have a favorable ratio. What is not yet certain is whether a middle-aged person who abandons the armchair for a pair of running shoes will be rewarded by a rise in HDL (some studies show the effect, others do not) or a longer life.

(3) Recommended dietary measures also have a familiar ring: reduce the intake of calories and of all kinds of fat, especially animal fat and cholesterol. Polyunsaturated fats can be *substituted* for other fats but should *not* be *added* to the diet as an extra. Cold-water fish seem to raise the level of HDL, as do garlic, brewer's yeast, and lecithin—but then so do chlorinated pesticides, which are

hardly recommended in the diet. As yet, *no evidence warrants a faddish use of any food or substance* to alter HDL-cholesterol levels.

Periodic measurement of the ratio can serve as a guide to the effectiveness of a diet-and-exercise program, but there is no solid proof at present that a middle-aged person can achieve instant salvation through such a program. Relatively long periods may be required to alter a physiological pattern that has been established over decades.

ONE FINAL NOTE Consumption of alcohol clearly raises the level of HDL and seems also to protect against heart attacks. Moderate drinkers (who consume no more than a couple of ounces of whisky a day or the equivalent) had a lower mortality rate than teetotalers in five out of six analyses conducted by the Framingham study. *More* than this amount, however, rapidly decreased life expectancy in direct proportion to the increasing intake. The difficulty many people have in controlling their alcohol consumption makes it unwise to encourage drinking for the sake of a small and uncertain benefit.

Reproduction and Child Care

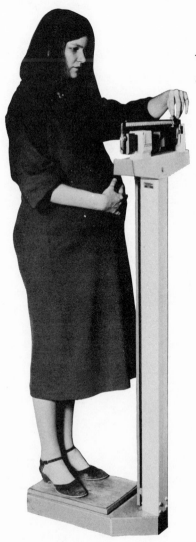

MYTH 3

Women shouldn't gain more than twenty pounds during pregnancy.

Contraception

Modern methods of birth control allow a range of choices that meets the medical and social needs of most people. However, a perfectly safe, effective, and acceptable method of birth control has yet to be devised. The following survey presents the relative advantages and disadvantages of the contraceptive methods currently available.

TRADITIONAL METHODS *Coitus interruptus* (withdrawal of the penis before ejaculation), *post-coital douche* (flushing of semen from the vagina after intercourse), and *lactation* (breast feeding) are time-honored methods of avoiding pregnancy. While they have the advantage of safety and no cost, they have the great disadvantage of a high probability of resulting parenthood. In short, none of these methods can be relied upon to prevent pregnancy.

RHYTHM METHOD Though also an often unreliable method of birth control, this method is used by many couples since it is the only method of contraception approved by the Roman Catholic Church. The method is based on the avoidance of intercourse during the fertile period in a woman's menstrual cycle—namely, from the time of ovulation (release of the egg from the ovary) until about three days later. Consequently, pin-pointing the time of ovulation becomes the key to success with this method. This pinpointing may be enhanced by the recording of basal (morning) body temperature—which rises about 0.5 °F–0.7 °F within 24 to 36 hours after ovulation. The rhythm method is difficult even in women with regular menstrual cycles and becomes almost impossible in women with very irregular ones.

183

METHODS OF INCREASED EFFECTIVENESS   The following
methods provide less effective control than "the pill," IUDs, and
sterilization, but offer other advantages for some people:

(1) Condom: Still the most commonly used method of birth control worldwide, condom use is second only to the pill in the United
States. It has the advantages of simplicity, minimal cost, and partial
protection against sexually transmitted diseases. The disadvantages
include psychological distraction, dulling of sensation, and rare mechanical failures (leaking and breakage).

(2) Spermicidal agents: There are a wide variety of vaginal
creams, jellies, foams, and suppositories which kill sperm directly or
present a physical barrier to their passage. Used alone, they are not
reliable, but used in conjunction with a condom worn by the male,
these preparations can be quite effective. The tablets and suppositories require several minutes for adequate distribution throughout
the vagina before protection is afforded. Some women will experience local tissue irritation from these agents. Recent claims for the
effectiveness of these agents alone, without diaphragm or condom,
are unfounded.

(3) Diaphragm: Used in combination with spermicidal preparations (jelly or cream applied to both sides of the diaphragm), this
method offers good protection. It has the disadvantages of requiring
careful fitting by a physician and insertion before love-making (or
the unwelcome interruption of such), and a degree of messiness associated with the use of the cream or jelly.

IUDs—SAFE OR NOT?   When IUDs (intrauterine devices) were
first popularized as a form of female contraception in the 1960s, some
advocates were almost euphoric in suggesting that IUDs were the
"ideal" form of contraception—safe and effective. Now, several decades later, the record clearly indicates that IUDs are neither perfectly safe nor completely effective in preventing pregnancy. However, recent public reports concerning the dangers of IUDs may also
create misleading impressions.

IUDs rank second only to the pill in practical effectiveness, but
they are not foolproof; about 3% of women using them will become
pregnant. However, that degree of effectiveness—combined with the

fact that no further action is required once the IUD is inserted—has made the IUD the contraceptive choice for between 15 and 20 million women worldwide.

The matter of safety can be put in perspective by pointing out that the overall risk of dying from pregnancy or delivery is about 20 times greater than that of dying from complications associated with IUD use. However, this "perspective" should not detract from the real dangers of IUD use, which include the following:

(1) Bleeding/cramping: While not life-threatening, these complications lead to the removal of the IUD in about one out of five women during the first year of use. In recent years, the addition of either copper or progestin (for added contraceptive effect) has permitted smaller IUDs to be designed. This should make insertion easier and cause less bleeding and cramping; however, because the medication gets used up, these IUDs have to be replaced periodically.

(2) Infections: In recent years, the increased risk for pelvic inflammatory disease has been highlighted by many studies which, on average, show a three to five times increased chance of infection in women using the IUD, versus nonusers. Fortunately, most of these infections can be treated successfully with antibiotics, but some infections may lead to subsequent infertility—and, *very rarely,* death. Because of the risk of infertility—and because infections are more likely to occur in younger women who have not had children—many experts advise other forms of contraception for women under age 25 and those who wish to have children at a future date.

(3) Perforation: The exact incidence of perforation (puncture of the uterus by the IUD) is unknown but is thought to be quite rare—approximately one per two thousand users. The reason that the incidence is unknown is that perforation—surprisingly—may cause no symptoms and go undiscovered until the next check-up; abdominal surgery to remove the IUD may be required.

In short, the IUD represents one of several alternative methods of contraception, none of which is ideal. Any woman considering the use of the IUD should be thoroughly informed of the risks and benefits—and should realize that the majority of women using IUDs find them to be, on balance, a quite acceptable method of contraception.

THE "PILL" Technically known as an oral hormone agent, this method of contraception remains the most popular one in the United States, despite recurring concerns about serious side effects. The only type of pill available today contains a combination of the two female hormones (estrogen and progestin) which exert a suppressive effect on the pituitary hormones that normally cause ovulation. (A sequential arrangement which offered 15 days of estrogen alone followed by five days of combined estrogen and progestin is no longer available in this country as a result of studies that showed a higher incidence of uterine cancer in women who used such a pill.) The original pill (released in 1959) contained amounts of estrogen and progestin much higher than are used in most preparations today. The reduction of the amount of estrogen used in modern pills is thought to be very important, since most of the serious side effects attributable to the pill are thought to be caused by estrogen content. These possible side effects include the following:

(1) *Strokes:* Most experts now accept the data which show a slight, but definite, increased risk in women who use the pill. Put in perspective, the over-all risk of death from blood clots in pill users is about 1.5 per 100,000 under age 35 and 4 per 100,000 over age 35—versus 0.2 and 0.5 respectively in those who do not use the pill. However, this must be weighed against the over-all death rate from pregnancy and delivery (*excluding* illegal abortions), which is about 22 per 100,000—and the fact that the pill, properly used, is the most effective method currently available in preventing pregnancy.

(2) *Heart attacks:* Data from British studies suggests that women over 40 using the pill are at higher risk for heart attacks—especially if traditional risk factors for heart attacks, such as smoking and high blood pressure, are present. However, other studies suggest that smoking is the major culprit and that the increased risk of a heart attack attributed to the pill occurs almost exclusively among smokers using the pill.

(3) *Tumors:* Animal and human studies have indicated that certain female hormones may cause changes in breast and uterine tis-

sue. However, there is no evidence to date that the combination birth control pill currently used causes cancer of either organ. Since estrogen-dependent tumors of the breast can occur, the use of birth control pills is not advised for women with a past history of breast cancer. There have been a number of reports concerning the occurrence of tumors (adenomas) of the liver in females who have been on long-term oral contraceptives. While these tumors are rarely malignant, they can be dangerous because of their tendency to bleed into the abdominal cavity. In some instances the bleeding has been fatal. The incidence of liver tumors is rare, but any woman taking the pill should be alert to the fact that onset of severe pain in the upper right abdomen demands prompt medical attention.

Many other side effects may be caused by the pill—including high blood pressure, obesity, mental depression, headache, nausea, and breast engorgement. Often these side effects can be eliminated by changing to a different pill. It is *generally agreed that women with the following problems should not use oral contraceptives:* strong family history of stroke, migraine headaches, evidence of vascular disease of the brain or heart, liver or kidney disease, thrombophlebitis, breast or uterine cancer, or uterine fibroids. Obviously, women should not start using the pill until a thorough history and physical examination have been performed.

More recently, two other forms of the pill have been developed. One is usually referred to as the "mini-pill" and is composed of small amounts of progestin alone. While the exact mechanism of pregnancy prevention is not known, this kind of pill is less effective than the IUD, but is an alternative for women who cannot tolerate estrogen. The only real disadvantage—besides a slightly higher pregnancy rate—is irregular bleeding and spotting in most women. Another version of the pill—known as the "morning-after pill"—involves the use of diethylstilbesterol (DES) for five days after unprotected intercourse. Most women develop nausea from these pills. And the current concern about the effect of DES on subsequent offspring suggests that a therapeutic abortion should be considered for those women in whom DES use does not prevent pregnancy.

Finally, it should be noted that injectable hormones—which offer contraceptive protection for at least three months—have not been approved by the Food and Drug Administration for contraceptive use.

STERILIZATION PROCEDURES   *Tubal interruption* in females (procedures that interrupt the continuity of the oviduct which transports the egg to the uterus) and *vasectomy* in males (procedures that interrupt the vas deferens which transports sperm from the testis) can be described as methods of "permanent contraception" (see diagrams). Though it is now possible to "reverse" (surgically restore continuity in) as many as 70% of vasectomies and 30% of tubal ligations, whether full-term pregnancy will routinely result from such restorations remains to be documented. In other words, persons undergoing these procedures should regard them as being permanent and should not expect reversibility. Both procedures are relatively safe, though bleeding and infection—possibilities in all surgery—do occur. In general, a vasectomy is a simpler and less costly procedure. There is no firm evidence of any long-term adverse physical effects from either procedure, though recent studies in monkeys suggest that vasectomy *may* increase the risk for vascular disease. Some males experience psychological impotence after a vasectomy until they can come to understand that the procedure does not involve

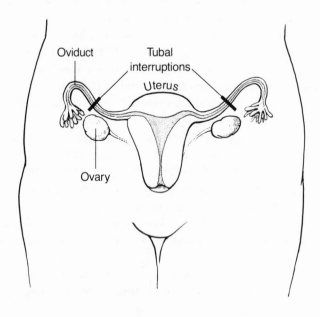

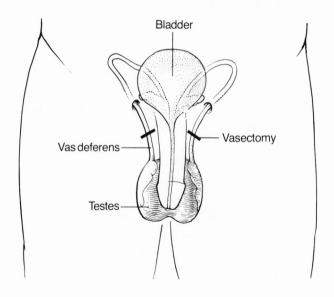

any impairment of male hormone levels or physical sexual performance, just as tubal ligation has no effect on female hormone levels.
Both procedures offer the great advantage of almost 100% effectiveness with no further concern about contraception.

IN SUMMARY   The above choices do not provide the ultimate
goal of contraceptive research—an effective method that is also
without danger. And there do not appear to be any breakthroughs
on the immediate horizon. A male pill seems unlikely because of unacceptable effects on male hormonal balance. However, careful attention to the needs of a given couple can usually result in a satisfactory choice from current alternatives.

Sexually Transmitted Diseases

Even as recently as the 1960s, the subject was considered straightforward. Venereal disease (so named for Venus, the goddess of love) encompassed five well-known diseases, the two most important clearly being syphilis and gonorrhea. The identification and treatment of these diseases—difficult for social reasons—was reasonably well understood from a medical viewpoint. The 1970s, however, produced a revolution in "venereology" to the point where even the suggested initials of designation changed: VD became STD—"sexually transmitted diseases," a phrase thought to be more to the point and less judgmental. More significant, our knowledge expanded dramatically during the past decade. Currently, over twenty different germs "associated with" sexually transmitted diseases have been identified. More important, the relationship of these organisms to problems other than immediate symptoms is increasingly emphasized; specific concern is now directed toward the role of sexually transmitted diseases in such problems as birth defects, infertility, and long-term disability. Indeed, the whole field of STD has become extremely complicated; this update will touch upon a few developments that deserve special consideration, with emphasis on some practical concerns relating to these diseases.

NEW DEVELOPMENTS   Among the many recent changes in our knowledge of STDs, the following merit particular attention simply because they potentially affect so many people:

(1) NGU (Non-gonococcal urethritis): In the late 1970s, NGU was widely highlighted in the public press as a "new" disease thought to be even more common than gonorrhea. The name derives from the common situation (particularly in males) in which infection of the

190

urethra (the passageway for urine from the bladder) is *not* caused by gonorrhea. Such a distinction—gonorrhea versus "something else"—is important for treatment: gonorrhea is almost always treated with penicillin, but non-gonococcal disease is best treated with antibiotics other than penicillin (usually tetracycline). In short—and from a practical viewpoint—NGU is a "diagnosis of exclusion," meaning that it is "discovered" when tests for suspected gonorrhea turn out to be negative. At that point, several other possibilities could be considered; indeed, it is now known that an organism called *Chlamydia trachomatis* is the causative agent in about 50% of cases of NGU. However, it is usually easier simply to begin treatment with antibiotics known to work in most cases of NGU— rather than spend the time and money pinpointing the actual offender. (It is also important that both sexual partners be treated to avoid reinfection.) In short, NGU is not so much a new disease as an entity increasingly recognized in cases when gonorrhea is not identified or when penicillin treatment for presumed gonorrhea fails.

(2) Asymptomatic and resistant gonorrhea: The two major STDs of past concern were syphilis and gonorrhea. Syphilis can be detected with a simple blood test. Unfortunately, and despite intensive research, no simple blood test for gonorrhea yet exists. Therefore, accurate diagnosis of gonorrhea requires obtaining material (via a cotton-tipped swab) from appropriate locations and then looking under the microscope or, particularly in women where microscopic examination is unreliable, growing the bacteria from specimens under laboratory conditions. Because of these more cumbersome diagnostic techniques, past practice often boiled down to treating suspicious symptoms (painful urination and milky discharge) with penicillin. However, this approach has been called into question by two developments: the emergence of strains of gonorrhea resistant to penicillin and the increasing realization that both men and women can harbor gonorrhea without obvious symptoms. Therefore, the safest course for sexually active men and women to follow is that of periodic screening for gonorrhea. Furthermore, it is critically important that persons treated with penicillin—or other antibiotics—be checked after treatment to make sure that the gonorrhea has been eradicated.

(3) Herpes simplex infections: As noted widely in the public press, the *Herpes simplex* virus is increasingly implicated as a com-

mon cause of STD. (A July 1980 issue of *Time* magazine titled an article in its medicine section as follows: "Herpes: The New Sexual Leprosy—Viruses of love infect millions with disease and despair.") First, a quick lesson in terminology. The herpes family includes many viruses. The two most commonly confused are *Herpes zoster,* which causes chickenpox in kids and shingles in adults, and *Herpes simplex,* which causes clusters of small red lumps that soon turn into painful blisters. These blisters are most common near the lips (where they are known as cold or fever sores) and in the genital area. The simplex viruses are further divided into two types: usually, type 1 is associated with blisters around the lips, while type 2 (HSV-2) is found in blisters on the genitalia and sometimes the buttocks and thighs.

Approximately 10 million Americans are estimated to harbor the HSV-2 virus, and it is easily spread by sexual contact. Indeed, HSV-2 now rivals NGU and gonorrhea as one of the most common sexually transmitted diseases in this country. However, unlike gonorrhea, which can be eradicated by simple antibiotic treatment, there is no effective cure for herpes. A variety of treatment programs have been tried, but to date nothing has been found to be both successful and safe. The best advice is to keep the skin clean and dry during a bout of herpes (in order to prevent additional bacterial infection) and to consult appropriate specialists (dermatologists, urologists, gynecologists) for difficult cases. Condoms are a help—but not a guarantee—in preventing transmission of this virus during intercourse.

HSV-2 has two additional implications for the female. Because herpes acquired during passage through the birth canal can cause severe, permanent neurological damage—and even death—in the newborn, a Caesarian section may be required if active herpes is present in the birth canal at the time of delivery. Also, it has long been known that cervical cancer is more common in women who have intercourse with many partners or from an unusually early age. Many researchers now think that HSV-2 is the missing link between sexual intercourse and cervical cancer. Women infected with HSV-2 are eight times more likely to develop such cancer than women not infected. Therefore, periodic Pap smears are particularly important for this group.

(4) Homosexual STD: The decade of the seventies has also pro-

duced an increased awareness that diseases not previously associated with sexual activity occur more frequently in male homosexuals. A variety of bacterial and parasitic infections of the bowel is one example, and hepatitis is another. Homosexual men—and physicians taking care of them—must suspect symptoms in throat or rectal areas as being caused by STD.

PRACTICAL CONSIDERATIONS   All of the above argues for the abolition of sexual activity; such a solution to the woes of sexually transmitted disease will, of course, never be acceptable to most members of the human race. Therefore, more practical approaches to preventing or minimizing the dangers associated with STD must be considered—including the following:

(1) Prevention: Short of total abstinence, emphasis on selective sexual activity ("know your partner") and the use of condoms remain valid suggestions. The importance—in most cases—of also treating sexual partners should be stressed as a method of preventing reinfection.

(2) Expertise: The diagnosis and treatment of STD is often no longer a simple matter, a medical item that can be handled by any and all practitioners. At the very least, whenever persistent symptoms occur—especially for persons who engage in extensive or unusual sexual activity—the skills of physicians specially trained in STD (dermatologists, urologists, gynecologists, infectious disease experts) should be sought.

(3) Periodic screening: While hard and fast rules are difficult to design, most experts feel that those who are sexually active with multiple partners should be screened periodically (at least yearly) for certain STD problems that might not otherwise be detected until more serious symptoms—or spread—occur. Such screening would include a blood test for syphilis, swab specimens for gonorrhea, and other tests as suggested by the individual's history or past medical problems.

(4) Pre-natal care: Since several STDs can be transmitted to a developing fetus or newborn, routine pre-natal care today should include a check for certain STDs. And, as mentioned above, it may be important to do a Caesarian section in order to avoid contamination of the newborn as it passes through the birth canal.

IN SUMMARY   Sexually transmitted diseases have always caused pain and anxiety. Unfortunately, the modern age has intensified these problems—requiring more thoughtful attention to these diseases by both health professionals and the general public.

Special Problems
of Women

VAGINAL INFECTIONS   These are among the more common annoying human afflictions. And, unfortunately, such infections are often treated inadequately or inappropriately—thereby causing unnecessary distress. The most important rule concerning the treatment of vaginal infections is to identify the exact cause—and then to treat it exactly. Too many infections are treated without any examination—often with applications that are ineffective or with "shotgun" creams that attempt to cover several possible organisms. (Recently, for example, two Food and Drug Administration advisory committees concluded that there is no adequate evidence that widely used sulfa creams are effective in eliminating the three organisms that most commonly cause vaginal infections.) Sometimes, a vaginal infection may be the first sign of diabetes. Rarely, underlying tumors may cause a vaginal discharge which is passed off as "just another infection."

In addition to the importance of exact diagnosis and treatment, the necessity of treating sexual partners should be recognized. Recurrent or continuing infections often can be traced to a woman's sexual partner who has never been treated and is a source of continued reinfection.

In summary, many ongoing problems with vaginal infections can be solved by careful diagnosis and exact treatment. There is usually no need to suffer the physical and emotional annoyance of prolonged symptoms.

MENSTRUAL CRAMPS   Millions of women suffer each month from severe pelvic pain related to menstrual periods; in the past, strong pain medications or birth control pills had to be used in some women to provide needed relief. In recent years, however, the ubiq-

195

uitous body chemicals known as prostaglandins have become implicated as a cause of some types of dysmenorrhea—the fancy medical word meaning "painful periods." And this discovery opens up the obvious possibility that drugs which act as "anti-prostaglandins" might decrease dysmenorrhea. In fact, there are many drugs now known which act as anti-prostaglandins, including several medications now used in the treatment of arthritis such as Motrin and Naprosyn. Recently, another of these drugs—Ponstel—was described in the public press as having demonstrated effectiveness in relieving the distress of dysmenorrhea in a study involving 46 women. All of these drugs have their share of side effects and must be used cautiously. But progress is being made in the understanding—and, therefore, the treatment—of one of humankind's oldest and most troublesome maladies.

ESTROGEN USE AFTER MENOPAUSE   The word "estrogen" refers to a class of compounds that exert certain specific biological effects, including the development of female sexual characteristics (body configuration, breast development, skin texture, genital maturation, and so on); the term is actually derived from the word "estrus" which refers to the sexual cycle of female animals. Since the 1930s when estrogen products became available commercially, their use in a variety of conditions has become commonplace. Between 1962 and 1973, estrogen sales quadrupled in this country into an $80 million per year industry. More recently, however, there has been considerable concern about the safety of estrogens, and the Food and Drug Administration has adopted regulations requiring that package inserts warning of dangers be given to all women using estrogens. We have asked Dr. Johanna Perlmutter, Assistant Professor of Obstetrics and Gynecology at the Beth Israel Hospital, Harvard Medical School, and a member of our Advisory Board, to respond to the following questions about estrogens.

Has it been conclusively proven that estrogens can cause endometrial cancer (cancer of the lining of the uterus or womb) in women who take them for relief of post-menopausal symptoms?

I would hesitate to use the phrase "proved conclusively," but there is strong evidence pointing to an association between the use of estrogens and endometrial cancer. We have known for a long time that estrogens can cause excessive proliferation of the cells that line the uterus. We have also known that estrogens can produce malignant growths in laboratory animals such as rats and mice. The most important evidence, however, comes from recent studies showing that women who used estrogens for the relief of various post-menopausal symptoms had a four- to eight-fold increased risk of developing endometrial cancer. Now, the "normal" risk for endometrial cancer in a post-menopausal woman not using estrogens is low—about one per one thousand women per year—so we are talking about an additional 3 to 7 cases per thousand women per year. In other words, most women using estrogens do *not* get cancer, but there does appear to be a definite increase in the risk. The greatest risk is apparently in those women on high doses of estrogen who use it over prolonged periods of time (greater than one year—with increasing risk as duration of use increases). While a few have argued that women found to have cancer while on estrogens really had *pre-existing* cancer that was unmasked by the estrogens, most gynecologists believe that estrogen use by post-menopausal women contributes to an increased risk of endometrial cancer.

What about other factors that might contribute to endometrial cancer?

Some have been clearly identified. For example, endometrial cancer is almost twice as frequent in white women as in blacks. Interestingly, Japanese women have a lower incidence if they live in Japan, as compared to Hawaii or mainland U.S.A.—indicating a possible environmental or dietary factor. Also, it has long been known that obese women are at greater risk; one explanation for this is the fact that fat cells can convert androgens (male hormones) produced by post-menopausal women into estrones, a type of estrogen that can predispose to endometrial cancer. Diabetes and high blood pressure also seem to be associated with an increased chance of developing endometrial cancer. So there is certainly more to the story of endometrial cancer than estrogen treatment.

What about estrogens and breast cancer?

Such a relationship is much less clear. Earlier studies had suggested a possible protective effect against breast cancer, but more recent ones conclude that estrogen use by post-menopausal women might lead to a slight increase in the risk of breast cancer. Thus, we can no longer say estrogens are protective, but whether or not they actually cause breast cancer is, I think, far from proven.

Given all these concerns, can anything good be said about estrogen use in post-menopausal women?

It is known that estrogens will retard bone thinning (osteoporosis), a process that accelerates after menopause and is most pronounced in women whose ovaries have been surgically removed at an early age. The bone thinning usually proceeds silently until fractures of the hip or wrist or severe back pain (from collapsed vertebrae) occur—a fate of approximately 25% of American women. While estrogen treatment can prevent bone loss, it cannot restore bone tissue nor can it correct deformities. Thus, for such treatment to be most useful, it must be started before significant bone thinning has occurred, and the hormone must be continued for its beneficial effect to be sustained. Thus, the dilemma is that of remaining on estrogens and decreasing the risk of bone problems, while at the same time increasing the risk of endometrial cancer. Each woman must evaluate the risks and benefits for herself. Conditions which predispose to disabling osteoporosis—early surgical removal of both ovaries; a sedentary life style; bones already affected by chronic arthritis, steroid drugs, or Paget's disease—might well prompt a decision for estrogens. (If the ovaries were removed at the same time as a hysterectomy, of course, the dilemma is removed, as cancer cannot occur in a uterus that has been removed.)

Claims that estrogens make women "feminine forever" are clearly nonsense. There is no good evidence that estrogens given before or after menopause will delay the aging process, prevent heart attacks, or promote femininity. The emotional problems which may occur during the time of life associated with menopause should not be treated with estrogens. The use of estrogens for post-menopausal symptoms should be confined to the treatment of vaso-motor symptoms (sweats, hot flashes) and the itching and pain (especially during intercourse) that might result from a drying out (atrophy) of the lining of the vagina. When these symptoms become serious enough to interfere with normal living, the use of estrogens under careful supervision is justified, in my opinion. Indeed, in such women, they may provide dramatic relief.

What do you mean by careful supervision?

Before estrogens are given, a careful examination should be done to uncover any reasons for *not* giving them—such as liver disease, suspicion of early breast or uterine cancer, or heart disease. When indicated, the estrogens should be used in as low a dose as possible for as short a time as possible. I prefer to give them on a cyclic basis—21 days on, 7 days off. Many physicians also add progestins at the end of each cycle to prevent estrogen build-up. A woman taking estrogen should be examined every 6 to 12 months for any sign of serious side effects. And, most important, any abnormal bleeding should be reported to her doctor immediately. Once the decision is made to discontinue estrogen treatment, it should be reduced gradually to minimize the recurrence of symptoms that necessitated estrogen use.

What about other dangers associated with estrogen use?

There is little doubt that the use of estrogens can be associated with an increased incidence of blood clots, heart attacks, and strokes. Other risks include liver tumors (usually benign, but potentially dangerous in terms of internal bleeding), high blood pressure, gallstones, and the unmasking of diabetes. The actual risk for these conditions varies considerably with age and use, but such effects must be kept in mind when estrogens are used (particularly in the form of birth control pills) for a long period of time. Fortunately, newer versions of the pill use much lower doses of estrogen than were used in early forms. And the current concern to keep the estrogen dose as low as possible in treating the menopausal symptoms described above is also a good trend.

Infertility

The birth of Louise Brown in 1978 not only aroused enormous interest in the frontier of conception research but highlighted, with momentary intensity, the on-going problem faced by millions of couples usually described as "infertile." While that word may be invoked too quickly by some couples with false expectations concerning the ease of conception (as women typically become less fertile after age 25), it is legitimately used to describe *a failure to conceive after one year of normal sexual relations without contraception.* While no one knows for sure how many are so affected, estimates suggest that 10–25% of American couples either cannot have any children or can only have fewer than they wish.

THE COURSE OF CONCEPTION   While the emotional and physical factors that make a baby possible are exquisitely complex, the mechanical details can be simply described. The male must produce sperm of adequate numbers and vitality and must provide pathways for the release of those sperm into the female. The female must produce an egg which can then be carried to a meeting with sperm, and must provide unobstructed pathways and a suitable chemical environment for sperm to migrate to the released egg. However, when one considers the number of psychological, hormonal, and anatomical factors that must properly coincide for conception to occur, it seems astounding that it ever happens. But it is precisely the detailed dissection of this event in recent decades that has provided treatment opportunities for infertile couples that were unknown (and unexpected) in preceding generations.

THE COURSE OF CORRECTION   It cannot be too strongly stressed that the approach to a fertility problem must involve the supportive concern of both partners; the notion that either one is at fault is inappropriate—and often destructive. Initial interviews will explore the general health, past medical history, and present and past sexual history of both partners. Occasionally, some relatively simple measures may emerge—such as increasing the frequency of intercourse (most experts suggest three times per week during days 3 to 20 of the menstrual cycle) or identifying drugs that may be interfering (excessive alcohol is notorious). More often, however, specific tests and therapy for either the male or female are in order.

MALE FACTORS   About 30–40% of the time, the male will be identified as the source of the problem because of abnormalities in:

(1) *Sperm production:* Analysis of sperm numbers, shape, and motility is standard in any fertility investigation; the absence of sperm—or very low numbers (less than 10 million per milliliter)—generally indicates a poor outlook for solution. More moderate deficits, however, may respond to a combination of measures such as reducing heavy alcohol and tobacco use; obtaining sufficient food, exercise, and rest; avoiding excessive testicular heat and pressure; and occasionally, attempting hormonal treatment. Varicose veins (varicoceles) in the scrotum may contribute to poor sperm production and can be surgically corrected.

(2) *Sperm transport:* Less commonly, sperm production is normal (as demonstrated by biopsy of the testicle) but transport is blocked in the system of tubes that ultimately discharge semen through the penis. Newer microsurgical techniques have improved the chances of correcting such blockages—especially those produced by previous vasectomy.

FEMALE FACTORS   The areas of investigation and possible therapy for the female partner are more complex and include the following:

(1) *Body fat:* Many women might be surprised to learn that extremes of body fat—either too much or too little—can lead to temporary infertility due to loss of ovulation (the monthly release of the egg from the ovary). This relationship has become increasingly recognized in our era of vigorous exercise and extensive dieting, both of which reduce body fat. Similarly, loss of ovulation occurs in *anorexia nervosa,* a condition seen mainly in young women who are

preoccupied by their body image and develop a tremendous aversion to eating. The exact reasons why loss of ovulation accompanies rapid loss of body fat is not clear. It obviously has something to do with changes in female hormones, particularly estrogens, since fat tissue is in part responsible for estrogen production. Whatever the cause, the resulting infertility is usually reversible with restoration of body fat to reasonably normal levels.

(2) Egg production: About 20% of female fertility problems will be traced to hormonal failure which can often be corrected today with drugs. The one most commonly used is clomiphene (Clomid) which acts to release eggs from the ovary; about 35% of females appropriately selected for this treatment will become pregnant. Clomid therapy should not be confused with the less common and more drastic therapy involving one to two weeks of daily injections of Pergonal (prepared from urine of post-menopausal females, which is rich in hormones that stimulate egg production), followed by timely administration of another hormone (HCG) to stimulate egg release. It is this latter course of therapy (Pergonal plus HCG) that is more often associated with multiple births, since the hormonal stimulation of the ovary may release more than one egg; multiple births—most often twins—occur in about 20% of women who respond. (Clomid, on the other hand, results in multiple births in only about one out of sixteen resulting pregnancies.)

(3) Egg transport: Problems with transport of released eggs via the oviducts (fallopian tubes) is the most common problem in female infertility. A wide range of congenital and infectious problems (such as gonorrhea) can account for malformation or malfunction of these tubes. A number of surgical approaches to this problem are now possible. Occasionally, the very methods used to diagnose tubal problems (passing carbon dioxide into the tubes or inserting dye for x-ray pictures) eliminate the blockage.

(4) Cervical environment: This phrase is used to suggest that less well understood factors may be involved in the environment of the vagina and cervix where sperm are ejaculated by the penis. This may include anatomic deviations (such as retroversion of the uterus), but more often refers to poor quantity or quality of the mucus produced by cervical glands during the time just before the egg is released. Sometimes this environment can be improved by small doses of estrogen or by correcting underlying infections. Occasionally, sperm are rendered ineffective by antibodies produced by

the female—and the temporary use of a cervical cap or a condom to prevent direct contact of sperm with female tissue may decrease antibody production. Tests for the adequacy of the cervical environment include examination of cervical mucus before ovulation and examination of cervical fluid for sperm numbers and motility after intercourse.

TEST-TUBE CONCEPTION   Further approaches to infertility include *artificial insemination*—using either sperm from the husband to bypass local "environmental" problems described above, or sperm from another donor when a deficiency of sperm is the identified problem. That term may also refer to the very rare procedure of using a husband's sperm to inseminate another woman—in effect using her womb and genetic contributions to produce a child. None of these methods qualify as "test-tube conception" but they do involve ethical considerations far beyond the typically employed fertility treatments.

The case of Louise Brown represents a very real technological advance—in which sperm and egg came from the legal parents but were united in a laboratory environment, with the resulting fertilized egg quickly placed in the mother's womb. Several observations are in order:

(1) This procedure does not describe a "test-tube baby," meaning the actual growth and development of the fetus outside the womb—a feat that is far beyond the range of present scientific capability. Rather, it represents a method of providing laboratory conception with subsequent natural human development. As such, it would seem to fit into the scope of fertility treatment—rather than bizarre science fiction.

(2) While this method of fertility treatment surely represents a potentially exciting approach to problems of tubal blockage in the female, it is very premature to translate the success of the Brown case into a standard expectation. Many experts feel it will be difficult in the near future to accomplish test-tube fertilizations routinely. And many questions concerning the ultimate outcomes for babies so conceived remain to be answered.

IN SUMMARY   The above glimpse into the present state of infertility treatment obviously suggests that technical expertise and wise emotional counsel are often required. Couples desiring infertility consultation should carefully seek available specialists. Many large teaching hospitals and specialty clinics provide a team approach that is often desirable.

Impotence—All in the Mind?

Standard medical wisdom has it that the vast majority of men suffering from impotence have underlying emotional problems as the cause of their inability to engage consistently in sexual intercourse. This bias often leads to the conclusion that any evidence of the physical ability to have an erection—such as early morning erections—indicates that the machinery is intact and the cause of impotence is clearly not physical. Against this background, therefore, a recent medical report (*Journal of the American Medical Association,* February 22/29, 1980) by researchers from the Beth Israel Hospital in Boston has generated considerable interest. They found that among 105 men who had the problem of impotence, 37 (35%) turned out to have unsuspected endocrine disorders when screening tests demonstrated abnormal levels of the male hormone testosterone. Subsequently, 33 of the 37 experienced restoration of potency with medical therapy.

The authors of the article also point out that some of these men with abnormal endocrine function had reported *occasionally* successful sexual functioning (including morning erections). Using appropriate caution, they go on to stress that their experience of seeing a selected, referred group of patients is probably not typical of a random sample of impotent men. But they do conclude that screening for blood levels of testosterone in impotent men would uncover endocrine abnormalities that "almost certainly will be substantially greater than is currently recognized." They emphasize that occasional sexual function or a normal physical exam does not exclude an endocrine abnormality as the cause of impotence.

While the above research experience needs to be repeated and verified by others, it does alert both those who have impotence and those who treat it to obtain male hormone levels in the evaluation of this problem.

Pregnancy

The more that we learn about pregnancy, the more apparent it becomes that the development of a fetus *can* be affected by many factors in its mother's environment. As with so many health issues, it's a matter of playing the odds: many babies seem perfectly healthy despite exposure to potentially damaging substances and events, but each exposure increases the risk that something will go wrong.

CIGARETTES, ALCOHOL, AND RECREATIONAL DRUGS
Cigarettes and alcohol are two agents known to injure a fetus (see pp. 77 and 88). Not only pregnant women but women who are planning a pregnancy should cut out smoking and drink little or no alcohol. Use of other "recreational" drugs, such as *marijuana* and *psychedelics,* is also likely to increase the risk of fetal injury. It is important to realize that the most vulnerable period is the first three months after conception; a woman should be avoiding alcohol, cigarettes, and unnecessary drugs even before she is certain she has conceived. We would also suggest that *caffeine-containing drinks* (coffee, tea, colas, and cocoa) be limited, although the evidence for caffeine's injurious effect on the fetus is thus far available only in animal studies.

By the way, potential fathers also should not take an entirely casual attitude toward their smoking, drinking, and drug-taking habits. Genetic damage to the sperm is possible and can be passed on to the baby.

MEDICAL DRUGS AND X-RAYS   Medically necessary or useful drugs create more of a problem. It is wise to consider whether their use can be curtailed or stopped during pregnancy—even though not many prescription drugs are known to have any effect on a fetus.

Similarly, nonessential medical x-rays should be avoided, especially those of the abdomen (see p. 162). *However, a woman should not endanger her health by giving up needed drugs or x-rays.* When a woman who regularly takes prescribed drugs is preparing for pregnancy—or when the need for drugs or x-rays arises during pregnancy—she should discuss her situation with her doctor and obstetrician and insist on a careful, thoughtful response from them on the balance of risks and benefits.

WEIGHT GAIN   It used to be considered an achievement to make it through pregnancy without anyone's noticing a large and protuberant abdomen: the less weight, the better. The last decade, however, has produced clear evidence that severe weight restriction during pregnancy can result in abnormally low birth weights which can be associated with serious developmental problems for the newborn. The *Standards for Ambulatory Obstetric Care* (published in 1977 by the American College of Obstetricians and Gynecologists) reflects this emphasis on adequate nutrition by stating that the total weight gain during pregnancy should be at least 22–26 pounds, with the increase being minimal during the first 12 weeks, but about a pound a week thereafter.

In short, it should no longer be fashionable (because it is not good for the developing child) to stay as thin as possible during pregnancy. Similarly, pregnancy is not the time to go on a weight-reducing diet. Those women who cannot afford nutritious food during pregnancy should take advantage of the federally funded WIC (Women, Infants, and Children) program, which provides counseling and food for those at "nutritional risk." (A call to your local or state health department will provide further information on this program.)

SEXUAL INTERCOURSE   One of the questions most commonly asked by couples during pregnancy is whether sexual intercourse is "safe" for both the woman and the developing child. Unfortunately, there are no good data on which to base a "scientific" answer to that question. The public press has given wide circulation to a study (November 29, 1979, *New England Journal of Medicine*) suggesting that intercourse one or more times a week during the last month of pregnancy was associated with a higher rate of womb infections and infant deaths as compared with abstinence from sexual activity during this time. However, these results come from data recorded between 1959 and 1966—when certain features of modern obstetrical care were not available. In an editorial accompanying the report, Dr. Arthur Herbst, Chief of Obstetrics and Gynecology at the University of Chicago, writes in part as follows: "Current data do not permit dogmatic statements about coitus and pregnancy outcomes ... A reasonable policy might be to recommend the avoidance of intercourse and orgasm in the third trimester in women with a poor reproductive history or in those who, on pelvic examination, have premature ripening of the cervix. More specific criteria and recommendations will have to await the results of prospective studies in contemporary populations." In short, we still don't have a firm answer to that question about intercourse during pregnancy.

TEENAGE PREGNANCY   Most in our society are accustomed to thinking of unplanned pregnancies as primarily a social problem. But when the entire phenomenon of teenage pregnancies (at least 80% of which occur out of wedlock) is considered, real medical dangers also exist. Partly—or even largely—this may stem from a social and psychological milieu that makes proper nutrition and regular pre-natal care difficult or unlikely. Whatever the contributing factors, there is now solid documentation that *teenage pregnancies result in a higher incidence of premature birth and low birth weight*—the two, of course, often related. The Alan Guttmacher Institute (the research division of the Planned Parenthood Federation) points out that 16% of children born to mothers under age 15 are of low birth weight. This, in turn, is associated with an increased risk for both immediate and long-term problems. Some studies indicate that the death rate during the first year of life for first babies is 2–3 times greater for children born to mothers under age 15 than for those born to women in their early 20s. There is also evidence that children born prematurely or with low birth weights have an increased risk for many medical problems—including cerebral palsy and mental retardation. *In short, the one million teenage pregnancies in this country each year represent a reservoir of very real medical problems.*

FETAL MONITORING   One of the "revolutions" that have occurred in medicine in the last decade has been the increasing use of electronic fetal monitoring during labor and delivery. This typically involves attaching a heart-rate recording electrode to the scalp of the fetus (while still in the womb) and simultaneously recording contraction patterns via a thin tube inserted into the womb. Although these procedures contribute to infection only rarely, they do lead to a higher number of Caesarean sections as "cause for concern" is picked up by the monitors.

Several studies have attempted to ask whether or not fetal monitoring is ultimately justified on the basis of decreased infant mortality. The August 17, 1978, issue of the *New England Journal of Medicine* describes the results of over 15,000 live births at the Beth Israel Hospital in Boston; almost 50% included fetal monitoring. The report concludes that "in the highest risk group, 109 lives might be saved for every thousand babies monitored." However, for the much larger lower risk group (full-term babies with no risk factors) only one baby per thousand monitored would benefit.

IMMUNIZATIONS   The increasing number of women of child-bearing age who have not been immunized against childhood diseases (including tetanus) and the increasing number of home deliveries (sometimes under less than ideal sanitary conditions) has caused worry about newborns developing tetanus (lockjaw). Indeed, several such cases have been described. The answer, of course, is to make sure that pregnant women are immunized against tetanus and that deliveries, wherever conducted, are as germ-free as possible. (See also the discussion of German measles, p. 232.)

Amniocentesis

Many people are now limiting the number of their children and delaying pregnancy until relatively late in life. As a result, they are increasingly concerned about the possibility that a baby will be born with a severe congenital defect. Drs. Richard Erbe and Wayne Miller of the Genetics Unit at the Massachusetts General Hospital and the Harvard Medical School answer questions about diagnosing congenital defects during pregnancy.

Why has the diagnosis of congenital defects become so prominent in obstetrical care?

There are two main reasons. First, the number of conditions that can be detected by available techniques has been increasing. Second, current diagnostic methods are generally so safe that they pose a relatively small risk to fetus and mother when family history or special circumstances indicate that prenatal assessment should be performed.

What techniques are now available?

The most frequently used one is *amniocentesis,* in which fluid is removed from the "bag of waters" surrounding the fetus. This fluid can then be chemically tested, or cells (always present in the fluid) may be grown in culture and studied for abnormalities of their chromosomes or metabolism. For example, when the fluid is examined, elevation of a protein produced by the fetal liver (alpha-fetoprotein) suggests one of several abnormalities, such as failure of the brain or spinal cord to close properly, failure of the abdomen to close, or in other cases, obstruction in the urinary system or the gastrointestinal tract. After several weeks, the cultured cells are examined under the microscope; they may reveal defects in the chromosomes—such as the extra chromosome associated with Down's syndrome. Finally, a variety of biochemical tests can be employed to identify about *seventy* inborn errors of metabolism.

Major malformations can be detected by *ultrasonography,* a process by which sound waves are used to outline the fetus. The picture that is formed resembles an x-ray somewhat, but it avoids the risks of x-ray damage to the fetus. The *fetoscope* is a long, very narrow fiberoptic tube which can be inserted directly into the womb. It allows direct visualization of the fetus, and a blood sample or skin biopsy can be taken directly from the fetus or placenta. However, it is still largely a research tool.

What are the mechanics, safety, and cost of amniocentesis?

Amniocentesis should be performed when a pregnancy is between its fifteenth and eighteenth week, a period when ample fluid is available for testing but time remains to terminate the pregnancy before the legal limit—twenty-four weeks. A 3 1/3-inch needle is inserted through the abdomen and advanced into the womb; through it, less than an ounce of fluid is withdrawn and sent to the laboratory, where fluid and cells are separated. The fluid is tested for alpha-fetoprotein and the cells are cultured in preparation for the requested examinations. Ultrasonography should always be performed concurrently with amniocentesis. This procedure, which does not involve radiation or penetrating the abdomen, gives important additional information concerning the age of the fetus, the presence of twins, and the existence of major malformations. It is especially used to guide the placement of the needle so that the fetus and placenta are not injured.

Estimates of serious complications from amniocentesis are somewhat at variance, but a widely quoted published estimate is a 1% rate of miscarriage after amniocentesis. Our experience suggests that the actual rate is less than 1 in 250. We therefore recommend that prenatal diagnosis be used only when the probability of finding a diagnosable defect is greater than 1 in 250.

The accuracy of testing is very high, better than 99%. However, a small risk of incorrect diagnosis remains, further reason for restricting the test to parents at relatively high risk of an abnormality.

Prenatal diagnostic testing is expensive. The usual charge for ultrasonography is $80-$120, for the obstetrician $50-$120, and for the laboratory work $300-$500. Insurance carriers vary in their coverage policies.

Who should have prenatal diagnosis performed?

For the "average" couple without known risk factors, the probability of a serious birth defect that can be diagnosed during pregnancy is very low. Because there is a small risk to the mother and fetus from amniocentesis and because the procedure is expensive, routine prenatal diagnostic testing cannot be justified. But the following situations—in our opinion—do justify considering testing:

(1) Mother over thirty-five years of age.

(2) A parent with a known translocation (abnormal arrangement) in his or her chromosomes.

(3) A previous infant born with a chromosome abnormality (such as Down's syndrome) or with a neural tube defect (such as spina bifida).

(4) A parent with any other known risk diagnosable during pregnancy.

(5) A mother carrying a sex-linked abnormality (such as hemophilia) that cannot be diagnosed during pregnancy but would affect only sons, whose sex can be determined by prenatal testing.

The main purpose of prenatal testing is to detect birth defects early enough to allow a pregnancy to be terminated. However, since approximately 95% of such testing results in no abnormalities being discovered, it also has the effect of enabling couples at high risk to proceed with a pregnancy without undue anxiety. Even when parents decide not to terminate, despite the presence of a defect, prenatal diagnosis may help in the management of a pregnancy and in preparing for the care of their child.

It is important to bear in mind that *prenatal diagnosis never guarantees a normal child;* currently, there is no way to test for all possible abnormalities. What it does accomplish is to inform parents with an unusually high risk of a *particular* abnormality whether that defect is present. But even after reassurance is provided that one abnormality is absent, a tested fetus, like all fetuses, runs about a 4% risk of other birth defects.

What are possibilities for the future?

Ultrasonography is becoming more informative thanks to technical progress and can even now be used to provide a kind of "movie" of the fetus. As yet only a few centers have the highly sophisticated equipment needed for this, but where the capability exists, many structural defects can be determined. Within a few years we expect that three-dimensional imaging will become possible, with a corresponding increase in accuracy of the method.

Fetoscopy, as mentioned, permits direct visualization of the fetus, but so far technical limitations have restricted its usefulness, and it carries a higher risk than amniocentesis. However, the fetoscope can be used to draw fetal blood samples for diagnosis of hereditary anemias, including thalassemia and sickle-cell anemia as well as the major form of hemophilia.

Direct study of genes through modern biochemical methods may increase the diagnostic power of amniocentesis. Because all genes are thought to be present in all cells, at least early in development, it is in principle possible to obtain any gene from the cells floating in amniotic fluid and, through a series of biochemical manipulations, determine whether the gene is normal. If this proves to be practical, the relatively simple technique of amniocentesis can be used to identify sickle-cell anemia or other blood disorders which now must be found by the riskier method of drawing blood through the fetoscope.

Breast Feeding

The "breast is best" movement is gaining a strong mouthhold in the field of infant nutrition. The American Academy of Pediatrics and the Canadian Pediatric Society have issued a joint statement to encourage all physicians to recommend breast feeding. We have asked Dr. Mary Ellen Avery, Physician-in-Chief of The Children's Hospital Medical Center in Boston, and Dr. Ilene R. S. Sosenko, Instructor in Pediatrics at Harvard Medical School (who has recently nursed a newborn), to answer some basic questions about breast feeding.

What are the benefits of breast feeding?

An increasing body of information suggests that significant advantages exist for the breast-fed infant. For example:

(1) Early and prolonged contact between the mother and her newborn infant are generally satisfying to both and this is enhanced by nursing.

(2) The breast-fed infant determines his own intake of milk, unlike bottle feeding when the mother may coax the infant to drink all that she has poured, which may be more than needed.

(3) The fats in human milk are better absorbed by infants than those of cow's milk. Also, the amino acid composition of human milk is particularly suited to the metabolic needs of the newborn infant, whose liver is relatively inefficient in converting some of the proteins found in cow's milk into forms the infant can use. However, some of the commercially available milk-based formulas have modified the proteins in cow's milk to resemble more closely those in human milk.

(4) Although iron content of milk from all mammals is low, the iron in human milk is better absorbed than the iron in cow's milk.

Thus, the iron in human milk is sufficient to meet the requirements of the breast-fed full-term infant for the first six months of life.

(5) The concentration of sodium and other minerals is somewhat lower in human milk and more suited to meet the infant's needs; many of the cow's milk formulas for infants have been modified to match the mineral concentration in human milk.

(6) The infant at birth must quickly develop immunologic responses in order to survive in the germ-laden outside world. Increasing evidence shows that infants acquire important antibodies to intestinal germs when fed human milk. The critical role of breast feeding in preventing gastroenteritis in infants in developing countries has been well documented. Not only gastroenteritis but respiratory infections, meningitis, and other overwhelming infections are less frequent among breast-fed infants. Human milk also spares the gastrointestinal tract from exposure to substances in foods that might be absorbed and cause sensitization. Some studies show a reduction in allergic problems (such as eczema) in breast-fed infants. Although rare, some infants manifest an allergy to cow's milk itself, with a wide range of symptoms that can include breathing problems as well as severe diarrhea and anemia.

(7) Breast feeding may aid in contraception, although it is not reliable in this respect. Generally, return of ovulation and menstruation are delayed up to at least ten weeks (and sometimes to six months) in nursing mothers.

(8) Even premature infants thrive on human milk when provided by their mothers. Protein concentration in milk of mothers of prematurely born infants is somewhat higher than that of milk produced at term, and this may meet the higher protein requirements of the low-birth-weight infant. It is not always possible to maintain full nutrition of such infants with breast milk, but it is increasingly being used as a source of nourishment for the smallest premature infants.

In the 1940s approximately 65% of the infants in the United States were breast fed, but by 1972 only 15% of infants were nursed as long as two months. Why did breast feeding fall into such disuse?

Surely social custom had much to do with it. Prepared formulas were available and are satisfactory for most infants. Some mothers received less than adequate encouragement and information, and quickly turned to formulas. Others may have given up too easily, thinking they didn't have enough milk. "Milk drying up" is not a reflection of a woman's ability to produce milk so much as a lack of awareness of ways to stimulate and improve milk production. Success at nursing is not a matter of breast size and is generally not dependent on nipple shape.

As the infant suckles, nerve endings in the nipples are stimulated and they, in turn, signal the brain to produce two hormones—prolactin and oxytocin. Prolactin is responsible for stimulating the breast to produce milk. Oxytocin causes the ejection of milk to the nipple, where it can be obtained by the suckling infant. As long as a breast receives stimulation by suckling, it will continue to produce milk; the more it is stimulated, the more milk is produced. This law of supply and demand enables a woman to nurse a growing infant with increased intake and caloric needs, to nurse twins, and, at times, even to donate "extra" milk to hospital milk banks. In fact, a little "home banking" is often helpful. One can express milk and store it, which allows the working mother the necessary hours away from home.

What does the infant need in addition to human milk?

Vitamin D concentrations in human milk are not sufficient to meet the needs of the infant beyond the first months of life. If the mother is deficient in vitamin D (as in the case of some on unusual diets), the infant may develop rickets during its first year. All infants should receive vitamin D supplementation (400 I.U.) daily. Nursing infants should receive fluoride in addition to vitamin supplementation. The question of introduction of solid foods causes much debate among pediatricians and mothers. The infant who is nursing well on human milk has no nutritional requirements for solid foods during the first six months. The early introduction of cereals and other prepared baby foods may increase the caloric intake and lead to overweight. On the other hand, some infants seem more satisfied when they have some solids, and there is no known medical reason for not introducing them at three or four months of age. (For more information on fluoride and solid foods, see below.)

What is your personal advice to new mothers?

Quite frankly, we think it is amazing, in an era of interest and emphasis on natural food, that less than half of new mothers undertake to nurse their infants—and even fewer persist for more than a few weeks. Ironically, those who can best afford prepared formulas are leading the new movement to a return to nursing their infants. If you want to, and know how to, you have a greater than 95% chance of success with breast feeding. Our advice is to give it a try.

Additional Notes on Infant Feeding

IRON SUPPLEMENTATION   Iron deficiency is the most common cause of anemia in children as well as adults. The risk of iron deficiency in infancy is greatest when iron stores received from the mother during pregnancy have been used up. This occurs at about 2 months of age in infants born prematurely and at about 4–6 months in full-term infants.

Both breast milk and cow's milk contain a relatively *low* amount of iron when compared to a general diet. Specifically, a general diet provides about six times the amount of iron available in an equivalent amount of calories provided by milk. The Committee on Nutrition of the American Academy of Pediatrics, which reported on the subject of iron supplements for infant feeding in *Pediatrics,* November 1976, makes the following points for all present or prospective parents:

(1) Although breast and cow's milk contain the same amount of iron, the iron in breast milk is much more efficiently absorbed than that in cow's milk. The report suggests that breast feeding is much less likely to result in iron deficiency than the use of cow's milk.

(2) Iron fortified formulas, used largely before age six months, and dry infant cereals, used before and after six months of age, are good sources of iron, as are iron drops. The committee recommends that one of these sources of iron be started by age two months in infants born prematurely and by age four months in full-term infants.

FLUORIDE SUPPLEMENTATION   In the January 1979 issue of *Pediatrics,* the Committee on Nutrition of the American Academy of Pediatrics proposed a revised schedule for fluoride supplementation which considers the important factors of age and existing fluoride levels (natural or supplemented) in the community's water supply. Accordingly, that committee has developed a table which is modified as follows:

	Concentration of fluoride in drinking water (parts per million)		
Age	< 0.3 ppm	0.3–0.7 ppm	> 0.7 ppm
2 wk–2 yr	0.25 mg/day	0	0
2–3 yr	0.50 mg/day	0.25 mg/day	0
3–16 yr	1.00 mg/day	0.50 mg/day	0

In other words, if the level of fluoride in the water supply is greater than 0.7 parts per million (ppm) no supplementation is needed at any age; if it is less than 0.7 ppm, supplementation is recommended as above. (The doses were chosen to correspond with amounts commercially available in drops, tablets, and vitamin combinations.)

While the above guidelines are intended to provide a simple approach to fluoride supplementation, they do not take into account the variability in the amounts of tap water ingested by children below age three—and in particular, the differences in the amounts of water that vary with the precise prepared formula diet that an infant receives. Thus, fluoride supplements should be worked out with one's doctor by considering the level of fluoride in the water and how much water is actually being consumed during the first several years of life.

These recommendations represent a lowering of the committee's previous dosage recommendations of 1972 to reduce the possibility of mild discoloration of teeth sometimes seen at higher doses. It is important for parents to check the fluoride levels in their water supply before giving supplements. However, there is no scientific doubt as to the effectiveness of appropriate amounts of fluoride in preventing tooth decay; we agree with the strong statement by *Consumer Reports* (August 1978): "The simple truth is that there is no 'scientific controversy' over the safety of fluoridation. The practice is safe, economical, and beneficial."

ON THE FEEDING OF SUPPLEMENTAL FOODS TO IN-
FANTS   This is the title of a report from the Committee on Nutrition of the American Academy of Pediatrics (published in the June
1980 issue of its official journal, *Pediatrics*). The title suggests a phil-
osophical essay as much as a scientific treatise—which is appropriate given the emotions that often surround the introduction of solids
into the life of an infant. Indeed, parental and family pressures—to
see rapid weight gain, to supposedly help the infant sleep through
the night, to take advantage of convenience foods—often dictate the
move to solids rather than considerations which may be best for the
child.

The committee's report re-emphasizes earlier recommendations
that solids not be introduced until 4 to 6 months at the earliest.
(Maybe we should remember that Mother Nature designed a system
capable of providing a fluid-only diet well beyond the first year of
life.) As pointed out in the report, various organs in the infant may
not be able to handle the challenge of solids: the kidneys may be of-
fended by the new and foreign proteins, and the neuro-muscular
system may not be able to manipulate the ingested solids.

The committee then goes on to offer some specific recommendations for adding solids, among them:

(1) Add only one food at a time at weekly intervals. Introducing
mixed solids not only provides more of a challenge to the infant but
makes the identification of any "food intolerance" obviously more
difficult; when mixed solids cause upset, it is hard to know which one
is the culprit.

(2) Increase fluid intake when solids are introduced. Added
fluid helps the kidneys handle the new load. Water offers the advantage of "no calories." It is important to remember that an infant cries
when thirsty—not just when hungry.

(3) Avoid adding salt to solid food. Salt is an acquired taste and
we shouldn't foist the bad habit on our kids, given what we now
know about the possible role of salt in the development of hypertension.

(4) Wait with certain foods that might be especially allergenic.
The oft-identified foods in this category include cow's milk, eggs, and
wheat.

(5) Remember that calories count for infants as well as adults. There is some evidence that excessive calories at an early age may pose lifelong problems with obesity.

The entire report is short, well-written, informative, and sensibly flexible. Those of you ready to introduce your infants to the wonderful world of solid foods may wish to read it in its entirety.

Bringing Up Baby

DIAPER RASH   Ammonia produced by bacteria is not the cause of most cases of diaper rash. Rather, simple moisture seems to be the underlying problem—which means that the commonsense measures followed by many parents (frequent changing, talcum powder, avoiding plastic pants when possible) do indeed make sense. However, cornstarch should probably not be used since it is a growth medium for troublesome fungi. When talcum powder is used, gentle local application is the rule, to avoid large puffs that might be inhaled by the infant.

BED WETTING   Recent medical journals have called attention to the dangers of antidepressants which are commonly used to treat bed wetting in young children. In Britain, these drugs have replaced aspirin and iron as the most common cause of fatal poisoning in children under age 5. The drug most often used for bed wetting in this country is imipramine (Tofranil). Most experts stress that it should not be given to children under age 6, and only in carefully prescribed dosage to older children, since overdosage can cause convulsions, coma, heart rhythm disturbances, and depression of respiration.

Since bed wetting is an embarrassing problem for the child affected, it is not surprising that he (or she, though girls are less likely to bed-wet) might be tempted to take more of the medicine which has been given to "cure the problem." Therefore, children must be warned about the dangers of taking extra pills in an effort to achieve extra control. Also, many physicians would advise using alarm devices and motivational methods ("gold-star charts") before resorting to drug treatment.

DIARRHEA Drugs for treating acute diarrhea in children are widely used; the affliction is annoying and worrisome, and both doctors and parents are anxious to try something to stop it. However, proof for the effectiveness of the drugs used is lacking. An article in the *Journal of the American Medical Association* reported on one study of four widely used drugs for childhood diarrhea—kaolin-pectate, kaolin alone, pectin alone, and diphenoxylate-atropine, which is better known as Lomotil. None of the drugs was demonstrated to be more effective than a placebo in reducing stool frequency or volume. (Lomotil is also known to be dangerous in children under two and has been reported as a cause of accidental childhood poisoning.)

The above is not to suggest that acute diarrhea in children is not a potentially serious problem. Fluids lost must be replaced; especially dangerous is any fluid loss in a young infant. But the above-mentioned study does point out that many drugs used today for a variety of conditions may lack solid scientific proof of effectiveness.

SUDDEN INFANT DEATH SYNDROME The April 1978 issue of *Pediatrics,* the official journal of the American Academy of Pediatrics, contains several articles and editorials that pertain to a problem that provokes fear in the hearts of all parents—so-called sudden infant death syndrome (SIDS). That journal also contains recommendations from the Academy's Task Force on a *related but not synonymous* problem known as *prolonged apnea.* In order to sort out some proposed answers to both of these problems, the following facts need to be considered:

(1) Sudden infant death syndrome refers to the catastrophic event of unexpected death (usually during apparent sleep) in a young infant—typically during the first six months of life. This tragedy strikes 2–3 of every thousand children born in this country. In up to half of such deaths, there is evidence of *mild* infection. SIDS is more common in infants who are non-white, who are of lower socioeconomic status, or who have been born prematurely. The risk is also somewhat higher in those with a sibling who succumbed to SIDS. Despite great interest and much research to date, no certainty as to the cause (and, correspondingly, the prevention) of SIDS

exists. The vast majority of such deaths are indeed sudden and unexpected.

(2) Another disorder observed in infants is known as prolonged apnea. The Task Force defines this condition as cessation of breathing for more than 20 seconds, or briefer episodes if they are associated with slow heart rate, cyanosis (blue color), or pallor. Such episodes must be distinguished from breathing problems that have identifiable underlying causes. According to one study, only about 5% of infants who die of SIDS have a history of prolonged apnea.

This last statement becomes important in light of the Task Force's recommendation that "24-hour surveillance is critical to the management of prolonged apnea." *This recommendation should not be taken to mean that most cases of sudden infant death could be prevented by careful 24-hour observation.* Nor should parents who have lost a child via sudden death be led to think that they might have prevented that death with such surveillance. The current facts of the matter are that the vast majority of sudden infant deaths could not have been prevented.

The Task Force does, however, recommend such 24-hour surveillance for those infants identified as having had episodes of prolonged apnea. They suggest that such observation can be done in the home by trained persons. They point out that the use of monitors *may* be useful but only under medical supervision. Finally, they emphasize that even careful 24-hour observation does not guarantee that death will not occur. Several accompanying editorials discuss these recommendations (and those of others) and stress the great monetary and psychological burdens involved in such monitoring—especially given the uncertain results.

Again, the current views are that (1) sudden infant death is seldom preventable and that (2) the small group of infants who have experienced prolonged apnea *may* benefit from careful 24-hour observation. (3) Siblings of a sudden-death infant should be evaluated routinely for the presence of prolonged apnea.

FEVER SEIZURES The sight of a child having a convulsion strikes terror into the hearts of most parents—even though they might realize that seizures due to a high fever are relatively common during childhood. Once such a seizure has occurred, there is understandable pressure from parents to "do something so that it won't happen again." Apart from giving fever-reducing medicine (aspirin or acetaminophen) and sponging a child when and if fever occurs, the most frequent recommendation for preventing further fever seizures involves giving a *daily dose* of phenobarbital. (Taking the medicine only when a fever strikes will not do the job.) However, there are side effects from long-term phenobarbital use—some potentially serious. All of which, in the past, has posed an obvious dilemma.

Fortunately, several recent studies have charted the natural history of fever seizures. The best data come from the Collaborative Perinatal Project which followed 54,000 children from birth to age 7. About 9% of these children had three or more fever seizures during the first seven years of life. However, follow-up showed that no deaths, no serious nerve damage, and no decrease in IQ occurred. There was a slight increase in the risk of developing later epilepsy, but 98% of those who had such seizures did *not*.

Given the usual lack of serious consequences from uncomplicated fever seizures—and the potential problems from continuous phenobarbital—most pediatricians today choose not to give phenobarbital as prevention, but do advocate early treatment of fever with aspirin or acetaminophen. The data support this as a wise decision—even though parents might push for additional medication.

ROCK, BANG, AND ROLL—KID STYLE   The October 1978 issue of the *Journal of Pediatrics* contains a study of body rocking, head banging, and head rolling in 525 apparently normal children. The prevalence of these movements was as follows: 19% for body rocking (especially when listening to music, less often when alone in the crib), 5% for head banging (most often when upset or tired or when alone), and 6.3% for head rolling (again most often when alone in a crib or playpen). In the November 9, 1978, issue of *Pediatric Alert,* Dr. T. Berry Brazelton (Chief, Division of Child Development, The Children's Hospital Medical Center, and Associate Professor of Pediatrics, Harvard Medical School) offers some useful comments on the study—including the following: "This is an interesting paper and I am sure it was written in part to reassure pediatricians and mothers about these all too common syndromes . . . many children do need some such pattern to handle their frustrations and to get themselves to sleep; these patterns are as comforting and as independent as thumb-sucking or loving a 'lovey' which satisfies many other children . . . I would hope pediatricians would not reinforce parents' guilt over these symptoms but rather will continue to be alert to them and their meaning . . . So this article makes one feel better about these rhythmic behaviors in normal children. I still wonder whether we shouldn't be rocking our children more, so they won't have to rock themselves. But who has the time?"

CONGENITAL HIP DISLOCATION   One of the more common orthopedic problems of childhood is congenital hip dislocation (occurring in about five of every thousand births) in which the upper end of the thigh bone (femur) does not fit properly into the hip socket. If this condition is detected in early infancy, treatment can be a relatively simple matter of diaper or pillow splints until the hip joint is restored to normal alignment. Treatment begun at a later age usually requires more restrictive casting and even surgery, and is less likely to be successful. Your physician probably routinely examines infants and young children for this condition, but parents may also notice signs suggestive of hip dislocation—including the following:

(1) Asymmetrical skin folds on the buttocks and thighs. (In other words, when the child lies on his tummy, you may notice that the skin folds of the two thighs are not symmetrical.)
(2) Apparent shortness of one leg.
(3) Difficulty in spreading one leg at the hip joint—often noticed during diapering.
(4) Diminished spontaneous motion of the affected leg.

All of the above may be perfectly normal, but if you notice them, you should ask your child's physician to re-check for congenital hip dislocation.

SMALL CHILDREN AND SMALL OBJECTS   Reports of children swallowing the button-sized batteries used in many cameras reminds us that these batteries contain potentially harmful materials that might be released when subjected to digestive juices. Another item to keep away from the kids.

"Body odor" may be caused by an unexpected "foreign body"—

such as a forgotten or unknown wad of paper stuck somewhere (nose, ear, for example) by a child. Small children love to poke things into their body openings . . . and leave them there.

Add toy rattles to the list of things that children can stick in their mouths and choke on. The Consumer Product Safety Commission has warned of several deaths caused in this manner. Anything small enough for a child to choke on should be kept away from an unsupervised child.

INFANT FURNITURE SAFETY The following safety tips are among those endorsed by the American Academy of Pediatrics' Committee on Accident and Poison Prevention (modified from a listing published by The Children's Hospital Medical Center, Boston). We offer them as safety reminders you might not think of—versus obvious ones such as not leaving safety rails down or not leaving an infant unattended on a changing table.

(1) Do not leave large toys or stuffed animals in a crib because an infant might use them as stepping stones to climb out.

(2) Straps on changing tables will not always hold an infant; an infant should not be left unattended on the presumption that they will.

(3) Young siblings may accidentally or purposefully tip over infant seats or lower safety rails; infants should never be left alone with young brothers or sisters.

(4) Cribs should not have slats more than 2 3/8 inches apart, since infants may stick their heads and necks through wider slats and strangle.

(5) A crib mattress should be the same size as the crib to avoid space around the mattress through which a child might catch an arm or a leg.

BURN PREVENTION Numerous reports point out that the majority of serious burn injuries in small children occur from scald injuries, usually in the kitchen. Hot liquids within reach (or eye view) of small children are life-threatening.

Dr. Jerold Kaplan, an Army burn specialist, in a report to the American Burn Association, suggested that many homes and hotels keep their hot water temperature too high. Many hot water faucets and showers were found to emit water at temperatures greater than 135 °F (57 °C). This can be a dangerous level, especially for infants or handicapped people who cannot react appropriately. And apart from the safety hazard involved, such temperatures waste energy. Many authorities suggest keeping the hot water thermostat set to less than 125 °F.

AUTOMOBILE SAFETY AND COMFORT   Everyone agrees in theory that children should be appropriately restrained during car rides—but few do it in practice. This is the case despite the fact that in the United States highway accidents are the leading cause of deaths in children between the ages of 1 and 14. Many of these deaths could be prevented with appropriate restraints. One of the reasons for lack of use is the assumption that children being held are safe from injury. However, studies show that head-on impacts at 10 and 30mph cause a newborn infant to become a "missile" weighing 200 and 600 pounds, respectively. Few persons are capable of re-straining such objects, even if the holder of the child is securely strapped. Studies also show that most auto accidents occur at *low* speeds *near* home—precisely the kind of driving that is not thought to be dangerous. If the above information motivates you to consider appropriate car seats for your infants and small children, consult your pediatrician or write the U.S. Printing Office, Washington, D.C. 20402, for booklet number 050-003-00052-3 entitled "What to Buy in Child Restraint Systems." By the way, it obviously makes sense for mom and dad to strap themselves in as well—not only to serve as "role models," but to remain around and intact for the years ahead.

Some families think twice about long car trips because of a very common problem: one of the children is prone to car sickness which routinely reduces happy family excursions to a series of quick stops by the side of the road. In a letter to the *New England Journal of Medicine,* Dr. Edward L. Schor describes a typical five-year-old girl who routinely developed car sickness in the back seat—but not in the front seat. However, when placed in a car seat in the back, no car sickness! Dr. Schor postulates that the elevation resulting from the car seat allowed the child to see out of the car and focus on more distant scenery—rather than having to look at a bobbing front seat with outside objects whizzing by. That hypothesis certainly agrees with the ancient wisdom concerning sea sickness—namely, that it is better to focus on the distant horizon than on nearby portholes. And this suggestion offers the additional advantage of having the child in a protective car seat—where children ought to be anyway when riding in a car.

VISION PROBLEMS IN PRE-SCHOOLERS   About one out of every twenty pre-school children has a vision problem. Of great concern is *amblyopia* or "lazy eye," which is caused by poorer vision in one eye that makes the child "turn off" the vision in the bad eye to avoid confusing the good one. Such disuse can result in permanent damage to vision if the underlying problem is not corrected by age six or seven. The earlier the problem is detected and treated, the better.

Sometimes there are obvious symptoms of eye trouble—such as excessive rubbing of the eye or a child's covering or shutting it. Often, alignment problems (cross-eye or wall-eye) are apparent. But in many instances, only testing can uncover an eye problem. This is why parents or guardians should insist on a vision check as part of any routine physical exam in a pre-school child.

Of great help to some families is the use of the Home Eye Test for Pre-Schoolers, developed and distributed by the National Society to Prevent Blindness. Available free in both English and Spanish versions, the test is based on having the child point out the direction of the "arms" of the letter E. The test comes in fold-out form and contains very clear directions; all that is needed in the home are a pencil, scissors, and paper cup to cover the child's eye during testing. Copies of the test can be obtained by writing to: The National Society to Prevent Blindness, 79 Madison Avenue, New York, New York 10016.

SHOE CONTACT DERMATITIS   Is nothing safe anymore? Now dermatologists are telling us that "occlusive" footwear (meaning shoes that don't allow for air circulation) can sometimes cause inflammation of the weight-bearing areas of the foot, leading to redness and pain accompanied by scaling and cracking. The problem of occlusive footwear is bad news for kids, and for those beloved running/tennis shoes that stay on day and, in some cases, night. The theory is that the sweating that occurs inside such shoes leads to the leaching out of chemicals within them, and this, in turn, sensitizes the skin—or results in actual contact allergies. Fortunately, the solution is mostly a matter of common sense—namely, avoiding wearing such shoes for prolonged periods, keeping the feet dry with an absorbent powder, and frequent changing of socks. Which presumes that you can get your child to part with those beloved Adidases, or whatever his or her brand happens to be. And, obviously, this particular problem must be distinguished from other kinds of foot skin problems—particularly athlete's foot, which is caused by a fungal infection requiring more specific forms of treatment.

SPORTS COMPETITION FOR GIRLS   As more girls enter interschool competition in non-contact sports (basketball, baseball, volleyball, etc.) some parents worry that their daughters might be uniquely prone to injury—just because they are girls. If your daughter(s) want to try out for teams this fall, you might be reassured to know that there is no evidence to suggest that they are at special risk as compared with boys. For example, a group of researchers at the University of Washington studied injuries during two years of interschool competition by girls' teams at four high schools. They found that the injury rate was no different than that for boys in similar sports. There were no injuries to breasts or genitalia. The survey did suggest that girls might experience some problems (such as tendon inflammation) as a result of poor general athletic conditioning; presumably better training for competition would help. In short, Moms and Dads, let your girls go out for the team. It's as good for them as for their brothers.

Immunizations

There is no preventive health practice with more payoff than that of immunizations. In recent years, several changes in the routine immunization schedule of childhood have been made—and several questions concerning some of the immunizations have been raised. This essay addresses those changes and questions.

THE SCHEDULE   The following schedule of childhood immunizations is currently recommended. Although it may be modified because of illness or allergy, an interruption does not necessitate starting all over again.

(1) DTP: The DTP shot combines protection against three diseases that were at one time childhood killers: *diphtheria* (D), *tetanus* or lockjaw (T), and *pertussis* or whooping cough (P). These vaccines can be given separately in special circumstances, but for the vast majority of children, the simplest plan is a combined DTP shot given three times during the first 8 months of life, again during the second year of life, and just before entering school. In other words, the DTP shot should be given *five* times before school to afford optimal protection.

(2) TOPV: This designation (as it often appears in immunization charts) stands for "trivalent oral polio vaccine." There are two forms of polio vaccine, the so-called *inactivated* form (also known as the killed or Salk or injectable vaccine) and the *attenuated* form (also known as the live or Sabin or oral vaccine). Since there are three types of polio viruses, protection must be achieved against all three. The most common method of giving protection against polio is the attenuated (oral) form, which contains all three in one swig. Like the DTP shot, the oral polio vaccine must be given *five* times

during childhood and it is usually given at the same time the DTP shot is given.

In the specific case of the live polio vaccine, there has been some concern about the danger of contracting polio from the oral (live, but weakened virus) versus the injected (killed virus) vaccine. Many European countries use only the injected vaccine, but since 1962 the official policy in this country has been to use the oral vaccine. Recently, the Institute of Medicine released a report addressed to this issue and these are its summary points:

The safety of both vaccines is outstanding. No cases of polio have been attributed to the injected vaccine. The risk for the oral vaccine is estimated to be about one case of polio for every 11.5 *million* persons vaccinated, with a further risk of one household contact case for every 3.9 *million* vaccinated. Only one death since 1969 has been attributed to the use of the oral vaccine—as compared with the hundreds or even thousands of deaths annually from polio before the vaccine.

Given the *very minimal* risk from oral vaccine versus no risk from injected vaccine, some ask why the injected vaccine is not recommended for the general population. The answer to the question involves some sophisticated theory which can be summarized by saying that the oral vaccine provides better immunity in the general population because the vaccine virus spreads to and immunizes some contacts of the vaccinated person.

Therefore, the Committee for the Study of Poliomyelitis Vaccines of the Institute of Medicine has unanimously recommended that the oral vaccine continue to be the vaccine of choice for routine immunizations in children. In addition, it recommends that children receive an oral polio booster before entrance into the seventh grade (age 11-12) to provide continued protection into adult years. Injected vaccine should be available for persons with immunological disorders which make them unusually susceptible to infections, for adults undergoing initial vaccination or traveling to areas where polio is a problem, and for persons who wish to receive this vaccine after understanding the issues described.

(3) Measles-Mumps-Rubella: These are the other three recommended immunizations of childhood. They have often been given separately, but increasing use is now made of a single shot which combines all three. Until recently, the measles shot was usually

given as a single vaccination at one year of age. That recommendation has now been changed to fifteen months following studies which demonstrated more protection if the vaccine is given then. Children who were previously vaccinated *before* 12 months of age or who received inactivated vaccine (used between 1963 and 1967) should be revaccinated. Persons who were born before 1957 are likely to have been infected with measles naturally—and therefore are usually protected. However, persons born after 1957 but vaccinated prior to 1968 with a measles vaccine of unknown type—or those born after 1957 who cannot remember having been vaccinated against measles—should now receive the current measles vaccine.

The above schedule can be translated into the following simple reminder:

At ages 2, 4, 6, 18 months and before school: A DTP shot plus oral polio vaccine.
At age 15 months: Combined measles, mumps, and rubella vaccine.

In other words, there are really only two things to remember and check on: the DTP and TOPV given at the same time five times during childhood and the measles-mumps-rubella combination given once. Simple! (P.S. You will note that small-pox vaccinations are no longer needed.)

ADDITIONAL COMMENTS   Because of current discussion about the vaccination programs for both regular measles and German measles, the following observations are in order:

(1) "Regular" measles (rubeola): Since the introduction of the live measles vaccine in 1963, the number of reported cases in the United States has dropped from about a half million per year to a low of 22,000 in 1974. More importantly, the dreaded complications of measles—including brain infections—have been drastically reduced as a consequence of vaccination. There is no question that this vaccine should be given routinely to children and the recent change in time recommendation (described above) should make it even more effective.

(2) German measles (rubella): The controversy over this vaccine concerns its timing, not its safety or effectiveness. Rubella is a mild disease in children but can cause severe damage to the developing fetus of a pregnant woman who contracts the disease. Therefore, the reason for immunization is not to protect children but to protect pregnant women from exposure. Some argue that the best way to do this is to achieve widespread immunity (so-called "herd immunity") among children—hence the official recommendations outlined above. Others argue that this approach will not work and we should instead concentrate on immunizing those at risk, namely girls, just before they enter child-bearing age. Despite the controversy, the key point is that each female who reaches child-bearing age ought to be protected against rubella. It is important to urge women of child-bearing age—preferably in early adolescence—to find out if they are protected against rubella by means of a simple blood test. (About 15% of adult women in this country do not have antibodies against rubella.) If not, a vaccination should be given. *An adult woman who is vaccinated against rubella must not become pregnant for three months, as the vaccine itself carries a small risk of harming a fetus.*

IN ADULTS While discussion of immunizations has been largely directed toward children, any of the above vaccinations that were not given during childhood (except pertussis, which is not given after the sixth birthday) should be considered for adults. Adults are especially advised to maintain immune status against tetanus—which still kills unprotected adults in this country each year—and diphtheria. The current recommendation is that routine boosters for tetanus (and diphtheria) should be given every ten years; an injury may require a tetanus booster before that time. If a physician feels that a tetanus booster is indicated at any time, it is helpful if combined diphtheria *and* tetanus vaccine (of the adult type-Td) is given, to make a further booster against diphtheria unnecessary for the following ten years.

Recommendations for flu shots and the pneumonia vaccine in adults are found in the chapter on colds and flu.

Strep Infections

Infections caused by the bacterium group A beta hemolytic streptococcus, hereafter referred to simply as "strep," are of special concern because they may lead to the major diseases known as rheumatic fever (which can cause permanent heart damage) and acute glomerulonephritis (which produces kidney damage).

These potentially serious complications can be largely eliminated by prompt and adequate antibiotic treatment of strep infections. While strep can cause infections in many sites, the two most common are the *throat* (pharyngitis, tonsillitis) and the *skin* (especially impetigo). The full details of the diagnosis and treatment of strep infections are unnecessary to remember, but the following information is essential:

(1) Though the clinical picture of strep throats (enlarged glands, fever, pus) may be suggestive, the only way to make a specific diagnosis is to take a throat swab for culture. Cultures are cheap and easy to perform, and they should be considered whenever a suspicion of strep infection exists.

(2) Once a strep infection has been positively identified, adequate treatment with antibiotics is mandatory. The drug of choice for strep infections is penicillin, but other antibiotics, such as erythromycin, may be used in persons with penicillin allergy. Penicillin can be given either by means of a single injection or via ten days of pills or liquid. If the penicillin is taken orally, *it is critically important that the entire ten day course be taken* because it often takes that long for group A strep to be eradicated from the throat. There is a great temptation to stop medication after a person feels better—which usually occurs within 48 hours—and this is why many physicians prefer to treat strep infections with a single injection of

233

long-acting penicillin, even though there is a slightly greater risk of an allergic reaction when penicillin is given in this manner. Some experts recommend re-culture to make sure that treatment has been effective.

(3) Once a strep infection has been identified in one member of a family, it is important to remember that close contacts are at high risk for infection, and cultures should be obtained if they develop any suggestive symptoms.

(4) Persons who have had rheumatic fever are at much greater risk for subsequent bouts of rheumatic fever if they get a strep infection. Therefore, such individuals are strongly advised to take penicillin (either by injection monthly or by mouth daily) on a continuous basis to prevent such infections. Whether such a practice must continue for an entire lifetime is a matter of some controversy and individualized advice must be sought.

The incidence of rheumatic fever in this country is decreasing. However, it is *still* a cause of childhood death and adult disability. The above measures are simple and well worth the effort in preventing serious complications.

Tonsillectomy and Adenoidectomy

There is suggestive evidence that removal of the tonsils (tonsillectomy) was performed as early as 3000 B.C. Yet even now, there is considerable controversy over the appropriateness of this operation—despite the fact that over one million tonsillectomies are performed each year in the United States at a cost of over $200 million. Even the few scientific studies that have attempted to compare surgical versus non-surgical treatment have been challenged as having biases in patient selection and treatment evaluation. Often, there is also a difference of viewpoint between surgeons and non-surgeons. A report in the *New England Journal of Medicine* (August 18, 1977) indicated that many physicians do not conform to guidelines developed by specialists for recommending a tonsillectomy.

Despite all this, most physicians believe that it is still possible to achieve a rational decision as to whether a tonsillectomy (and/or adenoidectomy) should be performed for a given child *if* parents and physicians jointly consider the clinical history, the results of physical and laboratory examinations, and the anticipated results as well as the potential hazards. We have asked Dr. Marshall Strome, Senior Otolaryngologist at The Children's Hospital Medical Center in Boston and a member of our Advisory Board, to respond to the following questions, in the hope that his answers will provide useful information for those of you who may face the decision of whether or not a tonsillectomy should be performed on *your* child.

What are the tonsils and adenoids and what are their functions—if any?

The tonsils are patches of lymph tissue (similar to lymph nodes) that are located on the side walls of the throat just behind the last

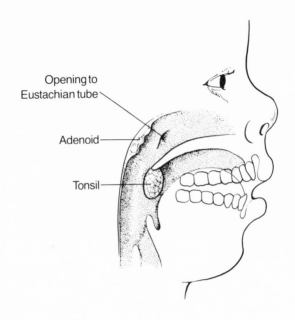

Opening to
Eustachian tube

Adenoid

Tonsil

molars; the adenoids are similar patches of tissue located at the very back of the upper part of the throat where the nasal passages end and the openings of the Eustachian tubes (which connect to the middle ear) are found (see diagram). It is important to recognize that the tonsils and adenoids are separate and distinct anatomically—especially when surgery is to be considered; they should never be removed together simply because they are somewhat near each other.

When the tonsils and adenoids function properly, they serve as "islands of defense" against infections. In other words, there is evidence that, unlike the appendix, they play a role in maintaining health. However, when these tissues become overwhelmed by infection or for some other reason do not function properly, they tend to cause more trouble than they prevent.

The tonsils can be associated with (1) repeated infections (including abscesses), (2) persistent enlargement leading to swallowing problems, speech difficulties, and abnormal dental development, and (3) blockage of the passage of air into the lungs (with *severe* enlargement).

The adenoids can be associated with (1) repeated infections (including sinusitis), (2) frequent middle ear problems (infections, fluid accumulation) due to blocked Eustachian tubes, and (3) mouth breathing when air flow through the nasal passages is blocked.

When should surgery be considered for these problems?

Emergency surgery is necessary only rarely, when sudden blockage of air to the lungs occurs or an abscess is not responding to medical management; otherwise, a tonsillectomy or adenoidectomy is an *elective* procedure that should occur only after careful evaluation of several issues—including the age of the patient and his chances of "outgrowing" the problem. By "outgrowing" I refer to the fact that these tissues normally reach their maximum size at about three to six years of age and then begin to shrink after age eight. Children also tend to develop increased resistance to infections as they grow older.

Bacterial infections should always be treated with antibiotics initially, although large tonsillar abscesses may require prompt surgical treatment. Recurrent infections constitute a "gray area" of judgment as to when the dangers and problems (absence from school, for example) posed by these infections warrant surgery. It should be remembered that surgery does not prevent further viral or bacterial infections in other areas of the throat. I often use the criterion of five documented episodes of infection per year for two consecutive years as a means of identifying those children who should be considered for tonsillectomy. However, individualization of the decision is always necessary.

Complications due to *blockage* by enlarged tonsils or adenoids are less common but usually easier to assess in terms of the need for surgery; x-ray examinations may be helpful in such an evaluation. Severe problems with breathing clearly caused by tonsil or adenoid enlargement can lead to oxygen deficiency which, in turn, can lead to heart and lung problems. Speech may also be seriously impaired. Very rarely, enlargement (especially if occurring on only one side) can be caused by a tumor which must be removed.

The decision to operate—as I said earlier—should be made only after a careful consideration of all the factors involved. The tonsils and adenoids should never be removed just because they are there and appear to be a problem or are thought to be enlarged.

What are the potential dangers of these operations?

The immediate surgical mortality (from anesthesia complications, uncontrollable bleeding, and so on) is estimated to be somewhere between one per 10,000 and one per 100,000 tonsillectomies. I should also mention the real problem of psychological trauma that may occur in any child. These factors cannot be overlooked.

Long-term dangers are less clear. Some scientists have proposed that removal of these defense tissues in childhood may lead to an increased incidence of disease in adulthood. For example, it has been suggested that adults without tonsils are more likely to get Hodgkin's disease than adults whose tonsils are present. However, I feel that there is no good evidence to support this argument against tonsillectomy.

Hyperactive Children

Rare is the parent who at one time or another has not been convinced that his or her child is hyperactive. Indeed, there are those who still maintain that the hyperactive child represents nothing more than the extreme end of a normal behavior scale. However, most experts now accept the designation "hyperactive" as useful in distinguishing *those children who exhibit behavior patterns that interfere with normal living and learning and who might benefit from professional advice and attention.*

DEFINITION   The words "hyperactive" or "hyperkinetic" (often used synonymously) refer to a collection of traits that typically include *overactivity, restlessness, distractability, short attention span,* and *impulsiveness.* Classically, the child is described as "constantly in motion" and unable to concentrate on a bedtime story or to complete a simple task without getting distracted. While all children may occasionally demonstrate these bits of behavior, they occur in a more severe and relentless manner in hyperactive children. The exact prevalence of such hyperactivity is not known; several school surveys suggest that about one of every twenty-five elementary school children could accurately be described as hyperactive. The condition is much more common in boys. Most often, hyperactivity is not detected until poor school function calls attention to the condition, but many parents, in retrospect, can identify behavior patterns in early childhood that were clues to later difficulties. Studies have also shown that problems associated with hyperactivity in early school years (low scholastic achievement, misconduct, and poor self-esteem) persist in almost half the cases into junior high school, again arguing that hyperactivity is worth identifying and treating.

CAUSE The cause (or causes) of hyperactivity are unknown. However, as is usually the case when specific knowledge is lacking, there are many hypotheses. One popular theory is that hyperactivity results from minimal brain damage or dysfunction (MBD) that is too subtle to be expressed in more obvious neurological symptoms. However, most authorities prefer to avoid these labels, given the absence of proof and the unfortunate consequences of labeling someone as "brain damaged." Another theory contends that sensitivity to food additives causes the heightened behavioral characteristics seen, but again, there is no solid proof for this conclusion, at least for most children. In short, at this time hyperactivity can only be distinguished by its behavioral manifestations and not by any known physical or chemical abnormality.

DIAGNOSIS As already discussed, the determination of hyperactivity is made by careful assessment of behavioral traits that interfere with normal living and learning. *It is critically important to rule out other physical or emotional causes of similar behavior patterns.* For example, a child with an unrecognized hearing or visual problem may manifest his frustration in behavior that is conveniently, but very misleadingly, labeled as "hyperactive." A child with a specific learning disability (such as inability to handle simple math) may similarly express his frustration. Therefore, before a child is labeled primarily as hyperactive—and started on treatment—he must be evaluated for contributing physical, emotional, and learning factors, both in school and at home. Because the problems in attention are more significant than the overactivity, the new diagnostic manual adopted by the American Psychiatric Association employs the term *attention-deficit disorder with hyperactivity,* for which the key features are inattention, impulsivity, hyperactivity, onset before age 7, and a duration of at least six months.

TREATMENT Most people are conditioned to think automatically of drug therapy in conjunction with hyperactivity. And while appropriate drug therapy is often a useful aid in helping the hyperactive child, *drugs alone never constitute an adequate treatment program.* Rather, all of the following elements must be considered in the therapy of a hyperactive child:

(1) Behavior modification—a fancy phrase for the kind of attention that rewards desirable behavior and discourages disruptive activity—can be, in the opinion of some experts, as effective as drug therapy in reducing hyperactivity. However, such an approach requires a kind of patience and skill that is often beyond the capacities of ordinary parents and teachers.

(2) Remedial teaching programs are essential to overcome or compensate for academic deficiencies. Neither drug therapy nor behavior modification have been shown to improve academic achievement per se, but they can create the opportunity for improved learning via special programs.

(3) Counseling for all involved with the child—parents, teachers, relatives—can be invaluable in creating an environment which allows the child to change by expanding his limits for overall emotional growth and achievement. And there are times when direct psychotherapy can prove useful for the distressed and unhappy child—as a means of restoring badly needed self-confidence.

(4) Special diets—free of food additives—are recommended by some allergists and endorsed by some parents, although good evidence for this treatment has yet to be provided. On the basis of published data, it seems clear that if the dietary method works at all, it works for only a minority of hyperactive children. There is as yet no way of identifying those for whom it might be suitable.

(5) Stimulant drugs—such as methylphenidate (Ritalin) or dextroamphetamine (Dexedrine)—are often an essential part of treatment programs for hyperactivity. While they do not cure the problem, they do allow reasonable control of behavior so that other functions can improve. (The fact that stimulant drugs result in *less* stimulated behavior and do not cause addiction is another example of drugs acting in children quite differently than in adults.) There is no good way of predicting which children will benefit from stimulant drugs or how long they might be needed; periodic reassessment of dosage and need is vital. Stimulant drugs may interact with other drugs; most important is the increased effect of phenytoin (Dilantin) seen in a child taking Ritalin. The most common side effects are insomnia and decreased appetite, but both usually decrease with time. A more worrisome possibility, suggested by some studies but not confirmed by others, is interference with growth. Children taking these drugs should be monitored for height and weight progression

and most experts suggest *stopping* the drugs during weekends and school vacations. Sedatives such as phenobarbital have no place in the treatment of hyperactive children.

Thus, while drugs are often essential in the treatment of a hyperactive child, they are only one component in what should be a total plan to help a child who happens to be, for lack of a better word, hyperactive.

IN SUMMARY   Hyperactivity is far from being fully understood, but has enough basis in school and home experience to be recognized as something other than normal exuberance. Drugs and behavior modification can be useful for symptom suppression but are insufficient in themselves. Close attention must be paid to school progress and family relations if the child is to be helped to develop normally.

Learning Disabilities

When parents become aware that their child is not performing adequately in school, they often wonder if a "learning disability" is the reason. Almost unheard of as a technical phrase earlier in this century, learning disabilities are frequently identified today as the cause of poor school performance; estimates of the number of children affected vary from five to as much as thirty percent of the school-age population. Yet many authorities (educational, psychological, medical) admit that techniques of evaluation and correction are still far from being scientifically precise and that labels are, therefore, more a matter of working definitions than foolproof diagnoses.

BASIC CONCEPTS   Normal learning requires several pre-conditions, including mental development appropriate for the tasks or subject matter, a reasonably stable emotional environment at home and in school, normal physical abilities (seeing, hearing, nervous system development), and adequate learning opportunities.

Educational dysfunction, defined broadly as school performance below what is expected for a given age, may involve problems in any or all of the above areas. Experts usually agree that mental retardation, physical handicaps, cultural deprivation, and emotional disorders should *not* be included under the umbrella of learning disabilities—though they may, obviously, interfere with learning. For example, so-called *hyperactivity* (hyperkinesis) may co-exist with a learning disability or may specifically interfere with learning, but it is not regarded as a learning disability per se.

Learning disabilities, therefore, refer to educational performance problems that cannot be attributed to gross physical handicaps, to mental retardation, to emotional upheaval, or to environmental factors. Rather, they are rooted in more subtle distortions in

243

the way in which images and thoughts are processed by the brain. Examples of such problems include deficits in short-term memory, disordered sequencing of events in time or objects in space, or specific language disabilities. While often associated with physical, intellectual, or emotional difficulties, these distortions and dysfunctions are separate and, as such, require special testing to discern.

EVALUATION   The typical evaluation of a child whose school performance is poorer than expected usually begins with an assessment of physical and emotional factors that may be contributing to the problem. More specific testing for learning disabilities is usually the next step and may include the following measures:

(1) Intelligence tests: While not a perfect tool, intelligence tests serve a useful function in assessing mental capacity and in providing a profile of specific strengths and weaknesses. For example, one of the most popular individual intelligence tests used today—the Wechsler Intelligence Scale for Children (better known as the WISC test)—measures two large skill areas: verbal and performance. Verbal tests include information, similarities, arithmetic, vocabulary, comprehension, and digit span; performance tests include picture completion, picture arrangement, block design, object assembly, coding, and mazes. Performance on some of the tests depends on environmental and cultural influences; others are more truly reflective of intellectual potential and the ability to solve new problems. Proper interpretation of these tests involves a healthy respect for the variability of results, particularly at younger ages. Nonetheless, the IQ remains an important factor in evaluating children with learning problems. And it is often the discrepancy between potential (as identified on IQ tests) and actual performance that raises the possibility of a learning disability.

(2) Achievement tests: These tests, which measure actual performance, translate into useful information concerning the child's proficiency at a given grade and age level, provide further clues as to more specific learning problems, and help in making recommendations for corrective measures. Traditional skills often measured include:

Reading: Reading (translating visual symbols into sounds) is the area most commonly affected by learning disabilities. (The word *dyslexia* has become somewhat synonymous with reading problems, though some argue for more precise definitions.) Various "errors" (such as reversing *b* and *d*) are common in normal first graders but become more significant signs of possible learning disability in older children.

Spelling: Spelling represents the translation of sounds into symbols. Reading and spelling problems often co-exist, though spelling ability typically lags behind reading ability.

Writing: This skill involves additional tasks including visual-motor coordination, use of syntax and punctuation rules, and so on. Specialized skill tests may be needed to sort out writing problems.

Arithmetic: More attention has been given to math skills in recent years, with a consequent "discovery" of more learning problems in this area. It is not unusual to find children with language problems who do well in arithmetic.

(3) Neurodevelopmental testing: These examinations are designed to evaluate the maturation of the nervous system and the different "processing" areas of the brain, rather than actual achievement levels. Analysis of various skills (visual and auditory perception, memory, sequencing, visual-motor integration) helps prepare a profile of a child's learning strengths and weaknesses which can be of use in planning individualized correctional programs. While some controversy remains concerning the overall value of this kind of approach, almost all agree that younger children (below eight) are better candidates for such testing.

RESOURCES   One of the most difficult questions to answer is the most obvious one: "Where can I find help for a child who is not doing well in school?" Traditionally, family physicians and pediatricians have provided counsel concerning any physical or emotional problems that may be involved. Quite frankly, though, most have not been well trained in psychological and educational evaluation, although pediatricians are increasingly acquiring such skills. In more recent years, school systems have developed resources to identify and test children with learning problems; national and state laws now make such capabilities mandatory. Many private sources of evaluation also exist. However, the competence of *any* of these sources is variable. A multidisciplinary approach, one which can use the special skills of psychologists, neurologists, educators, and others whose expertise may be brought to bear on the child with a learning problem, is most likely to avoid the bias inherent in any single emphasis. *At the very least, parents should be satisfied that their concerns can be answered in simple and understandable terms, that a formal approach to measuring possible learning disabilities is undertaken, and that steps to correction can be outlined.*

In addition to responding to specific educational recommendations, parents need to be in tune with the child's emotions and feelings about "being different" and not being able to "keep up" with other children. Most experts agree that parents should not become teachers and tutors in relation to actual learning disabilities. Rather, parents should provide general educational support, special emotional support, and loads of praise for the strengths and achievements (including non-academic ones) that can be found in any child.

IN SUMMARY   The label "learning disability" has taken on more precise definition in recent years and modern testing may disclose specific learning problems—and, more importantly, suggest appropriate corrective measures. However, it is important to recognize the lack of absolute precision in learning disability theory and practice. Second opinions should be sought if learning problems cannot be explained to the satisfaction of parents.

Diseases Mainly
of Adulthood

*People who are "hyper" are much more
likely to develop hypertension
(high blood pressure).*

MYTH 4

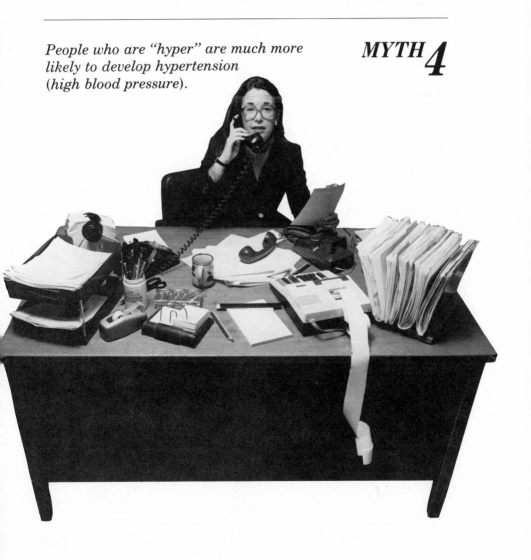

Heart Disease

Heart disease can take many forms, but the most dreaded by far is what is commonly called a "heart attack." This chapter will concentrate on coronary artery disease resulting from atherosclerosis—the underlying cause of the vast majority of heart attacks. But attention will also be given to coronary artery spasm and to a usually benign condition unassociated with the coronary vessels—mitral valve prolapse.

Coronary Artery Disease

Coronary artery disease (CAD) accounts for over 600,000 deaths per year in this country and for almost a third of all deaths occurring between the ages of 35 and 65. Since the coronary arteries supply blood to the heart, CAD may be understood as a "supply and demand" problem. When the blood flow through the coronary arteries (see diagram) to heart muscle falls below critical levels—or when demands on the heart increase beyond the available flow—the heart muscle cells do not get enough oxygen to do their job of pumping. This "decreased flow in relation to demand" may cause warning symptoms that range from chest pain to abnormalities of heart rhythm; sometimes the first—and last—warning symptom of decreased blood flow is a massive and fatal heart attack. Often, *reversible* symptoms precede the permanent damage of a heart attack. These reversible changes are usually due to *ischemia*—a temporarily decreased blood supply usually due to obstructed blood flow. The characteristic response of any muscle to inadequate blood supply is pain; when the heart muscle is so deprived, the resulting pain is known as *angina*. When the blood flow falls to a critical level in

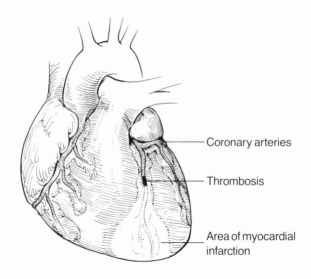

Coronary arteries

Thrombosis

Area of myocardial infarction

relation to a given demand, the muscle tissue affected may be permanently and irreversibly damaged or "killed"; this event is known as an *infarction* of the muscle tissue, and in the case of the heart as a *myocardial infarction* or heart attack. (The term *coronary thrombosis*—or simply *coronary*—is often used to describe this irreversible event because a blood clot, or thrombosis, in one or more coronary arteries is usually the cause of the blocked blood flow that leads to infarction.)

In short, coronary artery disease is a continuum of disease that ranges from insignificant symptoms to an infarction large enough to cause death. And in recent years, scientists have discovered a great deal about atherosclerosis—the underlying process which causes progressive narrowing of the coronary arteries.

ATHEROSCLEROSIS   In a normal artery, blood is strictly confined to the lumen (the central channel through which blood flows) by a smooth lining of flattened cells which are tightly joined to each other (see diagram). When kept in good repair, this lining (called the endothelium) permits blood to flow without sludging or clotting. Surrounding the lining is a relatively thin sheath of muscle cells.

The earliest change in atherosclerosis is believed to be the formation of *fatty streaks* along the inner lining of the artery. These streaks are largely composed of *cholesterol* that is deposited in and

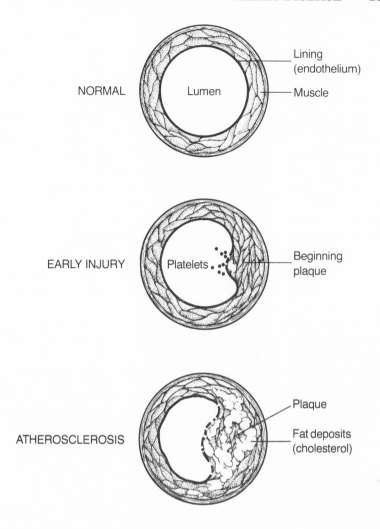

around muscle cells next to the lining. At a later stage, plaques begin to form and protrude into the channel. These plaques are made up of an overgrowth of newly formed muscle cells that become engorged with cholesterol. As plaques spread and thicken, they eventually make the artery wall so rigid that it can no longer dilate or contract in response to changing needs for blood. Also, the inner wall becomes roughened, and blood may begin to clot in reaction to the irregular surface. The eventual result is a narrowed artery.

What makes the artery's muscle cells start to overgrow? Answering this question has been extremely difficult because the earliest stages of atherosclerosis are hard to observe in animals and virtually impossible to study in people. But a consensus is emerging that some kind of damage to the endothelial lining cells of the artery is the first event. For example, a frequent cause of such damage may simply be wear and tear by excessively rapid or turbulent flow of blood in a particular area; thus high blood pressure may lead to atherosclerosis in part by increasing stress on the linings of major blood vessels.

Once the lining cells are damaged, blood penetrates into the arterial wall, which normally is shielded from direct exposure to the bloodstream. When this happens, at least two constituents of blood appear to harm the muscle cells in the wall—namely, platelets and low-density lipoprotein cholesterol (LDL-cholesterol).

Platelets are cell fragments that circulate in the bloodstream; they are, in effect, little bags of chemicals that initiate the clotting of blood. Platelets ordinarily do not stick to each other or to blood vessel walls, but when the endothelium is damaged, they gather in the area of injury. Once there, they stick to the injured surface and begin to release their chemicals, among them thromboxane, which stimulate other platelets to aggregate in the same neighborhood. Some very recent research indicates that while producing thromboxane, platelets manufacture a by-product which combines with LDL-cholesterol and changes its chemical nature in ways that make it very damaging to the artery's muscle cells.

LDL-cholesterol is a term for cholesterol attached to a complex protein (low-density lipoprotein). When LDL is modified by the platelet by-product, the resulting protein–cholesterol complex is chemically altered so that the muscle cells take it up very avidly. Unfortunately, once the cells have ingested cholesterol, they can dispose of it only very slowly; consequently, cholesterol accumulates and the cell begins to bloat with accumulated fat. The more LDL-cholesterol there is in the blood, the more rapidly this process takes place.

At the same time that the platelets are releasing the substance that modifies LDL-cholesterol, they also seem to release a factor that stimulates the muscle cells to proliferate. Thus, when part of an artery's lining is damaged, the underlying muscle cells are exposed to two abnormal influences: one stimulus to increase their numbers and another stimulus to gorge themselves on cholesterol. The result is a *plaque,* which now deforms the arterial wall and thus, presumably, creates additional turbulence in the flow of blood and even further damage to the artery's lining.

The above is but one model—rather neat in explaining many features of atherosclerosis. The story is undoubtedly more complex. But even though we do not yet know the exact chemistry of atherosclerosis, we can attempt to modify its progression by eliminating risk factors that have been shown by long-term studies to be associated with CAD. The list of possible risk factors is long—with new suggestions added every year—but the following summarizes the most important information as it now stands:

(1) Almost all experts agree that cigarette smoking, high blood pressure, and elevated cholesterol levels are the "big three" risk factors. And even though there is no *final* proof that reducing or eliminating these risk factors will decrease the incidence of heart attacks, most experts anticipate that conclusive evidence will eventually emerge. In fact, many believe that attention to these risk factors by large numbers of Americans (particularly males) accounts for the recent reversal of heart attack death rates. For more detailed information on risk factors, see p. 186 (birth control pills), p. 11 (obesity), p. 100 (stress), p. 265 (high blood pressure), p. 77 (smoking), p. 3 (exercise).

(2) The "big news" of recent years has been the rediscovery of the *apparently protective role of HDL (high-density lipoprotein)*— one of the five major fractions of cholesterol-containing lipid in the blood. This has been so convincingly established in the minds of some experts that they are recommending the measurement of HDL along with, or even in place of, the total cholesterol concentration. As a practical matter, strenuous exercise and a decreased intake of saturated fats seem to correlate with an increase in this protective cholesterol fraction. Much remains to be learned about HDL, but there seems to be little doubt that, unlike other cholesterol fractions, more is better. (See p. 177 for more information on blood fats in general and HDL in particular.)

THE DIAGNOSIS   A physician may use several tools to diagnose CAD or an actual heart attack:

(1) Blood tests: There is no simple blood test to diagnose CAD, although certain blood tests are useful in diagnosing increased "fats"

and cholesterol in the blood which may contribute to the development of CAD. Other blood tests, when taken at the time of chest pain, detect enzymes released from heart muscle damaged by an actual heart attack; they may be very useful in deciding whether an individual with chest pain has had a true heart attack as opposed to an "anginal" attack.

(2) Electrocardiogram (ECG): This familiar test involves the recording of electrical impulses from the heart on a moving strip of paper. It may be done with the person lying down—the "resting" ECG—or while the person is exercising (on a treadmill or a bicycle)—the "stress" ECG. Resting ECG's miss a significant amount of CAD that will be detected by stress ECG's, but even stress ECG's will miss some cases of CAD. The stress ECG—which requires sophisticated equipment and a physician in attendance—is used most often for the individual with suggestive symptoms in whom the resting ECG is normal. An ECG taken *during* an episode of chest pain may be particularly helpful; indeed, when angina or an actual heart attack is occurring, the resting ECG will often show definite abnormalities that help clinch the diagnosis.

(3) Coronary angiography: This technique—which involves injecting dye directly into the coronary arteries and taking x-ray moving pictures of the dye as it flows through them—has revolutionized the diagnosis of CAD. It is the only test which provides a direct look at the flow of blood through the coronary arteries and their branches. Since coronary angiography is such an imporant diagnostic tool, it is important to put its use in perspective. There are several reasons why this procedure is *not used on a routine basis.* First, it must be done under operating-room-type conditions with preparation for emergencies that can develop during the procedure; the cost in terms of equipment and personnel is considerable. Second, even under the best of circumstances, risks are involved; when done by experienced physicians, the risk of death is well under 1%, but other complications are possible. Therefore this important diagnostic procedure should be used selectively. Examples of patients who may benefit from angiography include:

> Those in whom the diagnosis of CAD is strongly suspected but cannot be proven and in whom a definite answer is important in terms of adjustment of life style, therapy, etc.

Those in whom coronary by-pass surgery (see below) is anticipated. Angiography is absolutely necessary before such surgery, since "seeing the arteries" allows one to know where narrowing is present and whether by-passing is possible.

Those who have become "cardiac neurotics"—that is, persons who have developed such fear of "heart disease" that angiography is justified to assure them that no disease exists.

(4) Nuclear cardiology: The ideal diagnostic technique for CAD would be one that combines the accuracy of coronary angiography with the safety of the ECG. Though such a technique is not yet available, great progress has been made in the field of "nuclear cardiology," which involves the injection of low-dose radioactive tracers into an arm vein followed by analysis of the distribution of the tracers within the heart.

One test in particular—the thallium scan—has become widespread in hospital practice and has been recently approved for diagnostic use by the FDA. A typical thallium scan involves the injection of the radioisotope thallium 201 while the patient is exercising on a treadmill and monitored by a continuous electrocardiogram. As the thallium circulates in the blood through the coronary arteries to the heart muscle, a gamma scintillation camera placed over the chest "picks up" the progress of the radioisotope. These signals are translated by computer into a "picture" of the distribution of thallium in heart muscle. An area of poor circulation of thallium to heart muscle, appearing as a "cold spot" in the computer picture, indicates blockage of the coronary artery supplying that area.

Aside from the fact that this test is non-invasive (except for the simple injection of thallium) and without known side effects (the radiation dose involved is little more than a chest x-ray), its appeal lies in its accuracy. Thallium scans are generally more sensitive than conventional exercise electrocardiograms in detecting disease. The only disadvantage compared to the exercise ECG is higher cost due to additional equipment and personnel.

While the thallium scan is not expected to replace the exercise ECG completely, it is being used increasingly in people with suspicious symptoms of coronary artery disease—and in those who need reassurance about the absence of such disease.

TREATMENT   The ideal treatment of CAD would be one which "melts away" existing blockage. While there is some evidence from animal studies that careful attention to risk factors may result in actual reversal of blockage in the arteries, such results cannot yet be routinely expected. Even if eliminating risk factors may not result in the disappearance of blockage, further progression should be lessened. It has been demonstrated, for example, that people who continue to smoke after a heart attack are at much greater risk for sudden death than those who quit smoking. Also, exercise rehabilitation after a heart attack can clearly aid in the recovery process—although it has not been shown to reduce the risk of another heart attack or of sudden death.

The treatment of the actual symptoms of CAD, of course, varies with the nature and urgency of the symptoms. The most important point to stress concerning *acute* (sudden and severe) constricting chest pain is the importance of seeking immediate medical attention. One of the major causes of death from heart attack is the development of abnormal heart rhythms in the initial hours after an attack. These rhythm problems can cause the heart to stop functioning even though the heart muscle may still be adequate to support life; adequate medical care during periods of temporary rhythm irregularity will improve chances of survival.

Many more people, however, are affected by chronic symptoms—usually chest pain on exertion—that are related to CAD after a heart attack or CAD not severe enough to cause an actual heart attack. The great majority of these people can be helped to live a near normal life with a judicious combination of life-style changes and medical treatment—including the following:

(1) Drug therapy: The two most commonly used medications in the treatment of CAD today are nitroglycerin and beta blockers. *Nitroglycerin,* which acts by dilating blood vessels, is typically used by placing a tablet under the tongue when angina occurs or before physical activity that might cause angina. This, and related, longer-acting versions are widely used in an effort to improve blood supply to the heart and reduce the work of the heart. *Beta blockers* (drugs which block the heart's response to stimulation by the sympathetic nervous system) cut down the work of the heart and thus cut down on its demand for blood.

Appropriate use of beta blockers (such as Inderal and Lopressor) in the relief of angina (as well as high blood pressure) has been one of the most important developments in the non-surgical treatment of cardiovascular disease during the past decade (see p. 272). Indeed, many people whose angina could not formerly be controlled can now lead relatively normal lives with the judicious use of nitroglycerin and/or beta blockers. In addition to these standard and widely used drugs, many others are in various stages of investigation or testing. There is considerable interest in the possibility that "anti-thrombotic" drugs—which suppress the activity of platelet blood cells that promote clotting—may be useful in protecting against heart attacks. Thus far, studies on persons who have survived a heart attack (and are thus at much higher risk for another) have not shown conclusively that aspirin, which has anti-thrombotic properties, is beneficial. A major trial using a different drug—sulfinpyrazone (Anturane)—seemed to show more encouraging results, in that a 74% reduction of death rate was noted in those taking the drug as compared to a placebo. Although these results have attracted much attention and have led to the recommendation of a number of leading clinicians that Anturane be approved for use after myocardial infarction, the FDA declined to do so because of concerns about some aspects of the design of the study. Thus, the Anturane trial yielded very promising results, but it seems advisable to wait until the controversies are resolved before this drug can be definitely recommended for heart attack survivors. Other anti-thrombotic drugs are also being tested.

(2) Coronary by-pass surgery: No development in the treatment of coronary artery disease is more dramatic—or controversial—than by-pass surgery. The technique is logical and straightforward: a vein, taken from the leg, is used as a conduit to literally by-pass an area (or areas) of blockage in one or more coronary arteries. Successful surgery often results in an immediate increase in blood flow and a dramatic relief of angina. So why the controversy? The basic reason is that disagreement remains concerning the extent to which such surgery will prolong life—even though it is usually very effective in relieving symptoms; many studies are now under way to determine more precisely when by-pass surgery might be reasonably expected to prolong life. There is already clear agreement that by-passing a major blockage of the left main coronary artery, which controls the

blood supply to a large area of the heart, will improve life expectancy. A large European study has also shown improved survival in angina patients with "three-vessel disease" who underwent by-pass surgery.

Given the uncertainty of just who might benefit from surgery, there are the added concerns of cost (at an average cost of about $15,000 per patient and over 100,000 operations per year in this country, this is no minor concern) and the demands of space and personnel in the midst of limited medical resources. However, there is no question that by-pass surgery is an important treatment tool—even a life-saving one—for the properly selected patient.

(3) Percutaneous transluminal coronary angioplasty: In plain English, these words mean the widening of the inside of a narrowed coronary artery via a device (see diagram) inserted through the skin. The "device" is a very thin balloon which is inserted in collapsed form into the artery of an arm or leg and then gently pushed through the arterial system of the body to the opening of the coronary artery in question—at which point (under x-ray control) the balloon is carried along by the flow of blood in the coronary artery to the point of blockage. Then comes the definitive step in the procedure: the balloon is inflated for several seconds, thereby opening up the passageway for blood.

Sounds simple—and, compared to the possible alternative of coronary by-pass surgery, it is—in terms of both financial and emotional cost. Angioplasty can be done under light sedation; the total time should be less than an hour. The obvious question: Why isn't this being done routinely (less than two thousand patients have been so treated thus far) in place of coronary by-pass surgery for those

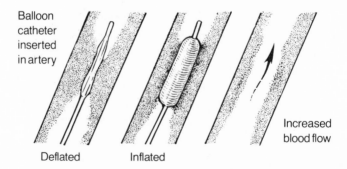

Balloon catheter inserted in artery

Deflated   Inflated   Increased blood flow

who are in need of a better blood flow to the heart? At this moment, there are several answers to that question:

The procedure is new (it was first performed on a human in September 1977) and is still experimental in terms of both safety and long-term results. The few patients who have been restudied after the procedure (with x-ray pictures to show dye moving through the coronary artery) continue to have an unobstructed flow of blood. But the real story will be told in years, not months.

Many patients are not candidates for balloon angioplasty for various reasons, including widespread blockage or blockage in the smaller parts of the coronary arteries and in areas "around corners" which cannot easily be reached by the device.

At present, the procedure is being done only in selected research centers. And even those most enthusiastic about its future expect it to be used in a relatively small number of patients with blockage; the majority of persons requiring more than medical therapy will still need by-pass surgery. But balloon angioplasty should be highlighted as a new procedure whose simplicity of technique and goal is appealing.

IN SUMMARY Coronary artery disease clearly causes more deaths and disability than any other single disease. However, dramatic strides have been made in all levels of our war against this disease.

Coronary Artery Spasm

Atherosclerosis, which results in a *fixed* obstruction to blood flow, has dominated our approach to the diagnosis and treatment of coronary artery disease since 1940 when classic autopsy studies showed blockage of coronary arteries by fatty plaques in conjunction with zones of destroyed heart muscle—a myocardial infarction or "heart attack." There is no question that atherosclerosis is the leading culprit in heart disease. However, during the past decade many research and clinical findings have highlighted the fact that not all angina pectoris—the pain caused by poor blood supply to heart muscle—can be explained by fixed blockage in the coronary arteries. As anyone reading the public or medical press knows, there is intensifying interest in the role of coronary artery spasm as a cause of angina and heart attacks. This update will summarize some of the current information and speculation concerning coronary spasm.

A BIT OF HISTORY   Coronary arteries contain a layer of smooth muscle cells that help regulate blood flow. The idea of spasm—a sudden narrowing of a portion of a coronary artery due to intense constriction of this muscular layer—has been around at least since 1910 when it was suggested in a lecture by Sir William Osler. In 1959, Dr. Myron Prinzmetal described an unusual variety of angina (now known as "Prinzmetal's," "rest," or "variant" angina), which is characterized by chest pain occurring *during rest*—rather than exertion—and by electrocardiogram findings almost opposite to those usually associated with angina. In 1970, Dr. Albert Kattus actually observed a coronary artery go into spasm during heart surgery. Since then, spasm has been seen during angiography when the coronary arteries are injected with dye to visualize blood flow through them; other studies have indirectly confirmed the phenomenon of spasm.

CURRENT CLINICAL IMPRESSIONS   While the evidence is still very preliminary, many distinguished cardiologists now believe that temporary spasms of coronary arteries not only cause variant angina, as described above, but contribute to the whole clinical spectrum of coronary artery disease—ranging from typical angina (chest pain with exertion) to actual heart attacks (permanent death of heart muscle) to the occurrence of sudden death in which no evidence of fixed blockage of a coronary artery can be found. According to this hypothesis, spasm may occur in an area of a coronary artery totally free of fatty build-up (atherosclerosis), or the spasm may be superimposed upon an area already ravaged by the fixed blockage of atherosclerosis. This kind of theory is attractive, since it provides an explanation for the wide range of cardiac problems that can occur with or without evidence of underlying permanent blockage in the coronary arteries. There is particular interest in spasm as an explanation for the statistically rare angina that occurs in younger women—a group normally free from symptoms of coronary artery disease. However, *experts caution that supporting evidence for spasm as a cause of more traditional manifestations of coronary artery disease is still limited,* and much experimental and clinical research needs to be done to pinpoint the exact role of spasm in the various problems that can occur when heart muscle does not get enough blood.

CAUSES OF CORONARY SPASM   While much uncertainty exists as to the exact physiological triggers that may set off coronary artery spasm, the following areas have received considerable attention in recent years:

(1) Platelets: When platelets clump together they release a substance known as thromboxane A2, which is a potent "vasoconstrictor"—a substance that causes narrowing of a blood vessel. Therefore, there is continuing interest in the role of aspirin and other agents that might interfere with this process.

(2) Smoking: Several investigators have reported dramatic decreases in the frequency of angina when cigarette smoking is stopped; it is postulated that this improvement is due to less coronary spasm.

(3) Stress: The clinical correlation between stress and heart pain in some people has long been noted—and current research suggests that spasm might be the connecting link. For example, taking a banana from a baboon—which is stressful to baboons—can cause demonstrable coronary artery spasm.

The final common pathway for all of the triggers that initiate spasm *may* be an increase in the calcium flow into the smooth muscle cells lining the coronary arteries. (This "calcium flow" has nothing to do with dietary calcium—or even the blood calcium level—but is instead a common part of the molecular machinery of all smooth muscle cells.) Based on this theory, drugs that specifically interfere with this calcium flow (see below) are now an important area for investigation.

DIAGNOSIS OF SPASM   As pointed out earlier, a good guess is that spasm may be part of the problem when "atypical angina" and/or characteristic electrocardiogram findings occur. However, more specific diagnostic techniques—known as provocative tests— are being used increasingly to pinpoint those individuals whose problems are caused by spasm. One such test involves injecting a drug (such as ergonovine) which is known to cause arterial spasm. If the drug produces symptoms similar to the person's complaints and can be shown to produce coronary spasm during angiography, the diagnosis is confirmed. Such testing carries some risk and should be done only by experts and only on highly selected patients, but it is increasingly helpful in sorting out those people who might benefit from therapy specifically directed at arterial spasm.

It is also worth mentioning that there are still a number of patients who have symptoms suggestive of coronary artery disease, but in whom neither CAD nor spasm can be demonstrated. The chest pain in these people is often somewhat atypical for angina. Although some of them may have undetected spasm, others probably have pain arising from causes outside of the heart. The outlook for this group is excellent.

TREATMENT   The question of specific diagnosis is becoming more important, because specific treatment for spasm is becoming available and because other traditional treatments may be less successful in people whose cardiac symptoms are caused by spasm. As mentioned above, several "calcium antagonist" drugs (such as nifedipine and verapamil) are now being reported to have remarkable success in some patients with angina. These drugs are currently undergoing trials in the U.S. and other countries. The use of known vasodilators (nitrates) is often very helpful in the treatment of spasm. However, two other traditional forms of treatment for coronary artery disease—beta blocker drugs and coronary by-pass surgery— may be less helpful if angina is caused primarily by spasm. Many other treatment approaches to the problem of spasm are under investigation.

IN SUMMARY   Coronary artery spasm is now a well-accepted explanation for so-called variant angina and is arousing increasing interest as a possible explanation (at least in part) for more traditional forms of ischemic heart disease—that is, symptoms caused by poor blood supply to the heart. While atherosclerosis is unquestionably the major culprit in most forms of coronary artery disease, spasm has clearly moved toward center stage in much current research.

Mitral Valve Prolapse

The above is the usual official name (MVP for short)—but the condition is also known as the "click-murmur syndrome" (to describe what the doctor might hear through a stethoscope) and as Barlow's syndrome (after the physician who in 1968 described its association with some potentially serious complications). Whatever the name—and we choose to use the MVP designation—this diagnosis is so common today that one can hardly attend a social gathering without finding at least one person with the label. This sudden epidemic of MVP is, however, not likely due to a new disease, but rather to the recent recognition of something that has probably existed for as long as the human race. So what is it, what does it mean, and is it serious?

(1) What it is: The mitral valve, located on the left side of the heart, keeps blood from going "backward" when the heart contracts and pumps blood through the aorta to the body. If the mitral valve does not close completely, the murmur of blood flowing backward will be heard through a stethoscope. The most common cause of this kind of valve problem was thought to be damage caused by rheumatic fever—but increasingly, briefer murmurs, sometimes following a clicking sound, are being recognized in otherwise healthy persons, particularly young women. Their mitral valves are not deformed by rheumatic fever, but some portion of a normal valve is pushed back too far (prolapsed) during heart contraction—causing the click and murmur.

(2) What it means: In the absence of any complications—such as chest pain or heart rhythm problems—the presence of a murmur or click sound signifying possible MVP probably means nothing. Indeed, many physicians are concerned that telling the person about the murmur or a possible underlying valve problem only leads to unnecessary worry. On the other hand, when symptoms are associated with MVP, it is important to recognize that they may be due to MVP so that the patient and physician do not ascribe them to potentially more serious causes.

(3) Is it serious? The answer in the majority of adult cases is "no." Even when there are associated symptoms, the risk of serious complications is small. However, because in rare cases prolapsed valves can become infected, persons with MVP are usually advised to have prophylactic antibiotics at the time of dental procedures. The simple truth is that while we currently think that the overall risk for complications is very small, we do not know exactly how small that risk is.

In short, MVP syndrome is a medical infant in terms of our understanding of its long-term course and complication rate. The earliest reports, coming as they did from major referral centers, focused mainly on MVP patients with symptoms that specifically brought them to the attention of specialists. Enough experience has been accumulated to know that most persons with this "condition" will live normal lives.

High Blood Pressure

It is well-known that high blood pressure is a common problem—one out of every five Americans is affected—and that persons with untreated high blood pressure have an increased risk for strokes, heart disease, and kidney failure. In fact, all of the recent publicity concerning the dangers of hypertension—so often referred to as the "silent killer" because it rarely produces warning signals—is based on clear evidence that effective treatment of hypertension reduces the risk of early disability or death. At present, almost all physicians recognize the importance of treating an otherwise healthy person whose blood pressure, on repeated examination, is or exceeds 160 over 105. But what about that gray area of milder elevations of blood pressure—or readings that are intermittently in the high range? Much of what follows is directed to those concerned that they "may" have high blood pressure and what this means.

TERMINOLOGY "High blood pressure," in strict usage, refers to the fact that at a given moment, one's blood pressure is "up" compared to the normal range for his age. As is now widely appreciated, such an elevation can frequently occur during moments of tension or even quiet concern (as is often the case when one's blood pressure is being checked). *The diagnosis of hypertension, however, should be reserved for a pattern of consistently elevated blood pressure* as determined by at least two separate blood pressure measurements by the same person using the same equipment under relaxed conditions—unless the initial blood pressure is so high as to indicate clearly an abnormality that does not need further verification. There is good reason for being cautious in labeling somebody as hypertensive, because this diagnosis usually leads to a recommendation for extended if not lifelong treatment, as well as to increased insurance premiums.

Blood pressure is expressed in numbers equivalent to the pressure exerted by a mercury column of varying height. (The original devices used to measure blood pressure contained actual columns of mercury. Indeed, some remain in use today because of their simplicity and accuracy.) Two numbers make up a blood pressure reading; they refer to the pressure within the arteries during the two phases of the heart cycle. The first number (the *systolic* pressure) designates the pressure during the period when the heart is actually contracting (systole), thus forcing blood into the arteries at a temporarily increased pressure. The second number (the *diastolic* pressure) designates the lower pressure which is present during the longer resting phase (diastole) between the heart's contractions. Two final comments related to terminology. The prefix "hyper" means, in this case, "higher than normal" and has nothing to do with personality type. Second, the term "malignant hypertension" refers to blood pressure elevation that is unusually severe and has nothing to do with cancer. Now to the more difficult issues.

SCREENING AND DIAGNOSIS   The key question is this: what level of systolic or diastolic pressure is high enough to be called hypertension—and to warrant treatment designed to prevent long-term complications such as heart disease, strokes, and kidney failure? The extremes are no problem; it's the territory in between that provokes disagreement. For example, the World Health Organization has placed the upper limits of normal at 160/95 (spoken as "160 over 95," meaning a systolic pressure of 160 and a diastolic pressure of 95). The Joint National Committee on Detection, Evaluation, and Treatment of High Blood Pressure report (1977) offered the following guidelines for verified average diastolic pressures:

(1) All adults with average diastolic pressure greater than 120 should be immediately evaluated and treated.

(2) Those in the range of 105–119 should be treated.

(3) Those in the range of 90–104 should be individualized for treatment.

However, the National Heart, Lung, and Blood Institute recently released data from a study of approximately 11,000 Americans which adds new support to the importance of treating blood pressures often described as "mildly" or "moderately" elevated. Specifically, the study suggests that by treating diastolic pressures (the *lower* number) in the 90–104 range, deaths from all causes can be reduced by about 20%. Even more dramatic were the reductions in death rates for those diseases most directly linked to hypertension—strokes and heart attacks. The study again pinpointed the special threats posed by hypertension to blacks—and the special benefit of treating blacks. In short, this report will probably encourage physicians to begin treatment for lesser degrees of high blood pressure than before.

Insurance companies have long been rigorous in setting upper limits of normal—given that their actuarial projections clearly show that even apparently mild elevations of blood pressure predict a reduced life span. (One actuarial example: a 35-year-old man with a blood pressure of 150/100 will have a shorter life span by 16.5 years if his hypertension remains untreated.) Not surprisingly, premiums are higher for persons with hypertension; for example, a 55-year-old man with a blood pressure of 165/105 has to pay $46.37 per $1,000 on a five-year renewable term insurance, as compared to $23.04 for a person with normal blood pressure.

Other factors must also be considered in dealing with the gray area of mild hypertension. Some of them are as follows:

(1) Systolic versus diastolic elevation: While both pressures are considered to be important, many experts make a distinction between them. For example, the systolic pressure is often elevated by "hardening" of the arteries as a part of the aging process—and most clinicians still allow for this factor (100 plus your age) before deciding that true systolic hypertension exists. Elevation of the systolic pressure alone can also be caused by other diseases, such as an overactive thyroid gland. Diastolic elevations, on the other hand, consistently mean hypertension in its traditional sense.

(2) Age, sex, and race: As already noted, mild pressure elevations have more serious meaning at a younger age. Also, there is general agreement that men are more likely to suffer from the complications of high blood pressure than women. The complication rates are also higher in blacks than in whites. However, the general trend in recent years has been to initiate treatment for consistent pressure elevations—regardless of race or sex.

(3) Other risk factors: In ultimately deciding whether a given level of pressure deserves treatment, many physicians will also consider the presence of other factors that tend to increase the risk of complications—such as smoking, diabetes, elevated cholesterol levels, and a family history of the complications of hypertension.

(4) Physician bias: Some doctors who are strongly prevention oriented are persuaded that the evidence at hand is sufficient to urge treatment for patients with very mild hypertension; they argue that even patients with borderline hypertension will, in time, develop more strokes than those in lower ranges. Other doctors are less convinced of the need to recommend lifelong therapy (with its attendant expense and inconvenience) to combat what they perceive to be a slight risk.

In short, the diagnosis and treatment of mild hypertension is a tricky business that requires thoughtful consideration of many factors other than just the numbers. The very uncertainty about criteria for diagnosis and treatment carries implications for screening policy. Persons should not conclude that they have hypertension on the basis of a single blood pressure reading taken on a drug-store machine or at a street-corner booth. While such screening programs may be valuable in alerting someone to the *possibility* of hypertension, the diagnosis must be confirmed under the conditions described earlier. This means a visit to one's physician—an important step toward getting a final answer.

Also, in our judgment it is neither necessary nor advisable to purchase home equipment for the purpose of "discovering" high blood pressure (though such devices can be extremely useful in monitoring the progress of treatment). Indeed, we have enough to worry about without getting our blood pressure checked all the time because of the possibility that "it might be up." Better to rely on periodic opportunities to have one's pressure checked by persons trained to do so.

CAUSES—PRIMARY AND SECONDARY HYPERTENSION
The overwhelming majority of cases of hypertension turn out to have *no* easily identifiable and remediable cause; these cases are referred to as *primary.* We know that hormones and nerve impulses may contribute to primary hypertension, and much research in

these areas points to exciting future breakthroughs. In addition, the following factors are of increasing interest in terms of their prevention and treatment potential:

(1) Salt intake: Evidence for the role of salt in the development of hypertension comes from both animal investigations and studies of human populations. For example, researchers can produce hypertension in certain animals simply by feeding them high salt diets. And human societies in which individual daily salt intake averages less than 4 grams (about two teaspoons)—versus the average American consumption of 12 grams—have much less hypertension. Few experts claim that salt is the sole cause of hypertension; rather, they describe salt as an important contributing factor in the 10–20% of Americans who are genetically susceptible to high blood pressure. And for such persons, the hidden salt in the processed food of the typical American diet is a real hazard. For example, one ounce of Corn Flakes contains twice as much sodium (the component of salt related to high blood pressure) as an equivalent serving of Planters Peanuts, and a Big Mac comes loaded with five times as much sodium as the one ounce serving of Corn Flakes. Salt is everywhere in the American diet, but it is a learned taste which our children can be trained to live without.

(2) Excessive weight: Many studies have now documented the fact that obesity heightens the risk for hypertension. Similarly, there is increasing evidence to show that substantial weight loss (20 pounds or more) can be effective treatment for high blood pressure. One striking example of the value of this approach comes from a study performed at the Tel Aviv University Medical School in Israel. In that study, persons treated *only* with weight loss (they were not salt restricted) experienced an average reduction of blood pressure of 26 points (mm of mercury) systolic and 20 points diastolic. In another group of persons with even higher blood pressure who were also taking medication, the drop during weight reduction was even more dramatic—averaging 37 points systolic and 23 points diastolic. A similar group treated with pills but not weight reduction did not show a significant reduction in blood pressure.

What about the rare person with hypertension who has an identifiable and correctable underlying cause—so-called *secondary hypertension?* Obviously, it is important to find these causes—such as an adrenal gland tumor or a narrowed artery leading to a kidney. In these instances, surgical correction can replace the lifelong drug therapy required in most cases of primary hypertension. The dilemma arises in deciding which persons with accurately diagnosed hypertension should be subjected to further diagnostic tests for secondary hypertension. The initial evaluation of all persons with newly diagnosed hypertension should include (in the opinion of most experts) a complete blood count, urinalysis, blood levels for urea nitrogen and/or creatinine, potassium, glucose, and cholesterol, and an electrocardiogram. These simple tests provide a baseline evaluation of the individual's heart, kidney, and "risk" status, but they do not really check out the possible causes of secondary hypertension. Additional studies looking for such causes are usually reserved for : (1) those with the onset of hypertension before age 35; (2) those with a rapid onset of hypertension and no family history of the disease; (3) those who have failed to respond to initial medical treatment; (4) those with unusually severe hypertension; and (5) those with symptoms suggesting an adrenal tumor. However, the majority of patients with moderate and uncomplicated hypertension can be treated without costly and potentially risky testing.

TREATMENT   The good news is that death rates attributable to hypertension have been considerably reduced (by as much as 35%) in the last ten years; with today's effective drugs, it is rare for a person to die of heart or kidney failure due to uncontrollable hypertension. Beyond this, many experts think that the recent decline in the death rate from heart attacks and strokes is largely attributable to the greatly improved treatment for hypertension developed during the past quarter century. Such treatment can be summarized under the following categories:

(1) Life-style changes: As mentioned earlier, salt restriction and weight loss may be all that is needed to control very mild elevations of blood pressure; in these cases, some would even quibble about using the term "hypertension."

(2) Behavioral therapies: Several studies have reported mild lowering of blood pressure using techniques of relaxation, meditation, and biofeedback. These approaches (particularly those that

involve no expensive equipment or investment) may be worthy of trial by themselves in cases of very mild hypertension and in combination with drug therapy for more severe cases.

(3) Drug therapy: Given the new data described above, most persons with diastolic blood pressure levels over 90 will be encouraged to take one or more drugs to bring it into a lower range. Understandably, the idea of having to take drugs, often for the remainder of one's life, is not appealing. Yet it is not an optimistic overstatement to suggest that the majority of persons requiring drug therapy will eventually (often very quickly) find a program of treatment that produces very little interference with normal living. Honesty also requires mentioning that some persons now taking anti-hypertensive drugs must learn to live with unpleasant side effects; it is anticipated that they will benefit from newer drugs with fewer side effects in the near future. The drugs used today can be categorized into three major groups:

Diuretics ("fluid" pills): The exact reasons for the effectiveness of these drugs, which promote increased urinary excretion of sodium, are not known. However, many patients require no other drugs. The long-term effectiveness and safety of diuretics is well established—with abnormally low potassium levels (easily corrected by diet or supplement) being the most common problem. The many different diuretics available today are roughly similar in effectiveness.

Sympatholytics: These drugs modify nervous system control of blood vessels in a manner that allows the vessels to dilate and thus decrease pressure; propranolol (Inderal) and methyldopa (Aldomet) are two of the more commonly used drugs in this category. More side effects typically occur with these drugs than with diuretics (with which they are often combined).

Vasodilators: These drugs widen blood vessels by acting on them directly. Like sympatholytics, they are usually combined with diuretics, and side effects may occur. Hydralazine (many brands) and prazosin (Minipress) are two commonly used drugs in this category.

The skilled use of anti-hypertensive medications requires thorough familiarity with the many kinds of drugs now available. In difficult cases, specialist care is required. For most patients, however, family physicians can provide adequate supervision.

IN SUMMARY The diagnosis of the disease called hypertension requires careful consideration of many factors. Once an accurate diagnosis has been made, effective treatment is available for the great majority of cases. Such treatment reduces the occurrence of heart disease, strokes, and kidney failure—complications that make hypertension the "silent killer." In short, it pays to know if you have hypertension—and to find effective treatment if you do.

The "Beta-Blocker" Drugs

One of the most important treatment breakthroughs of the past two decades has been the use of drugs known as "beta blockers" to treat angina, high blood pressure, and heart rhythm disturbances. Propranolol (Inderal) was the only such drug available in the United States until late 1978 when metoprolol (Lopressor) was approved for the treatment of hypertension by the Food and Drug Administration. Given the wide use of these drugs in medical practice today, a further review of how they act—and their dangers—is in order.

These drugs work because they bind to "beta receptors" present in various tissues, including the heart, and thereby block the body's own epinephrine (adrenalin) from attaching to these receptor sites. Ordinarily, the epinephrine produced within our bodies causes the heart to beat faster and pump harder and makes the smooth muscle of our breathing tubes (bronchi) relax. Thus, extra epinephrine in the body results in excessive heart activity (excitability, pulse rate, pumping force) and a widening of bronchi (which is why epinephrine drugs are so effective in the treatment of asthma). When beta blockers prevent epinephrine from exerting these effects, the result is *reduction* of heart activity and *narrowing* of the bronchi. While it is seldom desirable to constrict bronchi, decreasing the work of the heart *can* be helpful. Therefore, since its introduction in 1967, propranolol has been extremely useful in treating high blood pressure, heart rhythm problems, and anginal pain due to poor blood flow through the coronary arteries. However, the drug must be used with great caution—if at all—in persons susceptible to heart failure, who will be made worse if the pumping action of the heart is reduced. Patients prone to asthma may also be worsened by propranolol because of its constricting effect on the bronchial tubes.

Metoprolol is a beta blocker described as "cardioselective"— meaning that it acts more on the heart than on the bronchi. This makes its use safer for persons susceptible to asthmatic attacks. However, this selectivity is not complete and, particularly at high doses, bronchial constriction can still occur. Both propranolol and metoprolol can produce other side effects (fatigue, stomach upset, blood-sugar disturbances in diabetics, for example), and they should be taken only under the careful direction of a physician expert in their use. Moreover, it is now known that up to 5% of persons on prolonged propranolol therapy will experience serious heart problems if they *suddenly discontinue* the drug. These difficulties— which include rhythm abnormalities, severe angina, and even heart attack—have now come to be described as the "propranolol withdrawal syndrome." While the reason for these reactions on sudden withdrawal are not entirely understood, the message is clear: persons taking propranolol (or metoprolol) routinely should not stop it except under the guidance of a qualified physician.

Strokes

Strokes are the third leading cause of death in this country. Yet, most people have little understanding of the causes of a stroke and, more significantly, of what can be done to try to prevent a stroke.

DEFINITION   A stroke may be simply defined as a change in body function caused by interference with the blood supply to the brain. Since the major part of the brain is called the cerebrum, strokes are often referred to as CVAs—cerebral vascular accidents. Usually, the "accident" is rather sudden, and the resulting loss of function may range from a minor change in speech to severe paralysis or coma. While the possible causes of decreased blood flow to the brain are many, the vast majority of strokes are caused by one of three events:

(1) Thrombosis: This word means a "clot"—in this case, a clot or plug somewhere in the vessels of the neck or brain (cerebral thrombosis). Atherosclerosis—the villain that causes plugging of arteries supplying blood to the heart and thereby leads to heart attacks—also causes the narrowing that leads to "brain attacks" or strokes. Many of the same risk factors apply to both kinds of attacks.

(2) Hemorrhage: The breakage of a blood vessel in the brain (cerebral hemorrhage) can obviously interrupt blood flow to the part of the brain supplied by that vessel. Extensive bleeding can also cause direct damage to brain tissue. Hypertension (high blood pressure) may cause damage to blood vessels, thus setting the stage for rupture to occur.

(3) Embolism: An embolus is a piece of material, such as a blood clot, that dislodges from the heart or arteries leading to the head and

is carried into the smaller arteries of the brain, where it blocks the flow of blood (cerebral embolism).

PREVENTION The above explanation of the most important causes of strokes leads directly to a listing of some of the possible ways of preventing these events from occurring:

(1) Blood pressure control: Detection and control of high blood pressure is the single most important stroke prevention measure. High blood pressure contributes to both the process of atherosclerosis and the increased likelihood of weakened arteries rupturing. Hypertension is appropriately described as a "silent killer" because the initial damage to blood vessels occurs without warning symptoms. (For a more complete discussion of high blood pressure, see p. 265.)

(2) Other risk factors: Most experts also feel that the same risk factors that have been identified with an increased chance of a heart attack also contribute to strokes since the same process of atherosclerosis is often involved. Besides hypertension, this would include such factors as smoking and increased blood fats.

(3) Birth control pills: Studies clearly show that women using the pill are at higher risk for the development of strokes. While this increased risk is quite small, most experts would advise women with a family history of strokes or a history of other risk factors to seek another form of contraception. Especially worrisome is the combination of migraine headaches and pill use; most physicians feel such headaches should eliminate the pill from consideration as a form of contraception. Also, some women taking the pill develop hypertension while on it.

(4) Heart rhythm abnormalities: Persons with certain "arrhythmias" of the heart have an increased chance of emboli traveling to the brain, especially if they have heart murmurs or congestive heart failure. Such persons should be under the care of a physician and often require medicine (anti-coagulants) to minimize clot and embolus formation. Minor rhythm disturbances (such as occasional skipped beats) are not worrisome as stroke factors.

TRANSIENT ISCHEMIC ATTACKS (TIAs) An understanding of TIAs is now one of the most important aspects of stroke prevention. A TIA refers to a temporary (transient) episode (attack) of abnormal function caused by decreased blood flow (ischemia) to the brain. Obviously, the distinguishing feature of a TIA is that the loss of function is *temporary*—versus the longer lasting and often permanent damage of a stroke. *The significance of a TIA is that it may warn against an approaching stroke in time to prevent it.* Many TIAs are caused by a narrowing of the blood vessels in the neck (carotid arteries) where surgical correction is possible *if* the abnormality is discovered before a stroke occurs. When surgical correction of narrowed vessels is not possible (as in arteries in the posterior part of the neck), anti-coagulant medicine may be useful. Obviously, it pays to know more about TIAs, as follows:

(1) The most common *symptoms* of a TIA are temporary changes in vision or language function (reading, writing, or speaking) or in limb movement or sensation. *Visual symptoms* may vary from transient blurring or dimming ("a shade coming down") to total blindness. (Should visual problems occur, the individual should alternately cover each eye to determine which one is involved since that information may later be very useful.) Some types of double vision may also be caused by TIAs. *Language changes* may range from the subtle (difficulty in pronunciation) to the obvious (inability to recognize written or spoken words). *Body changes* may vary from tingling around the mouth to loss of movement in an arm or leg. Particularly suggestive of a TIA is a *combination of symptoms on the same side*—for example, both arm and leg or arm and face involved. Dizziness is a particularly difficult symptom to evaluate since the vast majority of dizzy spells are not significant. However, when dizziness is combined with other symptoms—or when in doubt—a physician should be consulted.

(2) The *response* to a possible TIA should be first and foremost to recognize that something is wrong and to head for a competent physician—possibly a neurologist, the medical specialist in diseases of the nervous system. Once in the care of a physician, tests are available—if necessary—to determine if narrowing of a blood vessel in the neck is responsible for the reported symptoms. The most accurate of these tests is angiography—the injection of dye into the blood vessels while x-rays are taken. This test is not without risk, though dangers are minimized when done by experienced medical

personnel. Many newer, less invasive methods of analyzing blood flow to the brain are now available and may be used in place of—or along with—angiography.

(3) A subject of great interest is screening for blood vessel narrowing (*before* symptoms occur). Several methods of detecting decreased blood flow are being used by some physicians. At the very least, palpation (feeling) and auscultation (listening with a stethoscope) of neck vessels should be a part of a physical exam in persons over age 50.

(4) It has long been known that certain *drugs*—including ordinary aspirin—interfere with the role of blood platelets in forming clots. Intensive interest in the use of these antiplatelet drugs to prevent clots associated with heart attacks and strokes has led to several important treatment trials. In 1978, the Canadian Cooperative Study reported striking results concerning the use of aspirin to prevent strokes in those at risk (*New England Journal of Medicine,* July 13, 1978). The Canadian study involved the use of aspirin (four regular tablets per day—a total of 1200mg) *in persons who had experienced a "threatened stroke"* (their phrase for a TIA). In other words, the effect of aspirin in persons who had not experienced warning symptoms was not studied. (It is also important to point out that persons with ulcers were excluded from the study and that coated aspirin was not tried.) Five hundred eighty-three persons who had experienced at least one threatened stroke during the previous three months were given either a placebo, aspirin, sulfinpyrazone (another anti-platelet drug), or sulfinpyrazone and aspirin together. No reduced risk for subsequent stroke could be attributed to sulfinpyrazone, but *males taking four aspirin per day—during an average follow-up period of 26 months—demonstrated a reduced risk for stroke or death of 48% as compared to males not receiving aspirin.* There was no substantial benefit for females.

The obvious question is this: Who should take aspirin? The study itself would justify recommending aspirin only for males who have had one or more warning episodes. (The reason why women did not respond is not clear.) It should also be stressed that some persons with warning episodes can be shown to have plugging of blood vessels in the neck that can be treated surgically. When diagnostic studies and surgery can be done without complications, the results, in terms of symptom relief and stroke prevention, may be better than with any medication—including aspirin. In other words, *persons who experience warning symptoms should not simply start popping aspirin but should see a specialist (usually a neurologist) to learn what treatment is most appropriate*. However, aspirin may be an effective treatment in some cases and the Food and Drug Administration has now approved it for use in men who have experienced TIAs.

What about persons without symptoms who think about taking four aspirin a day "just to be safe"? Obviously, it will not be safe for everyone to take aspirin—though most persons without known ulcer disease or bleeding tendencies can take this amount of aspirin without side effects. In fact, most experts are reluctant to recommend daily aspirin for a person who has not had warning symptoms of a stroke. Thus far, most of the thoughtful doctors we know are not taking aspirin themselves as a preventive measure.

Blood Clots

The words "blood clot" usually bring to mind visions of serious and even fatal illness. And not without justification, since certain kinds of blood clots can indeed set the stage for significant medical problems. However, these words are also used to describe situations that are not medically serious. The following describes some of the most common kinds of blood clotting and their implications.

BLOOD CLOTS IN VEINS   The veins of the extremities are anatomically divided into two systems—a set of superficial veins which can be seen as blue vessels beneath the surface of the skin and a set of larger veins that lie deeply hidden beneath muscle layers. Blood clots can form in both of these systems and commonly do so in the veins of the leg without any apparent cause. There are situations, however, which clearly predispose to clotting—including immobilization; pregnancy; abdominal, pelvic, and hip surgery; congestive heart failure; trauma; and use of birth control pills.

In general, blood clots (thrombi) which form in the superficial veins are not dangerous in terms of sending fragments of the clot (emboli) through the venous system to the lungs (pulmonary emboli). Superficial vein blood clots may feel bad (pain, tenderness, local heat) and look bad, but unless they extend into the deep venous system, they are seldom life-threatening. Still, medical attention can be useful in reducing symptoms and looking for contributing causes.

Conversely, blood clots in the deep venous system are much more likely to pose the danger of blood clots to the lungs. There is, therefore, enormous interest in the prevention, early diagnosis, and effective treatment of deep venous thrombi. The "bedside diagnosis" of deep clots is notoriously difficult in those cases where classical signs (pain, swelling, and heat) are absent. Therefore, other tests (x-ray dye, radioisotope, and ultrasound studies) are often employed in situations of high suspicion. Currently, injections of low doses of heparin (an anti-clotting agent) are being widely used to prevent clotting in high-risk surgical patients. Early ambulation—getting the patient on his feet as soon as possible after surgery—is also designed to prevent these deep vein blood clots from forming. Similarly, anyone—and especially pregnant women—should avoid long periods of sitting or standing in one position since these positions promote pooling of blood in leg veins which increases the chances of clotting.

EXTRAVASCULAR BLOOD CLOTS   In contrast to the above circumstances in which a blood clot forms *inside a vein* (and therefore has the potential to travel through connecting veins to the lungs), blood also forms clots when it escapes into tissues *outside of blood vessels* as a result of an injury. Such clots are usually referred to as *hematomas* or extravascular blood clots. The most common example of this is a bruise, which is a collection of blood that has leaked from broken blood vessels. These blood clots may look bad, especially as they change color during the healing phase of days to weeks when the old blood is reabsorbed by the body.

Initially, hematomas may cause pain due to local swelling and pressure. But unless these clots are so large as to represent excessive blood loss or unless they occur in critical anatomical areas, such as brain tissue, they are not life-threatening. Standard initial treatment for bruises includes elevation to reduce leakage and cold application to promote constriction of the leaking vessels.

IN SUMMARY   Deep vein blood clots are potentially very serious and should be treated vigorously. Other clots—especially those outside blood vessels—are rarely of major consequence.

Anemia

Anemia is sometimes much more serious than the colloquial phrase "tired blood" implies. Indeed, fatigue is poorly correlated with anemia and most fatigue is not due to "low blood." The diagnosis of anemia requires appropriate blood tests; anemia *cannot be accurately diagnosed by a quick look at the color of palm lines or the lining of eyelids.*

DEFINITION   The word "anemia" means a decrease in the number of red blood cells (or their hemoglobin content) that results in reduced transport of oxygen to the cells of the body. It is crucial to note that there are many possible causes of anemia—some potentially serious. For example, anemia can be due to diseases of the bone marrow (where red blood cells are produced), to deficits of certain nutrients necessary for red cell production, to "hemolytic" problems in which such cells are rapidly destroyed in the circulation after they are released from the bone marrow, or to bleeding that exceeds the ability of the bone marrow to send out new red cells.

In other words, "anemia" is not a specific disease; it describes a state of affairs, the cause of which must be sought. Thus, the discovery of anemia on a simple blood test (hemoglobin or hematocrit) should lead to further studies to determine the type of anemia and the underlying cause. In addition to anemias due to specific problems with red cell production and survival, "secondary anemias" may be caused by illnesses such as liver disease, rheumatoid arthritis, hidden infections, or thyroid disease. In all, the list of possible causes is almost endless. In some cases, an anemia discovered during a routine blood test may be the *first* sign of disease.

IRON DEFICIENCY   As it turns out, the most common type of anemia in this country is an iron-deficiency anemia. The cause is rarely a diet deficient in iron—though the steady tea-and-toast fare of some elderly citizens is an example of the kind of diet that might contribute to iron deficiency. Rather, *the vast majority of iron-deficiency anemias are caused by blood loss.* (When blood is lost from the body, the iron in that blood is also lost, thereby resulting in an iron-deficient state.) An iron-deficiency anemia should be assumed to be caused by blood loss somewhere in the body until proven otherwise. The following additional points should be made:

(1) In men, the occurrence of an iron-deficiency anemia must be taken as a sign of intestinal blood loss until proven otherwise. Initial testing for hidden blood in stool specimens is mandatory. If positive, further studies (such as barium x-rays and sigmoidoscopy) are needed to search for potential sources of bleeding such as tumors or ulcers.

(2) In women, the most common cause of blood loss is menstruation. Therefore, in otherwise healthy women still menstruating, it is not unreasonable to assume that an iron-deficiency anemia is due to menstrual blood loss. Such an assumption is obviously not valid in a post-menopausal woman. And even in a woman still menstruating, care must be taken not to overlook other and potentially more serious sources of bleeding.

(3) In infants, the most common cause of iron deficiency is inadequate dietary intake. Milk alone is not sufficient after 4–5 months of age, when rapid growth results in infants exhausting their iron reserves. Foods or drops containing iron should be introduced at about the third month of life, although there is more leeway for breast-fed infants, who absorb more iron.

If a benign form of blood loss—such as menstrual bleeding—is diagnosed, an iron supplement is often started. Iron pills (or rarely, iron injections) are much more effective than any over-the-counter tonic. *If iron deficiency does not exist, iron supplements are useless.* Unnecessary iron may even be dangerous in rare instances.

VITAMIN B-12 DEFICIENCY   Like iron deficiency, vitamin B-12 deficiency (which can lead to the very serious anemia known as *pernicious anemia*) is rarely caused by a lack of vitamin B-12 in the diet. (But total or "vegan" vegetarians—those who also avoid milk products—are at higher risk for a vitamin B-12 deficiency because of their diet.) In typical pernicious anemia, the deficiency is caused by the absence of so-called "intrinsic factor"—a substance normally made by the stomach that enables the intestine to absorb vitamin B-12. When intrinsic factor is absent, vitamin B-12 cannot be absorbed and pernicious anemia develops. If untreated with B-12 shots (taking pills will not do any good, since absorption in the intestines is the problem), this anemia can lead to permanent damage to the nervous system and eventual death. Several further points should be stressed:

(1) Vitamin B-12 shots are appropriate only for those conditions in which this vitamin cannot be absorbed through the intestines— that is, for pernicious anemia caused by the absence of intrinsic factor or poor absorption secondary to intestinal disease. For such people, vitamin B-12 shots are life-saving. For people *not* deficient in vitamin B-12, such shots are an unnecessary pain in the pocketbook and the muscles of the posterior parts.

(2) Many unnecessary B-12 or "liver" shots are given for "tired blood" or as a vague "pep tonic." The only anemia for which B-12 shots are appropriate is pernicious anemia. This is a relatively rare anemia which can be diagnosed only by sophisticated laboratory tests.

IN SUMMARY   The most important point to remember about an anemia is that it is a condition for which a cause must be found. Management of anemias requires more than a simple hemoglobin or hematocrit count and the announcement that you have "low blood" or "tired blood." If you are told that your blood count is low, you should ask why!

Hypoglycemia

"Hypoglycemia" means "low blood sugar"—nothing more or less. However, in our society, this word has become the focus of intense controversy; some organizations and physicians claim that low blood sugar is the cause of many unexplained ills of the human race, while others insist that the condition is overdiagnosed and falsely blamed for symptoms that are more often due to emotionally related problems. The purpose of this essay is to sort out the fact from the fiction that surrounds the problem of hypoglycemia.

CLASSIFICATION—FASTING AND REACTIVE HYPOGLYCEMIA   In most of us, several body systems (the intestines, liver, and endocrine glands) constantly interact to ensure that our baseline blood sugar (glucose) levels stay within a normal range—about 70–110 milligrams per deciliter (mg%). When we challenge these systems—either by excessive carbohydrate ingestion or by fasting—the body's reaction to the challenge can be measured. If blood-sugar levels go too high after carbohydrate ingestion, we say the person has hyperglycemia—the most common cause being diabetes mellitus. If blood-sugar levels drop too low, we say the person has hypoglycemia; however, the exact definition of what is too low—and the reasons for the drop in blood-sugar levels—are sometimes matters of debate.

To understand the usual classification of low blood-sugar states, one must appreciate the following sequence. If no calories are consumed during an overnight fast, the body will normally respond by releasing glucose from liver stores; even after days of starvation, when liver stores are depleted, other metabolic responses will keep the blood glucose from falling to dangerously low levels. However, in people with certain diseases (insulin-producing tumors, liver disease, alcoholism, and so on) and in some with no discernible physical explanation, the blood sugar will gradually drop to abnormally low levels during fasting and produce such symptoms as fatigue, headache, inability to concentrate, forgetfulness, and sleepiness. This state of hypoglycemia is known as *fasting hypoglycemia* and requires a careful search for underlying diseases.

If, on the other hand, a person consumes a large amount of carbohydrate—as is the case when 75–100 grams of glucose are gulped in the "oral glucose tolerance test" (OGTT), the blood-sugar levels will begin to rise immediately. (The *extent of the rise*—time and amount—is sometimes measured to check for mild diabetes.) Following the expected increase in blood sugar, there is a period of decreasing blood sugar; if there is an overshoot to below normal range, adrenalin is released and produces symptoms such as palpitation, sweating, and tremulousness. Since the usual OGTT for the diagnosis of hyperglycemia (diabetes) is often stopped after three hours, the period of continued decline is often missed. However, in the person with suspected hypoglycemia, the OGTT must be extended to five hours (with blood levels checked each half-hour and at *any* time that symptoms are reported) in order to detect an abnormally low level of blood sugar. This abnormally low level in response to ingested carbohydrate is logically referred to as *post-prandial* (meaning "after a meal") or *reactive hypoglycemia*—and it is this type of hypoglycemia that is so controversial.

REACTIVE HYPOGLYCEMIA   Now that we have focused our attention on reactive hypoglycemia—the type that develops rather suddenly several hours after eating carbohydrates—we can examine the key question that surrounds this phenomenon: how low is too low? This may sound like a simple question to answer, but it turns out not to be because *some people report no symptoms when sugar levels are quite low; others experience suggestive symptoms in the face of normal blood-sugar levels, usually a consequence of anxiety and not hypoglycemia.* Therefore, in order to make a diagnosis of a problem truly caused by low blood sugar, it is essential to correlate the simultaneous occurrence of low blood sugar (most authorities insist on levels below 50mg%) and the onset of symptoms (palpitations, sweating, anxiety, hunger, tremulousness). In other words, it is presumptuous to make the diagnosis of symptomatic hypoglycemia on the basis of blood tests alone—or the report of symptoms without simultaneous blood tests.

Many people have been told—or have assumed—that they have hypoglycemia without this correlation of symptoms and blood-sugar measurements. Such conclusions are often understandable—given the desire to "explain" troubling symptoms with a physical cause— and if the resulting dietary treatment (see below) produces improvement, it is hard to argue with the approach. If, however, such unproven assumptions lead to inappropriate medical practice (repeated blood tests, injection treatments, costly prescriptions)—or to postponing correct treatment for other underlying physical or emotional problems—unnecessary harm may result. Beware especially of doctors who claim to "specialize" in hypoglycemia.

When reactive hypoglycemia is judged to be the cause of symptoms, the usual treatment consists of dietary modification—smaller but more frequent meals that are relatively free of simple sugars; this reduces the stimulus for an overreaction of the body's blood-sugar regulating system. In some cases—particularly those caused by rapid passage of blood after ulcer surgery—medications to slow down the gastrointestinal tract may be useful.

IN SUMMARY   The term "hypoglycemia" is often used inappropriately to explain non-specific symptoms which may or may not be due to low blood sugar. To make an accurate diagnosis of true reactive hypoglycemia, a glucose tolerance test should be used to show a clear correlation between symptoms, and abnormally low sugar levels should be demonstrated.

Diabetes

More than 50 years ago, Canadian researchers gave extracts of the pancreas to a 14-year-old diabetic boy otherwise destined to die as so many others had before. Following his dramatic recovery, diabetes mellitus was thought to be a simple problem of the pancreas being unable to produce insulin, thereby causing the blood sugar (glucose) to reach extreme heights which, in turn, would trigger a series of disastrous metabolic derangements certain to lead to death. Today, however, diabetes is perceived as far from simple, and this essay will consider some of the questions concerning its cause, diagnosis, and treatment.

CAUSE   The underlying problem in diabetes is an inappropriately elevated level of blood sugar—hyperglycemia—which, when severe, can lead to a state of coma and extreme dehydration. Persons with diabetes who are predisposed to coma generally produce little or no insulin, the hormone released from the pancreas to help sugar get into the body's tissues and which, therefore, keeps the blood-sugar level within normal range. Diabetes beginning in childhood (juvenile diabetes) is almost always due to severe insulin deficiency. But diabetes that first appears in adulthood (adult-onset diabetes) may be associated with *normal* or even *elevated* levels of insulin that are not doing the job. Indeed, the terms "juvenile" and "adult-onset" are being supplanted today by the phrases "insulin-dependent" and "insulin-independent"— indicating that these two different forms of diabetes can occur at any age and that the type of diabetes, rather than the age, becomes the most important factor in treatment and prognosis. The reason why the pancreas stops making insulin, or why a given amount of insulin is less effective at other times, remains poorly understood. *Genetic factors* clearly play a role, as diabetes tends to run in families. However, the pattern of inheritance is far more complicated than was previously thought, thereby making it impossible to predict with certainty whether parents with diabetes will transmit the disease to any of their children. *Viral factors* have recently attracted widespread attention following reports that one particular virus (the B-4 Coxsackie virus) can trigger diabetes in genetically susceptible mice. While such research raises hope for a vaccine against viruses that might play a role in bringing on diabetes, such a vaccine is not likely in the immediate future. In short, the cause (or causes) of most cases of diabetes is unknown.

There are times, though, when hyperglycemia can be traced to specific causes, including: *pancreatic diabetes,* in which the cells of the pancreas are destroyed by disease (such as chronic pancreatitis); *endocrine diabetes,* in which the overactivity of various glands (thyroid, adrenal, or pituitary) raises blood-sugar levels; and *drug-induced diabetes,* in which hyperglycemia is caused by drugs such as steroids, diuretics (water pills), or even birth control pills in some women.

RECOGNITION   The most common symptoms of *severe* sugar elevation include excessive thirst and urination around the clock, increased appetite in the presence of weight loss, and profound weakness. These symptoms are usually associated with diabetes due to extreme insulin deficiency; they are the usual ones experienced by juvenile diabetics. Adult-onset diabetes is often diagnosed on the basis of a routine blood-sugar test that turns out to be elevated in persons who have no symptoms at all. However, certain complaints (itching, blurred vision, or excessive thirst and urination) may suggest the need for a blood test.

The diagnosis of diabetes is relatively simple in someone with typical symptoms and a greatly elevated blood-sugar level; in this case, a single blood-sugar test is sufficient to establish the diagnosis. However, in the more common situation, where sugar is detected in the urine or when mild hyperglycemia is discovered during routine testing, one must not hastily diagnose diabetes without considering other possible causes for the increased sugar.

SCREENING   The dilemma concerning screening for diabetes (searching for elevated blood sugar in the absence of symptoms) can be understood by contrasting its likely value with that of screening for high blood pressure. Since it is known that treating high blood pressure, even in the absence of symptoms, pays off in reducing serious complications of this "silent killer," screening for elevations in blood pressure makes sense. However, such certainty about diabetes does not exist because it is not known whether the treatment of mild, asymptomatic hyperglycemia will prevent the serious complications sometimes associated with diabetes—heart problems, kidney damage, and eye disease. Therefore, experts disagree as to how vigorously persons *without* symptoms should be checked for elevated blood sugar because there is uncertainty about how vigorously persons should be treated if *mild* elevations in blood sugar are found.

The following tests are often used in the screening and diagnosis of diabetes:

(1) Urine tests: Urine tests for sugar have been popular in the past because of their simplicity and the fact that they avoid any kind of "needle stick." However, they are often unreliable and *they should never be used to make a final diagnosis of diabetes.*

(2) Single blood tests: Both *fasting* and *one or two hour post-prandial* (after eating) blood tests are widely used to screen for and diagnose diabetes. Many experts think that a significant elevation in either of these tests is all that's needed to make the diagnosis. The blood-sugar level considered to be abnormal will depend upon various factors, including the age of the patient and the chemical method used in the testing: 170 (mg/100ml) at one hour or 120 at two hours are often used as upper limits of normal.

(3) Glucose tolerance test (GTT): This test involves drinking a sugar solution, followed by repeated blood tests during the next 3–4 hours. The result of the GTT can be affected by previous diet, age, and other diseases. Since this test is even more sensitive, borderline results are difficult to interpret. Most experts agree that the GTT is not necessary if the single blood tests described above are clearly abnormal.

Tests are obviously indicated in persons with symptoms suggesting diabetes. They are also advocated in high-risk persons—those from families with a history of diabetes, adults who are obese, and women who have given birth to large babies (over ten pounds).

But whether or not screening of *all* persons is wise remains a matter of debate.

TREATMENT   Once a diagnosis of diabetes has been made, there is a tendency to react with a vision of lifelong insulin shots and serious complications. While both of these consequences are possible, many people with diabetes face neither. Those with insulin-dependent diabetes *will* require insulin, but the majority of adult-onset diabetes patients will not. For them, careful attention to diet and weight control may be all that's needed to restore the blood sugar to an acceptable level.

(1) Weight control: It is clear that adult-onset diabetes is more likely to occur in persons who are obese and that elevated blood-sugar levels will often return to near-normal levels with simple weight loss. Therefore, *the initial and often most important therapy for obese persons with adult-onset diabetes is a combination of calorie restriction and exercise that will help attain ideal body weight.*

(2) Diet modification: Initial diet recommendations of the American Diabetes Association (ADA) set forth in 1949 stressed a reduction in carbohydrates and a consequent increase in fats and proteins. However, criticism arose over both the difficulty of rigid restriction of all carbohydrates and the possible dangers of excess fats causing atherosclerosis (hardening of the arteries)—a disease to which persons with diabetes are already prone. These concerns led to a revision in the dietary recommendations of the ADA (made in 1971) which now include the following emphases:

> *Fat* (at least two-thirds unsaturated) should be restricted to 35% or less of total calories.
> *Carbohydrates* (breads, potatoes, rice, and so on) may be increased to as much as 40–50% of the total calories as long as refined sugars (as in candy, molasses, icing) are avoided.

Given these changed guidelines and the many dietary aids available for those on insulin (exchange lists and special cookbooks, for example), most persons with diabetes can lead a very normal and satisfying culinary life.

(3) Oral drugs: In the past, many adult-onset diabetics were almost automatically treated with sugar-lowering drugs, while the im-

portance of weight control was inadequately stressed. Today, however, just the opposite should be true. Much of this de-emphasis of oral drugs stems from recent information concerning their dangers.

Sulfonylureas (trade names Orinase, Diabinese, Tolinase, Dymelor) act by stimulating the pancreas to release insulin. These drugs have become the subject of great controversy since a major report in 1970 suggested they are associated with more deaths from cardiovascular disease (such as heart attacks) than would otherwise be expected. This report—which emerged from a large multi-center study known as the University Group Diabetes Program (UGDP)—prompted the Food and Drug Administration to recommend a new package insert warning that oral drugs to lower blood sugar may be associated with increased deaths when compared to diet alone or diet plus insulin. While legal action and ongoing debate among diabetes specialists have delayed implementation of this recommendation, many experts suggest that these drugs be prescribed only for those who do not respond to dietary management and who *cannot* take insulin, such as persons with deforming arthritis or blindness.

Phenformin (marketed in this country as DBI and Meltrol) was also implicated in heart disease in the UGDP study. However, this drug—which lowers blood sugar in a different manner than the sulfonylureas—has been *banned* from general use in the United States. The specific concern about phenformin that led to this ban is its propensity to provoke a serious and often fatal metabolic complication known as "lactic acidosis." While estimates of the degree of risk vary, almost all experts agree that the risk is not worth taking—given the fact that phenformin is not essential in the treatment for the vast majority of patients with diabetes. For those very rare patients who may really need it, phenformin is still available by special arrangements.

(4) Eye disease in diabetics: Recent advances in the treatment of diabetic retinopathy (new blood-vessel formation, bleeding, and scarring of the retina) are offering new hope for the diabetic patient who develops this eye problem. Two new treatment methods have proven to be effective for many patients:

Photocoagulation with both laser and arc light has been used successfully for many years in the treatment of retinal changes that develop with diabetic retinopathy. The National Eye Institute has reported results of a continuing ten-year study of photocoagulation which have confirmed the effectiveness of this form of treatment in properly selected cases.

Vitrectomy is a surgical procedure involving the removal of vitreous, a semi-solid material that fills the posterior two-thirds of the eye globe. It may be indicated in those patients who have had bleeding into the vitreous gel as the result of diabetic retinopathy. This technique has produced dramatic results in some cases in which bleeding has not spontaneously cleared, but it is still regarded as experimental.

Both of the above procedures require careful eye examinations and advice from a specialist in eye disease of diabetics. Individuals with evidence of diabetic eye disease should consult an ophthalmologist (eye physician) recommended by their doctor.

(5) Insulin: For persons with diabetes characterized by insufficient insulin, insulin injections are mandatory and life-saving. However, giving *too much* insulin poses its own danger in the form of hypoglycemia (low blood sugar) which can cause coma and even death. Attempts to give enough insulin to reduce blood-sugar levels to the *normal* range will invariably increase the risk of producing hypoglycemic coma. A critical—and largely unanswered—question is whether "meticulous" control of blood sugar by insulin injection pays off in preventing or reducing the major kinds of complications of diabetes. At present, all would agree that the blood sugar should be lowered so as to avoid the symptoms of excessive urination and thirst, and most experts find it prudent to keep the blood sugar as close to normal as is possible without causing undesirable side effects—particularly hypoglycemic coma.

Because injected insulin cannot reproduce the minute-to-minute release of insulin of a normal pancreas, there is increasing interest in achieving a more "natural" insulin control as a possible means of reducing long-term complications. There are two basic approaches to better blood-sugar control now under intensive study. One involves the transplantation of normal pancreatic tissue (or the specific "islet cell" tissue of the pancreas responsible for insulin production) into the body; such transplantation creates predictable problems of tissue rejection, and the results of long-term transplants in humans are disappointing to date. However, animal studies continue with some interesting leads.

The more immediately promising approach involves the use of mechanical devices developed to achieve more complete control of blood-sugar levels. One variety is described as a "closed-loop feedback" system because it is designed to continuously measure blood-sugar levels and then to release appropriate amounts of insulin—much in the manner of a normal human pancreas. However, problems with the "sensing system" have thus far been difficult to overcome.

The other type of mechanical system is described as "openloop" because it is not designed to sense ongoing blood-sugar levels. Rather, it releases insulin in a pre-programmed pattern which can easily be adjusted to the anticipated needs of a given patient. Specifically, insulin is *continually* injected in minute doses through a thin tube inserted into the skin; a small, lightweight pump is worn about the waist. Several investigators have reported great progress with this kind of system in terms of blood-sugar control and improvement in other aspects of metabolism—including blood fats. As is stressed by all researchers in the field of mechanical devices, more testing is needed before such systems become widely available to persons requiring insulin. But the use of open-loop systems now seems much closer than before—most likely a matter of a few years.

Of even more immediate interest to insulin-taking diabetics are several recent reports that have suggested considerable variability in insulin absorption from different injection locations. For example, a recent study from the Yale School of Medicine (*Annals of Internal Medicine,* January 1980) describes short-acting insulin absorption from the abdominal wall as 86% greater than from the leg and 30% greater than from the arm; blood-sugar levels are correspondingly different based on the injection location. Other reports have demonstrated that the absorption from an arm or leg subsequently exercised is more rapid than when the limb is not exercised. Obviously, these factors can have important implications for the control of blood-sugar levels. For example, it might be important—at least in some persons whose diabetes is difficult to control with insulin—to use only one anatomical area for insulin injections and vary the locations of injections only within that area in order to achieve more stable insulin absorption patterns.

IN SUMMARY   Very careful control of blood-sugar levels does not guarantee that complications will not develop. However, the reasonable goal of treatment for any person with diabetes would seem to be a lowering of blood sugar to avoid symptoms and a life-style (diet, exercise, weight control) which avoids major fluctuations in blood-sugar levels.

Cancer

The ancient Greeks called the spreading growths "the crablike disease"—*karkinos*—which translates through Latin into the word "cancer." No word in our language has greater emotional impact. Many regard the diagnosis of cancer as an automatic death sentence. The facts of the matter, however, are different:

(1) Of the approximately 800,000 persons in the United States with newly diagnosed cancer each year, *one third will survive* to lead a normal life for many years—many with permanent cures.

(2) While the exact number is difficult to determine, it is estimated by experts that well over 100,000 persons die needlessly of cancer in this country every year because of late diagnosis or inadequate treatment.

(3) It is true that certain cancers—such as pancreas and lung cancers—are very difficult to diagnose early and treat effectively. However, many other common cancers—bowel, breast, cervix, skin—can often be detected early enough for a permanent cure.

It is essential to understand that *cancer is not one disease, but hundreds of different diseases* which share in common only one feature—unregulated cell growth. Various cancers are different in terms of cause, diagnosis, and treatment. Most experts feel it is highly unlikely that there will ever be a single cure for all cancers; rather, the war against cancer will likely be fought continually on many fronts.

WARNING SIGNALS Most of us cannot easily remember the seven warning signs of cancer. However, we can and should remember that *any persistent (more than two weeks) change in body ap-*

pearance or function is cause for concern—concern which should prompt an immediate visit to a doctor. Usually it's not cancer, but various studies indicate that most of us wait a foolishly long period of months before checking on changes that are obviously abnormal. Sometimes part of the rationalization for this is the idea that we can wait for our routine yearly physical—which then keeps getting postponed. *An immediate investigation of symptoms has a much greater pay-off than routine checkups.* The latter should never be considered a substitute for the former.

The following are some common and important warning signs:

(1) Skin changes: Any significant new growth or change in a previous skin growth or marking should be investigated—by a dermatologist (skin specialist) if a satisfactory explanation is not given by your usual source of medical care. And don't forget the "skin" inside your mouth.

(2) Change in bowel habits: This is a tough one because most of us experience occasional upsets in bowel habits, the *vast majority* of which are *not* due to cancer. However, any persistent change—more than two weeks—should be reported to your physician. It is your doctor's responsibility—not yours—to decide whether it is worth further study.

(3) Abnormal bleeding or discharge: Any bloody material that is coughed up or vomited is clearly abnormal, as is any vaginal bleeding in a post-menopausal woman or any discharge (bloody or otherwise) from the breast. More confusing is *minimal* bleeding from the rectum (often due to hemorrhoids) or in the urine (often due to infection). Also confusing is unusual bleeding in a woman still menstruating. Again, the only safe advice is to report such changes to your physician and make the matter his responsibility.

(4) Lumps and bumps: Most important is a lump found in the breast. Other lumps, however, should not be ignored even though most turn out *not* to be cancer—including 80% of all breast lumps.

(5) Coughing and hoarseness: These two common complaints usually are secondary to inflammation of the vocal cords. However, hoarseness of more than two weeks duration may be a very useful warning sign of cancer in the voice box. Unfortunately, coughing is not a useful *early* warning symptom of lung cancer.

Again, the above list is only partial. The bottom-line rule is always this: any persistent change in appearance or function should be reported to your physician.

Prevention and Detection

Even though cancer is a distinct second to cardiovascular disease (including heart attacks and strokes) as a cause of death in this country, it is clearly the most feared of all diseases. Much of this fear stems from the often incorrect image of long and lingering death associated with malignancy. Part of it comes from a feeling of helplessness about how to avoid cancer which, in its various forms, will afflict one in four of all Americans now living. We are constantly bombarded by messages suggesting that almost everything in our environment—external and internal—has the potential to cause cancer. Not surprisingly, many give up when it comes to thinking about a personal program of cancer prevention. Yet, the startling fact of the matter is that there are effective methods of prevention or early detection for all of the five most common types of cancer in this country. The following summarizes briefly some of the measures all of us can and should be taking in terms of personal cancer control. (The figures following each cancer below are the American Cancer Society predictions for 1980.)

LUNG CANCER (117,000 new cases; 101,000 deaths)   While new measures for the detection and treatment of lung cancer report limited success, the current overall rates for diagnosis and cure are dismal—as reflected by the fact that lung cancer kills almost twice as many persons as the next leading cause of cancer deaths. Chest x-rays, while simple and relatively safe, seldom detect lung cancer early enough for a cure. That's the bad news. *The good news is that we know the cause of at least 80% of the cases of this leading cancer killer—cigarettes.* What we do about this knowledge may be a commentary on our intelligence and resoluteness as individuals and as a nation.

COLON-RECTUM CANCER (114,000 new cases, 53,000 deaths) Cancer experts say that two out of three persons with cancer of the large intestine might be saved by individual attention to suspicious symptoms and the proper use of existing screening and diagnostic tools. Suggestive symptoms worth paying attention to include rectal bleeding (assumed to be due to cancer until proven otherwise) and persistent (more than two weeks) changes in bowel habits or abdominal distress. *The single most important screening tool available is an annual check for occult (hidden, microscopic) blood in the stool of persons over 40.* This should be done as part of a routine physical; the doctor obtains a stool specimen during a rectal exam, which also allows detection of growths within reach of the examining finger. Such screening can also be done with home kits which can be mailed to a doctor or clinic for interpretation. *The finding of hidden blood should lead to x-ray studies and direct visual inspection* by sigmoidoscopes (10 inches) or flexible colonoscopes (the entire length of the large intestine). Persons with a past history of polyps or ulcerative colitis may need these latter studies on a regular basis. More recently, much attention has been devoted to the role of nutrition in preventing colon cancer. While the role of diet in the prevention of colon cancer is not settled, it is known that populations with a high red-meat consumption have a high incidence of colon cancer. Whether a high dietary fiber content is preventive is far from proven, but there is no harm—and maybe some benefit—in increasing such fiber. (For a more complete discussion concerning dietary fiber, see p. 27.)

BREAST CANCER (109,000 new cases; 36,000 deaths)   When breast cancer is discovered in a localized stage, the five-year survival rate is about 85%. *Self-examination* (monthly) is still the most important method of detection; most breast lumps are discovered in this way. Much attention is being focused currently on methods of discovering abnormal areas of breast tissue that cannot be felt. *Mammography* offers an excellent method of such detection, and newer technology considerably reduces (often to one-tenth) the radiation exposure associated with older equipment; the benefit of mammography lies primarily in high-risk women—those with previous breast cancer; suspicious symptoms such as discharge, pain, lumpy breasts; strong family history in female relatives; infertility or no child before age 30. In our judgment, such high-risk women should use mammography on a regular basis beginning in their thirties; after age 50, the increased chance of breast cancer justifies more routine use of mammography. *Thermography* as originally conceived has fallen into disuse, but newer variations on the theme may prove beneficial for screening. The use of *ultrasound* is also being investigated.

PROSTATE CANCER (66,000 new cases; 22,000 deaths)   A thorough rectal examination in males still offers the most feasible method for the early detection of prostate cancer; about three-quarters of all such cancers are located in the posterior lobe of the prostate gland—readily accessible to the examining finger through the front wall of the rectum. (Note: The rectal exam thus represents a "triple threat" in males—detection of rectal cancer, occult blood in the stool, and prostate cancer.) Possible warning symptoms of prostate growth—mainly difficulty in urinating—are most often due to *benign* prostatic enlargement, which is extremely common in elderly men. Symptoms of advanced prostate cancer—bone pain in the pelvis or lower back—reflect a stage where the cancer has already spread, as do increases of certain blood enzymes originating in the prostate or bone. So, *routine rectal examinations still represent the "bottom line" in early detection for prostate cancer.* (For a more thorough discussion of prostate ailments, see p. 380.)

UTERINE CANCER (99,000 new cases; 11,000 deaths)   The phrase "uterine cancer" refers to two very different cancers which both originate in the womb. Important prevention and detection information for the two can be briefly summarized as follows:

(1) Cancer of the cervix: If cervical cancer is detected early enough, the cure rate approaches 100%. The Pap smear is a very easy and reliable means for early detection of this cancer—which is more common in women for whom sexual intercourse begins early or who have multiple partners. The American Cancer Society has recently recommended that a yearly Pap smear is not necessary for women between the ages of 20 and 40 who have had two previous negative smears a year apart; a 3-year interval for Pap smears was proposed for them. However, an extended period between tests might get women out of the habit altogether. Moreover, they miss out on other checks (such as blood pressure and breast exams) that went along with these yearly visits to "get a Pap."

(2) Cancer of the lining of the uterus (endometrium): The Pap

smear does *not* reliably detect cells from inside the uterus. There-fore, attention to early warning signs is important—*and the single most important warning sign is any vaginal bleeding in a post-menopausal woman, which must be considered to be due to cancer until proven otherwise.* Endometrial cancer usually occurs in women over 50 and is more common among those who have a late meno-pause, who are overweight, and who have been treated with long-term use of estrogens. Such women should have careful pelvic exam-inations (yearly after age 50), and periodic sampling of the lining of the uterus to look for microscopic changes should be considered.

OTHER MEASURES   Several other themes of cancer prevention and detection should be mentioned as safe and effective:

(1) *Skin cancer:* avoidance of excessive sun and early check on suspicious lumps, areas of increasing pigmentation, or chronic bleeding.

(2) *Oral cancer:* careful visual inspection—especially in heavy smokers (including cigars and pipes) and drinkers—for. unusual white or red areas within the mouth.

(3) *Voice-box cancer:* visual inspection (by a tube inserted under light anesthesia) in persons with persistent hoarseness (more than two weeks).

(4) *Testicular cancer:* self-examination for lumps every three months.

(5) *Industrial chemicals:* avoidance of known carcinogens (such as asbestos, aniline dyes, vinyl chloride) and checking on the safety of continued or concentrated exposure to any chemicals.

(6) *Urinary tract cancer:* investigation of blood in the urine (he-maturia)—again, cancer until proven otherwise.

Breast Cancer

Dr. Rita Kelley, Associate Professor of Medicine at the Massachu-setts General Hospital, Harvard Medical School, and a medical spe-cialist in cancer, has been asked to respond to questions that deal with suspected or proven breast cancer.

When a suspicious breast lump is found,
what are the next steps in diagnosis?

In the past, the standard approach was a total removal (excisional biopsy) of the lump under general anesthesia in the operating room. The woman was told beforehand that if the lump proved to be cancer (by frozen section) a radical mastectomy would be performed immediately. She would awaken in the recovery room, reach to see whether her breast was present or absent, and thus learn the diagnosis. Undesirable psychologically, this approach also deprives the woman of the opportunity to consider the various choices now available in treating breast cancer. While excisional biopsies are still the diagnostic procedure most commonly done, they are now performed in "out-patient" operating rooms under local anesthesia, with the woman discharged to await the pathologic diagnosis and a review of the consequent options for treatment.

An alternative approach is the needle biopsy, which can be performed in the surgeon's office on the first visit if the lump is sizable enough to allow it. Adequate tissue can be obtained without the risk of spreading disease if specific therapy is undertaken within a short time of a biopsy showing cancer.

What are the options for therapy once the diagnosis
of cancer is established?

It is important to realize that breast cancer is a dangerous disease not so much because of its growth within the breast, but because it has usually been present for a considerable time before it is found and therefore has had time to reach other areas of the body. This means that a careful search for distant spread (metastases) should be done with appropriate x-rays, scans, and blood tests *before* extensive local treatment is undertaken. Current controversy about therapy for cancer apparently confined to the breast exists because such "confinement" cannot be accurately ascertained. Following are the types of local treatment most commonly undertaken:

(1) Standard radical mastectomy: For many years, this was the only kind of therapy considered adequate regardless of the size, location, or tissue characteristics of the cancer. This operation in-

volves removing the breast, the two large muscles anchoring the breast to the chest wall and shoulder, and all of the lymph nodes in the armpit. It leaves a considerable cosmetic defect, but in certain types of disease—when tumor is located very close to and possibly penetrating the muscles—it may still be indicated. Fewer and fewer standard radical mastectomies are being done by surgeons as evidence mounts to show that the removal of so much tissue is generally not necessary—and as cancers are being diagnosed earlier due to improved diagnostic techniques.

(2) Modified radical mastectomy: This is similar to the standard radical except that there is less removal of chest muscles, leaving less of a cosmetic defect. The operation is subject to considerable variation in the amount of tissue removed, depending on what "modified" means to the individual surgeon, and this is the chief criticism leveled against it. The surgeon must be meticulous in removing as many of the armpit nodes as possible or the surgery may be self-defeating. As yet there is no evidence from carefully compared series that the modified radical mastectomy, now the choice of most surgeons, has a poorer survival outcome than the standard radical. A *simple mastectomy* removes only the breast tissue without node removal and is inadequate for most patients unless followed by x-ray therapy.

(3) Tumorectomy (or "lumpectomy") and x-ray therapy: This refers to total surgical removal of the breast lump followed by radiotherapy to the breast and the lymph drainage pathways. Lymph node sampling should always be done to establish whether the disease has spread beyond the breast. This type of treatment is based on the concept that modern x-ray therapy can kill all residual cancer cells that may be left in the breast or the drainage tracts, while preserving the woman's breast. It is a reasonable choice for the young patient with a small cancer and negative nodes, a person who has a good chance for cure by whatever type of primary therapy is offered. In the studies to date of patients treated in this way, follow-up data are comparable to radical mastectomy for those with negative nodes, but a little poorer for those with positive nodes. The cosmetic results are excellent. The major objections to this approach offered by its detractors are: (1) that cancer remaining after the removal of the major lump may not be totally destroyed by x-ray and may recur

years later, and (2) that the later effects of such high-dose radiotherapy given to young patients are as yet unknown.

Until long-term results exist for modified radical mastectomy or tumorectomy with x-ray therapy, the patient is in the quandary of trying to make a decision with insufficient information. But at least we have reached a position where optional pathways can be discussed. It is the natural role of the physician to provide his or her most enlightened judgment as to which is most suited to the individual patient. A single approach to all breast cancer is no longer tenable.

Why is it so important to know whether there is disease in axillary (armpit) nodes?

The patients at greatest risk for trouble with recurrent breast cancer are those who have disease found in the axillary nodes at the time of initial treatment. The more nodes that are positive, the greater is the probability that cancer has already spread beyond them. In the past, such patients were given post-operative x-ray therapy routinely, but this only protected the patient from local recurrence; it did nothing to suppress the possibility of distant disease or to increase longevity. The use of post-operative x-ray therapy is now limited to specific types of cases where it is clearly indicated.

In the past few years, patients with positive nodes have been placed on a variety of drugs (chemotherapy) singly or in combination in an attempt to kill any cells which may have escaped surgery. It is known that this type of treatment (adjuvant chemotherapy) is not as effective for post-menopausal women; but because their disease is apt to be slow in its growth pattern, this may not be a serious concern. For women who have not reached menopause, however, the figures so far available for the largest series show impressive protection for those with positive nodes who received adjuvant chemotherapy. Chemotherapy has unpleasant and sometimes serious side effects and it is not always easy for patients to undergo, but the benefits so far appear to outweigh the toxicity of prolonged intermittent therapy. Programs are being changed and improved all the time, and in the hands of qualified medical oncologists, they can be administered with maximum protection for the patient.

Cancer and the Immune Response

Recently, a lot of attention has been focused on experimental efforts to improve cancer therapy by harnessing the body's immune response. The hope is that this natural means of defense against infection can be used to identify and destroy cancer cells.

THE PROBLEM   Cancer is a difficult disease to treat in part because the body's own cells are the enemy. Cancer cells often differ from normal ones only in very small ways, so any attempt to identify and kill them is likely to injure normal cells as well. When cancer is caught early enough, it can be removed with the surgeon's knife, but many tumors scatter cells ("metastasize") to distant parts of the body before they are big enough to be noticed. Once they spread, cancers may be treated with radiation or drugs, but sooner or later, in most cases, they resist treatment. Meanwhile, the risk of hurting normal tissue limits the amount of therapy that can be given.

What is needed is a way to home in on cancer cells while leaving their normal neighbors unscathed. For a long time scientists have thought of ways to exploit immunity—the body's natural ability to fight foreign invaders—to combat cancer. A brief explanation of immunity will help to put this in perspective.

SEARCH AND DESTROY   The immune response is based on a system of surveillance, memory, and attack. When foreign material of certain types enters the body, the immune system recognizes it as "strange." Usually, germs (bacteria, viruses, and so on) or their products trigger the immune response, but under proper conditions a huge variety of chemicals can also cause the body to react in a manner that will neutralize or destroy what is foreign to it. And once a strange substance has been encountered, the immune system generally remembers it for months, years, or a lifetime. Then, if the body is again exposed to this material, its immune system reacts in either of two ways:

(1) Antibody production: Antibodies are a little like rubber darts; they are proteins with a kind of suction cup that sticks to the foreign object. But the suction cup is highly specific; it won't stick to just anything. Instead, it fits quite precisely against one kind of molecule and no other. So, when invaded, the body rummages through its box of darts to find the sort that work against the particular invader. It then reproduces as many of the right darts as possible and sends them through the bloodstream to hit their target. When an antibody becomes stuck to the surface of a target, it serves as a handle onto which search-and-destroy cells can grab. These cells contain chemicals that help to disable and kill the invader, which has first been marked by antibodies.

(2) Direct cellular attack: In this instance, antibodies are less involved. Instead, the "suction cup" is already attached directly to a kind of search-and-destroy cell that goes to the target and does its own work. Usually, this process is slower than the first.

Most day-to-day immune reactions occur silently, but if an intense immune response takes place near the skin, we can see the effects in the form of inflammation. Blood vessels dilate, making the area red and warm. There is also swelling as fluid and cells pour into the region. Then, pus (debris left from the microscopic battle) may be formed. If the defense succeeds, inflammation subsides and everything returns to normal.

CANCER AS AN INNOCENT BYSTANDER   This battlefield can be a pretty rough place. Potent chemicals are released that can injure *any* cell, not just the invaders. But some of the substances released (either by invaders or by the body) have the amplifying effect of stimulating the immune system to work even harder; thus, they intensify the struggle. The earliest use of immunity to combat cancer (in the 1890s) was based on this amplifying effect. It was found that tumors located at the site of an immune reaction would sometimes shrink. Presumably, in this case, the tumor was merely an innocent bystander. Some of its cells (but never all of them) were "accidentally" killed in the surrounding battle. In the past thirty years, many attempts have been made to use this "innocent-bystander" effect to shrink tumors. The best results have been obtained with small skin cancers. These tumors can be either painted with chemicals that evoke an immune response or injected with weakened bacteria such as "BCG" derived from the tuberculosis germ. So far, the method has made localized tumors shrink for a while, but it has not proved effective against cancers that have spread.

Meanwhile, the amplification concept has been carried further. Especially in the last ten years, attempts have been made to stimulate the *whole* immune system with substances such as BCG which make it respond more rapidly and intensely than usual. These treatments have indeed succeeded in raising the activity level of the immune system, but so far they have done little to slow the growth or spread of tumors.

More recently, considerable enthusiasm has been expressed for a protein known as *interferon*. In addition to its well-known function of combating viral infections, interferon stimulates the immune system. One such effect is to convert inactive immune cells into an active form known as "natural killers." These killer cells seem to attack tumor cells directly, at least in animals, but little is known about how they work or how important they normally are in fighting cancer. Information on the situation in humans is even sparser. A few clinical trials have begun, and there are some encouraging reports, but it is far too early to know what the results mean.

There are reasons for doubting that general immune stimulants, such as interferon, will provide the key to treating advanced cancer. The immune system can be pushed only so hard; once entrenched in the body, an invader is usually able to resist even a heightened immunological attack. Recent evidence indicates that there are natural regulators within the immune system, so that attempts to activate it beyond a certain point will tend to switch on a set of dampening responses. This form of regulation is especially important in protecting the body from attack by its own immune system.

CANCER AS THE TARGET   As normal cells change into cancer cells, they may also change their chemical "appearance"; they begin to "look" somewhat foreign to the immune system rather than looking like normal parts of the self. Under the right circumstances, then, the cancer might be attacked as though it were a foreign invader.

Indeed, there is evidence that we are sometimes protected from early cancer by just such a process.

Efforts to make the immune system identify cancer cells as alien have intrigued scientists. At times, a vaccine can be prepared from an animal's—or a patient's—own cancer cells. The vaccine can be made more effective in some cases by chemically modifying the cancer cells it contains in a way that emphasizes their differences from the normal. Such vaccines can be very effective at protecting experimental animals from tumors transplanted into them by scientists, but they have not been very successful for treating established cancers. Attempts to use vaccines in cancer victims have, so far, achieved very little. This disappointing result is not surprising; although some cancer cells differ slightly from normal in their chemical appearance, most of their surface probably looks very normal to the immune system.

Another potential strategy is to use "loaded" antibodies to destroy cancer cells. Antibodies to a human cancer can be produced in an animal; then, anti-cancer drugs or radioactive chemicals can be attached to them. When these antibodies, with their attached payload, are injected into the patient's bloodstream, they stick to the cancer and expose it to high levels of drug or radiation, while normal cells receive a much lower exposure (see diagram). This method

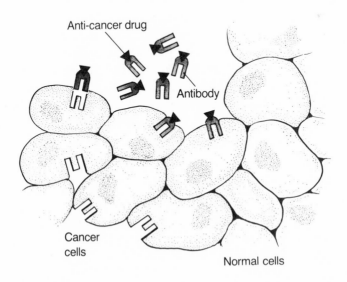

holds much promise, though it is still in its very early stages and many problems must be solved before it can be widely used.

IN SUMMARY   At present, all uses of immunity to combat cancer must be regarded as experimental. So far, stimulation of the immune system as a whole plays a very minor role in cancer treatment, and use of specific antibodies has an even smaller part. But it seems likely that help will come from basic research on the relationship between cancers and their hosts and from further study of how the immune system decides when and what to attack. One conservative guess is that by 1990, "immunological engineering" will provide important weapons for our anti-cancer armory.

Environmental Chemicals and Cancer

In the past few years a scary drama has been playing to a packed audience of television viewers and newspaper readers. The cast includes some old standbys, such as saccharin, cyclamate, and methpyrilene (best known for its role in Sominex, Nytol, Sleep-Eze, Compoz, and other over-the-counter sleep medications). Other less familiar names are tris-BP and furylfuramide. What brings them all together in one script is that they are carcinogens (cancer producers) for laboratory rodents. Because nobody knows whether they will cause cancer in humans, nobody can say how the story will end, as comedy or tragedy. This cancer concern is not just a media event; it serializes a real problem whose plot line can be hard to follow, mainly because experts genuinely disagree about what is going on. Thus, there are no simple or final answers to the question of whether these implicated chemicals produce cancer in humans. But it is important to understand the reasons for asking the question, and the methods being used to make educated guesses when final answers are impossible.

THE PRESENT FOCUS   Why the spotlight on chemicals? It has been known for well over a hundred years that certain chemical exposures *could* cause cancer in humans and in laboratory animals. Still, as recently as ten years ago, many authorities thought that hereditary factors and perhaps viruses were the major causes of cancer. Since then, newer information has pointed ever more strongly to natural or synthetic chemicals (including those in tobacco smoke) as producing the majority of human cancers.

Most of the evidence (much of it accumulated only in the last twenty years) comes from studies of the frequency of various cancers in different human groups. For example:

(1) The prevalence of the various kinds of cancer differs from one part of the world to another, but when people migrate from their home culture to a foreign one (for example, Japanese moving to the United States or European Jews to Israel), they acquire the cancer pattern of their adopted country within a couple of generations, even without intermarrying.

(2) By now there are perhaps two dozen known settings in which cancer has arisen from occupational exposure to chemicals such as dyes, asbestos, certain solvents, and plastic components.

(3) And there is the most powerful evidence of all: the death rate from lung cancer. Between 1900 and 1950, American men increased their consumption of cigarettes by about ten-fold and their death rate from lung cancer went up nearly a hundred-fold. (Women, who began smoking in earnest around World War II, are now making history repeat itself.) As John Cairns, a prominent cancer researcher, has said, "It is almost as if Western societies had set out to conduct a vast and fairly well-controlled experiment in carcinogenesis bringing about several million deaths and using their own people as the experimental animals."

While epidemiologists have been sorting out these facts about how cancer is distributed in our population, clinical and laboratory investigators have been exploring the biology of human and animal cancer. Viruses have proved to be extremely useful in producing laboratory cancers, but by now they seem unlikely to be primarily responsible for causing any of the common human cancers. As for heredity, it is important in establishing a person's susceptibility to cancer, but other factors are undoubtedly involved in causing the disease. Certainly, the common tumors are not "inherited" in very straightforward fashion.

Thus, the focus of attention is shifting to chemical causes. At this point, however, it is easy to lose perspective. The chemicals responsible for most of the cancers occurring today probably do not come from chemical factories. Even though the number of man-made chemicals in the environment has markedly increased, the overall frequency of cancer has not changed very much in the last fifty years (after lung cancer is subtracted and a statistical correction is made for the increasing proportion of older people in our population). Other chemical culprits may be natural substances, contaminants such as molds in our food, or even chemicals that are produced from food by bacteria present in our large intestine. The way food is cooked may also make a difference; charcoal broiling, for example, has been implicated in creating carcinogens.

INDUSTRY AND CANCER   Next to lung cancer, which is caused by chemicals in cigarette smoke, cancers of the colon (large intestine) and breast account for the greatest mortality, and these two diseases have hardly changed in frequency for decades. Changes in other types of cancer have occurred, however. Stomach cancer has been diminishing for several decades—nobody knows why. The death rate from cancer of the cervix has also fallen in the past thirty years. On the other hand, more deaths are being caused by cancers of the pancreas and nervous system. The leukemias increased in frequency from 1930 to 1950, but have not changed much since then. These facts suggest that changing environmental influences are at work, but they do not support the notion that our increasingly industrialized environment has, so far, produced an epidemic of new cancers in the general population.

But just because epidemiologists do not yet see evidence of a big rise in cancer deaths does not mean that it can't happen. Experience has taught us that there is a delay period; as a rule cancer usually appears ten to thirty years after exposure begins. A potent carcinogen brought into our chemical environment today would probably begin to show up as cancer deaths in the year 2000; a carcinogen introduced in 1960 could start to reveal itself any time now. The only way to be truly certain that a new chemical is carcinogenic for people is to find out over a period of time that it causes cancer. However, if the chemical were to produce cancer at fairly low rates, its effect on people might be undetected because so many other causes can contribute to the development of cancer.

TRYING TO SAFEGUARD THE FUTURE   What can be done to ward off potential epidemics? In the early years of coal mining, it is said, the miners brought canaries with them into the tunnels. The birds, being more sensitive than the men to deterioration of the atmosphere, would collapse in time to warn the miners to seek safer air. Obviously, we would all be a great deal more comfortable in making decisions about chemicals that we swallow, inhale, or rub on our skins, if we had a warning system of this kind. This is the principle that underlies present-day testing for carcinogens. Instead of canaries, modern researchers use mice, rats, hamsters, guinea pigs, or, sometimes, larger animals.

ANIMAL TESTING   For each chemical to be tested, about 500 animals are needed, of which half are not exposed while the other half receive the suspected agent in various doses. In a test of this sort, which costs about $250,000 when properly conducted, between 200 and 250 animals are put at risk. In other words, each animal is "standing in" for a *million* Americans. If animals and people were equally sensitive to the chemical, the test could easily miss carcinogens capable of causing many deaths, unless some method was used to increase the frequency of cancers in the animals. To compensate for this statistical disadvantage, the animals are usually given the highest daily dose of the chemical that they can tolerate without ill effects (other than the development of tumors). The other alternative would be to expose more animals to lower doses. But the cost of such an approach would rapidly become prohibitive, especially in light of the fact that there are as many as 63,000 chemicals in common use in the United States and of these some 5,000 have been identified as prime candidates for testing. The National Cancer Institute only has funds to test about 100 substances a year using present methods.

There is a misconception that high doses of virtually anything will produce cancer sooner or later and, thus, that the high-dose approach is bound to "invent" carcinogens which really are not injurious at common levels of exposure. In fact, many chemicals appear incapable of producing cancer at any dose compatible with life. (As scientists are becoming more knowledgeable about carcinogens in general, they are able to predict more reliably the chemicals that should be tested.)

ANIMALS AND HUMANS   When the announcement is made that a substance has been shown to produce cancer in rats or mice, a natural question is whether the same will hold true for people. The best answer to date appears to be, "Yes, maybe." Certainly, the reverse appears to be true; chemicals known to cause cancer in people also produce the disease in animals. It seems likely that people will almost always be susceptible to carcinogens that work in animals. But, and this is a big "but," people may be either more or less sensitive than the test animals. For example, the chemical 2-naphthylamine, formerly used in dye and rubber manufacture, is a potent carcinogen in people and dogs, but not in rats, mice, guinea pigs, or rabbits.

The most crucial and highly controversial question about the high-dose technique of testing for potential carcinogens is whether the ability of a substance to cause cancer changes in direct proportion to the amount an animal (or person) is exposed to. (It's like asking: If a hundred men can paint a house in one hour, how long will it take one man? A hundred hours? Maybe not. He might work faster without all the others to stumble over, or he might get frustrated and never finish. Simple arithmetic doesn't always give the right answers to real-world problems.) Some people have argued that a carcinogen may be completely ineffective below a certain level because there is a "threshold" below which it cannot cause cancer. Other scientists even theorize that an agent may be proportionately more potent at low doses because of differences in the way the body handles small amounts of a chemical. The problem has not been resolved, and because the answer has enormous economic implications, the debate has been fairly heated.

The government's position has been that nothing may be added to food if it has been shown to cause cancer in a well-conducted animal test (this is a provision known as the "Delaney clause"). The official rule is based on the assumption that thresholds do not exist, that is, lowering the dose of a carcinogen may result in fewer cancers but some people are still going to get cancer from even a low level of exposure. The policy implicit in the Delaney clause is that no exposure in food additives is worth the risk.

OTHER SCREENING TECHNIQUES   Crude as they may be, animal tests are expensive and time-consuming; they present a formidable barrier to anyone hoping to test the thousand-odd chemicals introduced each year, not to mention those already in use. New systems for evaluating carcinogens may help us out of this bind. They are based on the fact that chemical carcinogens produce their effects by damaging DNA in cells of the body. In other words, they produce mutations. If a mutation occurs in a sperm or egg cell, one's offspring may be affected by the genetic damage. If the mutation occurs elsewhere, that cell may begin to behave abnormally within the body and go on to the kind of unregulated growth that we call cancer.

Capitalizing on the fact that carcinogens act by producing mutations, researchers have developed several tests that use bacteria or cultured animal cells to display such mutations. The best known of these is the Ames test, named after its developer, Bruce Ames, of the University of California, Berkeley. In this system, slightly abnormal bacteria are placed under conditions in which a mutation is required for them to thrive and grow within their carefully controlled environment. When they are exposed to a chemical that causes mutations (a carcinogen), the bacteria begin to multiply, which would mean a positive test. If no growth of bacteria occurs, the test is regarded as negative.

The Ames test is much less expensive and much more rapid than animal testing, yet its results appear to correspond rather closely to the results obtained in animal tests. It may become possible by using the Ames test to identify prime suspects in the world of chemicals and then, if need be, subject them to further testing with animals. There is even some hope that the relative potency of various carcinogens can be determined in this system.

IN SUMMARY   Improved techniques will not, in the end, make decisions about carcinogens for us. To be sure, poor or insufficient testing may lead to either excessively restrictive or inappropriately lax policies. Because animal testing is cumbersome and subject to human error, there have been frequent disputes about results obtained with relatively weak carcinogens, such as saccharin. Even with very good testing, however, certain questions may always remain unanswered: How comparable are animals and people? How much of a threat are low doses of a "proved" carcinogen? Is it possible that one low-risk chemical will interact with others in the environment to increase the threat it poses to people?

And there are other questions that cannot be scientifically answered because they are matters of economic and moral choice. Is the benefit from, say, an artificial sweetener worth the potential risk that it poses? What reason is sufficiently compelling to allow a potential carcinogen into the human environment? Should a policy of absolute prohibition in food and drugs be modified, and whose interest is served by doing so? Unfortunately, there are no easy answers when scientific uncertainty coexists with disagreements on values.

Cancer Chemotherapy

Chemotherapy has become a familiar term to many people, but it is often misunderstood. Dr. Sheldon D. Kaufman, Associate Clinical Professor of Medicine, Harvard Medical School, and a medical specialist in cancer at Massachusetts General Hospital, tells us what chemotherapy has accomplished and how it is changing.

What is cancer chemotherapy?

In general, cancer can be treated with surgery, radiation, hormone therapy, or chemotherapy. Surgery is used to remove localized cancer with the goal of cutting the entire tumor out. X-ray or other forms of radiation are used to destroy a cancer when it is too widespread for the surgeon to reach all of it or when it is in a location that is too dangerous to approach via an operation. For the treatment of some tumors, radiation is the first choice. Hormones, or synthetic substances resembling them, can be used to suppress the growth of certain tumors.

Chemotherapy, as the name implies, refers to chemicals that are used to kill malignant cells. Although these drugs may also shorten the lifespan of normal cells, their greatest effect is on the cancerous ones. It is a common misconception that chemotherapy means a single drug or group of drugs used for all types of cancer. In reality, some 45 to 50 different agents are available. Although they may be given singly, they are increasingly used in various combinations. Not only is each type of cancer treated by a specific drug or group of drugs, but two people with the same kind of cancer may be treated with different programs because the details of their illnesses differ.

Has there been a major breakthrough in chemotherapy?

Not in the sense that a single wonder drug has swept everything else aside. Rather, there has been a substantial increase in the number of helpful drugs, although each of them has limitations. The variety of such agents now available and the strategy of using them in combination have made it possible for us to treat an ever-increasing number of cancers with chemotherapy. Many types of cancer that now are successfully treated weren't touched by drugs available five years ago. In each of these diseases it is not just one "magic bullet" that works. If a tumor is sensitive to chemotherapy in the first place, usually more than one drug can be used for treatment. But in some cases of advanced or resistant cancer, the benefit of chemotherapy is very brief or nonexistent.

The successes, nevertheless, have been real—though to date the best results have been achieved in relatively rare cancers, such as acute leukemia in children. The outlook for this disease has gone from being uniformly fatal—months after diagnosis—to being highly treatable. Patients can now expect to be free of the disease for long periods and usually without significant discomfort from the side effects of treatment. In many cases this form of cancer has been *cured* by chemotherapy. Hodgkin's disease was once uniformly fatal but now is highly treatable with intensive radiation or chemotherapy. Cancer of the testis also responds well to chemotherapy and can sometimes be cured. These diseases, although uncommon, usually affect young and otherwise healthy people, so cures save many productive years.

Many of us feel it is only a matter of time until we begin to make progress with more common cancers also. Recently there have been exciting reports of dramatic responses of one type of lung cancer, the so-called oat cell carcinoma. This is one of the most aggressive of tumors and accounts for about one-fifth of all lung cancers. Lung cancer itself is so common that new patients with the oat cell type of cancer number nearly 20,000 a year. Now this cancer can be treated with chemotherapy and, in a few cases, cure seems possible. What made the difference was a willingness to use combinations of agents in doses high enough to eradicate the disease even though toxicity was considerable.

It is important to bear in mind that progress in cancer treatment has not come about as a result of looking for a cure as soon as a new treatment is introduced. The first evidence of an advance comes from temporary disappearance of tumor masses in patients who already have advanced disease. Once that kind of response is obtained, then long-term control or possible cure becomes a plausible goal.

Do patients receiving chemotherapy always suffer from side effects?

Patients often expect chemotherapy to make their hair fall out or to have effects that make people miserable. But it's important to realize that there are many types of treatment in which the side effects are truly minimal. Hair loss, for example, doesn't always happen, even in cases where we expect it, and it is always temporary.

Other undesirable effects occur, to be sure, but they are extremely variable. Many of the drugs and drug combinations, but not all of them, produce nausea and vomiting. The patient may be nauseated for a while right after a treatment, but treatment is almost always given at weekly or longer intervals. On average, patients lose an hour or a few hours to discomfort—not days. Nausea lasting more than a few hours might be a clear signal to alter the dose or the program. Also, we are better able to control nausea with medication than we used to be, and tetrahydrocannabinol (THC, the active ingredient in marijuana) appears particularly promising. Chemotherapy has other, potentially more worrisome, effects; these include suppression of the blood-forming tissue and of the ability to fight infection. The extent to which these effects are acceptable depends largely on the goals of treatment. If the stakes are high—for example, potential cure—intense or prolonged reactions may be acceptable to both doctor and patient.

Despite a common belief, most patients do not have to be admitted to the hospital for chemotherapy. In 90% of cases, it can be administered in a doctor's office or other outpatient setting with the proper staff. To be sure, treatment often can't be given at home because many of these drugs must be given by injection, usually into a vein. But a great effort is now being made to keep patients at home, working, and living their lives with a minimum of interference from their treatment programs.

Is chemotherapy always a "last-ditch" measure in cancer treatment?

Definitely not. Chemotherapy is now often used as an early treatment. It is even used as a precautionary measure. In breast cancer, for example, a patient may be at high risk for later recurrence even though surgery (or radiation) has apparently been successful. In such a case, adjuvant chemotherapy is often given as a measure against potential recurrence. Such treatment is employed intermittently over a long time—a year or two—and almost without exception, patients carry on their normal activities.

Thyroid Abnormalities

The thyroid gland weighs less than an ounce and occupies a butter-fly-shaped space below the Adam's apple—straddling the windpipe with "wings" on each side (see diagram). But from this prominent command post, this delicate gland secretes hormones that literally control the pace of metabolism in the cells of our body. And that metabolic rate, if abnormal, can in turn cause upheavals in body function ranging from life-threatening heart disease to dramatic emotional disturbance. Despite the importance of the thyroid to continuing good health, it remains shrouded in mystery for many. This essay, therefore, describes briefly the major problems that can develop with thyroid function—with special emphasis on early recognition of possible thyroid troubles.

AN OVERVIEW   The thyroid gland produces its hormones (under the control of the hypothalamus and pituitary gland of the brain) by extracting iodide from the bloodstream, converting it to iodine, and hooking it to amino acids; the resulting hormones are carried on proteins to the cells of our body. Once there, these hormones function in several ways not yet fully understood to promote the process by which cells transform nutrients into energy. Apparently, the thyroid is the only tissue in the human body that uses iodine. And even though the gland's daily requirement for iodine is minimal, the absence of iodine in the diet can lead to real trouble—expressed visibly by the growth of excessive thyroid tissue (known as a goiter) in the front of the neck. Such growth represents the gland's frantic attempt to capture iodine. The widespread use of iodized salt today compensates for diets lacking in iodine, but there are still many areas of the world where enlarged necks are a common result of diets deficient in iodine.

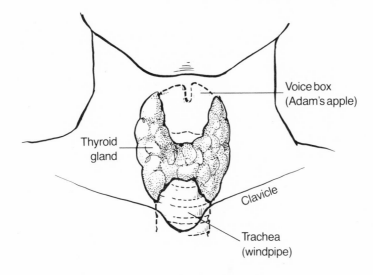

Voice box
(Adam's apple)

Thyroid
gland

Clavicle

Trachea
(windpipe)

Until the 1960s, the most common method of checking thyroid function was to assess indirectly the effects of thyroid hormones by various crude and cumbersome determinations of the so-called BMR—basal metabolic rate. Today, physicians have many more direct tests of thyroid function available, including measures of actual thyroid hormone. A discussion of these many tests—and their appropriate use—is far beyond the scope of this essay; suffice it to say that thyroid experts (usually the sub-specialists in gland diseases known as endocrinologists) can almost always pinpoint the many different kinds of thyroid troubles that may occur. And for purposes of our survey, we will describe these troubles under four categories.

HYPERTHYROIDISM This word refers to any condition in which the thyroid gland produces more thyroid hormone than the body needs. The most common form of an overactive thyroid gland is known as Graves' disease, a condition in which the entire thyroid gland enlarges and produces too much hormone. And while the exact causes of this condition are not fully understood, its recognition and treatment are well established and can be briefly described as follows:

(1) Symptoms: The classic picture painted throughout the body by an overactive thyroid gland is well known—excessive sweating

often accompanied by heat intolerance; palpitations of the heart; nervousness, irritability, insomnia; hand tremors; and weight loss despite a good appetite. In other words, the body is "revved up." Often these symptoms are accompanied by eye changes resulting in a "bulging" appearance; when very severe, these eye problems can lead to actual visual loss. A careful physical exam and selected tests of thyroid function can usually quickly confirm the presence of an overactive gland. Sometimes excessive thyroid function results in symptoms more limited to one system, such as the onset—or worsening—of heart problems in the elderly, the development of muscular weakness, unexplained weight loss, or major personality changes. Again, however, the wise use of thyroid tests—and a high degree of suspicion—should uncover these less typical cases of hyperthyroidism.

(2) Treatment: Once the diagnosis is established, three methods of reducing thyroid hormone production are available. Several effective and relatively safe *drugs* are available which act to interfere with hormone production by the gland. These drugs are usually given for about a year, after which they may be totally discontinued in about 30% of patients; the remainder need continuing drug therapy or other forms of treatment. *Surgical removal* of enough of the thyroid gland to reduce function to a proper level has the advantage of being a more permanent solution; however, such operations should be performed by surgeons experienced in this area because complications (including damage to vocal cord nerves) can be serious. *Radioactive iodine* is widely used today as a method of nonsurgically destroying thyroid tissue. Though there is no evidence that such treatment causes later malignancy, many physicians still prefer to reserve radioactive iodine for persons over age 40, minimizing the number of years during which malignancy might develop. The choice of treatment will depend very much on the specific condition and wishes of a given patient. Regardless of which treatment method is used, *a lifelong commitment to periodic check-ups is critical* since all treatment methods eventually lead to a significant number of "over-treatment" results—in which thyroid function swings to the other extreme of too little hormone.

HYPOTHYROIDISM This label refers to the consequence of having too little thyroid hormone; there are many underlying causes such as diseases of the brain areas (hypothalamus and pituitary) which regulate the thyroid gland, actual destruction of thyroid tissue by inflammation or excessive therapy for hyperthyroidism (see above), and reduced gland function due to insufficient iodine in the diet. These many different causes usually lead to a similar constellation of symptoms which should point to the possibility of low-thyroid hormone levels—and lead to tests to clinch the diagnosis.

(1) Symptoms: The classic symptoms of hypothyroidism include cold intolerance, dry and sometimes thickened skin, hoarse voice, constipation, slow speech, weight gain, general apathy and fatigue, and emotional changes easily confused with depression. (The extreme form of these symptoms—including possible coma—is often referred to as myxedema.) However, like hyperthyroidism, thyroid hormone deficiency may show only mild or isolated symptoms that could easily be mistaken for other problems; the classic—and often tragic—confusion is that of hypothyroidism "written off" as depression or dementia. Often the progression of hypothyroidism is so gradual that close friends and family may not notice it; sometimes a comparison of present appearance to an old picture provides dramatic evidence of the long-term change.

(2) Treatment: Treatment for hypothyroidism—which consists of giving either synthetic or natural thyroid hormone (from animal sources)—is both simple and safe. Indeed, hypothyroidism is one of the easiest human diseases to treat; it is tragic if someone suffers unnecessarily from this problem. Treatment involves a lifelong commitment to periodic check-ups to discover changing medication requirements. It is also important to stress that many persons in the past (before more precise tests for thyroid function were available) were thought to be "low" in thyroid function and then placed on thyroid replacement without firm documentation of actual hypothyroidism. Such persons may now be taking thyroid medication without need and usually without jeopardy—although larger doses can produce symptoms of hyperthyroidism. Obviously, anyone who suspects this possibility should check with a competent physician.

THYROID NODULES   Both "hyper" and "hypo" gland function can result in generalized thyroid enlargement. Thyroid glands can also become enlarged in the absence of abnormal function. These "simple goiters," as they are sometimes called, are generally harmless unless they grow to such a size that they compress the windpipe—in which case surgery may be necessary for relief. Of more concern—and usually more difficult to diagnose and treat—is the development of an isolated area of enlargement known as a "nodule." The basic question is whether or not such an isolated enlargement is benign or malignant. And the answer usually demands the special skills of a thyroid specialist, who may resort to several diagnostic techniques (including scanning and ultrasound studies and often requiring actual biopsy) before deciding whether or not surgery is appropriate. Fortunately, the vast majority of thyroid cancers are slow-growing, usually allowing discovery in time for adequate treatment. In recent years, special emphasis has been placed on the long-term risk of thyroid cancer resulting from irradiation treatment to the head and neck area (common in previous years for conditions ranging from acne to tonsillitis). While some recent data suggest that this risk may have been overemphasized, most experts believe that the link between irradiation and thyroid cancer is real and consequently advise that persons with a known history of such irradiation be carefully examined at least yearly.

CONGENITAL HYPOTHYROIDISM   Studies now indicate that approximately one of every 5,000 children is born with abnormally low thyroid function which, if not quickly corrected, can result in the devastating physical and mental retardation known as cretinism. Fortunately, such problems can be minimized by routine screening for thyroid function in all newborns—a practice now required by many states. Hypothyroidism may also develop later in infancy or childhood with symptoms similar to those of adults; again, early detection and treatment are essential in preventing developmental abnormalities.

IN SUMMARY   Thyroid abnormalities can usually be accurately diagnosed and adequately treated—*if* symptoms are recognized and proper screening (especially of infants and adults with a history of irradiation) is instituted. Persons who have been treated for excessive (hyper) or decreased (hypo) function require lifelong follow-up to detect possible changes in thyroid function.

Ulcers

Peptic ulcers are erosions of the surface lining of the gastrointestinal tract and are roughly comparable in appearance to canker sores of the mouth. Ulcers can occur in any area exposed to stomach juices, but the vast majority of ulcers occur in two locations (see diagram)—in the first part of the small intestine (duodenal ulcer) and, less commonly, in the stomach itself (gastric ulcer). While the symptoms of these two kinds of ulcer are generally similar, their implications are significantly different—as described below.

CAUSES   Our understanding of why ulcers form, as they do in approximately 10% of all Americans at some time in their lives, is only partial. We know that stomach acid is necessary for ulcers to occur—and that, in general, persons with *duodenal* ulcers tend to secrete more acid than normal. Yet, many such patients do not have excessive acid, so other factors (such as decreased tissue resistance or cigarettes, which inhibit the flow of neutralizing juice from the pancreas) must also be considered. Many patients with *gastric* ulcers may actually have diminished amounts of acid secretion; substances that damage the lining of the stomach—such as aspirin, alcohol, and bile—probably make the stomach more vulnerable to the effects of the reduced acid that is present. It is accepted by most physicians that personality plays a role in producing or prolonging duodenal ulcers, but mysteries remain. For example, many tense people never get ulcers, while many placid people do. There is no good evidence that special foods—spicy or hot—are more likely to cause ulcers; as one wag put it, "It's not what you eat but what eats you." All of this boils down to the fact that there is very little honest advice to be given as to how to avoid an ulcer—other than the generally useless recommendation to "take it easy."

323

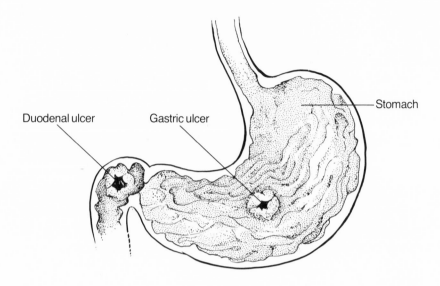

SYMPTOMS   The characteristic symptom of an ulcer is upper abdominal pain which occurs when the stomach is empty and which is relieved by ingesting food or bland liquids. Thus, the typical pattern is pain several hours *after* a meal (when the stomach has emptied) and during the wee hours of the night—between midnight and 2 A.M. Surprisingly, pain before breakfast is unusual in ulcer disease. (Note that this pain pattern differs from that of typical gallbladder disease, which may be triggered, rather than relieved, by eating.) However, many people with ulcers have distress that is not typical and might be more accurately described as "aching" or "gnawing." At times, *gastric* ulcer symptoms may even be worsened by eating. *Any* persistent discomfort is worth checking out.

DIAGNOSIS   Once a physician suspects an ulcer, standard diagnostic tools are available for confirmation. Most common is the famous "upper GI series" in which barium is swallowed while x-rays are taken to outline the stomach and small intestine. Such x-rays will clearly demonstrate a "crater" in about two-thirds of patients. When an actual crater cannot be shown, other x-ray signs may strongly suggest ulcer disease. Occasionally, further studies—such as stomach-acid analysis—may be helpful, but in the majority of duodenal ulcers, an upper GI series is all that's required. But this is not true of most gastric ulcers. Unlike duodenal ulcers, a small percentage (approximately 4%) of gastric ulcers are in fact cancers that *look* like ulcers by x-ray. Therefore, malignant disease must be first ruled out when a "gastric ulcer" is seen on x-ray. Most experts believe that anyone with an initial diagnosis of gastric ulcer should have gastroscopy performed; this involves the insertion of a flexible and lighted tube (fiberoptics makes this possible) into the stomach to visually inspect the ulcer directly and to obtain tissue and cell-washing samples. Such additional study greatly improves the chance of accurately determining whether a stomach ulcer is benign or malignant. Again, it must be stressed that most gastric ulcers are not malignant. But the fact that some might be makes gastroscopy advisable in most cases.

TREATMENT   A vast number of diets and programs for treating ulcers have been advocated over the years. However, their value cannot be assessed until we agree on what is meant by healing; in many cases, the ulcer may persist even when symptoms are relieved. Also, ulcers tend to get better on their own, in the absence of any specific therapy; the natural behavior of the disease may be responsible for the improvement falsely attributed to one or another treatment program. Nevertheless, the following comments will provide some overview on ulcer treatment:

(1) Diet: While "milk and cream diets" seem to be effective in relieving severe symptoms at the peak of an ulcer attack, there is no evidence that continuing such feedings are important in healing the ulcer. (Indeed, there may be mild risk to prolonged high-fat diets in those prone to coronary disease.) Frequent small meals—on the average of six a day—are recommended when an ulcer is "active." But once the symptoms have subsided, there is little reason to remain on a restrictive dietary program other than to avoid any particular food or beverage that causes distress.

(2) Antacids: It is common experience that antacids relieve stomach distress, and antacids have been shown to accelerate ulcer healing when they are taken frequently in large amounts (for example, 2 tablespoons seven times a day). Some of the most effective antacids contain magnesium, the active ingredient of milk of magnesia; thus, diarrhea is often a complication of high-dose treatment.

When antacids are used in smaller amounts, they are most effective in preventing symptoms when they are taken 1–2 hours after completing a meal, and when liquid (rather than tablet) preparations are used. Calcium-containing acids should be used sparingly, if at all; large amounts ingested over prolonged periods can cause kidney damage. Moreover, calcium actually stimulates the stomach to secrete acid.

(3) Cimetidine (Tagamet): Cimetidine is the exciting new drug that many physicians now turn to first in treating active ulcers. Unlike the traditional antacids, which act by neutralizing the acid secreted by the stomach, cimetidine actually inhibits the acid from being secreted in the first place. It has been shown to accelerate duodenal ulcer healing, and has relatively few side effects when taken on a short-term basis. However, like all new drugs, its dangers will not really be known until it has been widely used for many years. The recommendation that cimetidine be used on a short-term basis (for example, 1–2 months), rather than chronically, is prudent at this time.

(4) Other drugs: A variety of other drugs, including minor tranquilizers and the so-called anticholinergics, are still used in ulcer treatment. For selected patients, they may be of some value. A relatively modest dose of the anticholinergic drug propantheline has been shown to be just as effective in reducing acid formation as larger doses that so often produce prominent side effects.

(5) Surgery: While the majority of ulcer patients will never need surgery, complications may occur in approximately 15% of such patients that make an operation necessary. These include severe or repeated bleeding episodes, perforation (where the ulcer breaks through the wall of the stomach or duodenum), and obstruction of flow out of the stomach (due to scar tissue). Most difficult to assess is the patient with "intractable pain"—pain that continues even in the face of intensive medical treatment. Since such a problem is not immediately life threatening, careful consideration must be given to all factors before surgery is recommended. Several types of operations are available for ulcer disease. They are reasonably safe (with mortality rates below 1%) and effective in relieving symptoms, with recurrence of ulcer disease ranging from 2 to 10%. However, surgery can cause other digestive problems such as diarrhea and weight loss in some patients, so that there is good reason to use caution in the decision to operate.

IN SUMMARY   Ulcers are common and usually easy to diagnose and treat. Though ulcers tend to recur, most persons will not need surgery. Gastric (stomach) ulcers—unlike duodenal ulcers—are malignant in a small number of cases and must be investigated thoroughly.

Heartburn and Hiatus Hernia

Nearly everyone has experienced heartburn at one time or another; its description as a glowing fire beneath the sternum (breastbone) is familiar. But for those who are plagued by frequent heartburn, concern about a "hiatus hernia" arises. When this is reported to a physician, his concern may turn to "reflux esophagitis." The purpose of this essay is to make sense out of these terms and, most important, to describe how heartburn sufferers can relieve their misery—which has nothing to do with the heart.

A BIT OF ANATOMY   The story of heartburn must focus on the lower end of the esophagus (foodpipe) just above the point where it leaves the chest by passing through the diaphragm to join the stomach (see diagram). Normally, the opening (hiatus) through the diaphragm is tight enough to prevent the stomach from slipping up into the chest cavity. When that hiatus is too wide, a portion of the stomach may ride up into the chest; the anatomical result is described as a "hiatus hernia." This, in itself, need not be associated with heartburn. Rather, another structure—the *lower esophageal sphincter (LES)*—seems to be more important. *The LES is that area of "muscular squeezing" by the wall of the lower esophagus that determines whether or not irritating stomach juices will back up into the esophagus.* When the LES is too weak, backflow will occur. Irritation of the lower esophagus by acid stomach juices is termed *reflux* (meaning "a backward flow") *esophagitis* (meaning "inflammation of the esophagus"). In brief, heartburn is best understood as a symptom caused by excessive backflow of stomach juice—due to a *weak* LES.

Here the plot thickens—because a weak LES can occur independently of a hiatus hernia. Thus, heartburn may occur in the ab-

328

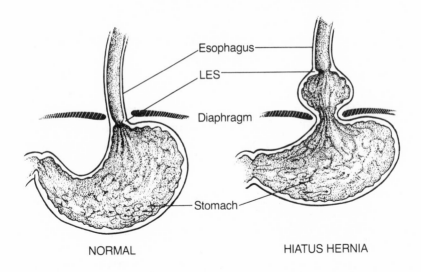

Esophagus

LES

Diaphragm

Stomach

NORMAL HIATUS HERNIA

sence of a hiatus hernia. Conversely, hiatus hernias (when looked for) can be seen on barium x-ray in so many *normal* persons—up to 50% in some series—that it is evident they often cause no problem whatsoever. In short, there is no sure correlation between the presence of a hiatus hernia and a weak LES. Although heartburn occurs more often in persons with hiatus hernias, even in them it is usually due to a lax LES.

DIAGNOSIS OF REFLUX   Often heartburn is described in classic form—a burning feeling under the breastbone after eating a large or spicy meal and accentuated by lying down or bending over. In this instance, many doctors would not even bother with further testing before initiating treatment. At other times, though, reflux can produce more confusing symptoms, such as sharper pain that may radiate to the jaw or arms mimicking angina caused by coronary artery disease. In such cases, it is obviously essential to distinguish reflux esophagitis from angina. Certain points may be helpful—such as the fact that anginal pain is exercise-related and the discomfort produced by reflux occurs after meals and is worsened by lying down. However, there are times when special testing may be needed to pinpoint the cause of the pain. Tests aimed at evaluating reflux include barium x-rays, direct inspection of the lower esophagus with a flexible optic tube (endoscope), and the use of swallowed tubes to measure LES pressure or acidity within the lower esophagus. But these are not necessary for most patients with "garden variety" heartburn.

TREATMENT   Once it is understood that heartburn is essentially a problem caused by backflow of acid juices into the esophagus, the rationale for various treatment approaches becomes evident. These include:

(1) Decreasing backflow: Anything that reduces reflux is useful in treating heartburn. Mechanical measures include the avoidance of large meals that overdistend the stomach; remaining in an upright position for several hours following a meal; eliminating tight-fitting belts and girdles; and using six-inch bedblocks under the bedposts at the head of the bed. Weight loss, for obese persons, is also helpful. Substances that are known to weaken the LES should also be avoided: tobacco, alcohol, chocolate, garlic, onion, coffee, and even peppermint are notorious offenders. The use of bethanecol, a drug that *strengthens* the LES, has proved helpful for some persons. On the other hand, estrogens—which *decrease* the "tone" of the LES— may *aggravate* heartburn. (Therefore, pregnant women have two reasons for heartburn—increased abdominal pressure and higher estrogen levels.)

(2) Antacids: Neutralization of stomach acid by conventional antacid drugs reduces the tendency of refluxed juices to irritate the esophagus. Similarly, cimetidine (which blocks the production of stomach acid) relieves heartburn and related symptoms.

(3) Surgery: When heartburn coexists with a hiatus hernia, repair of the hiatus hernia will very often relieve the symptoms. This is because the modern and more successful techniques of hiatus hernia repair have been shown to result in a *strengthening* of the LES. So once again, although the hernia may "be there," it's probably an abnormal sphincter that's the culprit. However, surgery for heartburn is advisable only after all of the non-surgical approaches described above fail. Less than 10% of persons with typical reflux esophagitis should ever need an operation. Those who develop severe bleeding or critical narrowing of the esophagus are more likely to require surgery. Aside from the cost, discomfort, and risk, late after-effects (such as "trapped gas" problems) can be more troublesome than the

symptoms that prompted the operation. Seeking a second opinion about proposed hiatus hernia surgery is a good idea, especially when the proposal comes before all non-surgical measures have been adequately tried.

Bowel Disease

Our society has sometimes been described as "bowelcentric." Indeed, some people can recount a history of recent bowel patterns better than they can remember their spouse's birthday. Obviously, we do not mean to belittle legitimate concern about changing bowel patterns or other symptoms suggestive of important disease. Fortunately, existing diagnostic tools—combined with a careful "listen" to the patient's story—can almost always sort out a serious underlying problem from temporary changes in bowel function. This essay focuses on inflammatory bowel disease, the irritable bowel, and diverticulosis—three disorders of the intestines (the terms *bowel* and *intestine* are synonymous) which are often confused with one another in terminology and significance. The territory involved is portrayed in the diagram. It is worth noting that:

(1) The first part of the intestinal tract, named the *small intestine* because it is narrow compared to the large intestine, consists of about 20 feet of coiled tubing responsible for absorbing nutrients as food passes through; the last segment of the small intestine, which connects to the abdomen, is known as the *ileum.*

(2) The five-foot long *large intestine* (or *colon*) functions mainly to absorb water and thus convert the waste from the small intestine from liquid to solid. It ends in a twisted portion (in the left lower part of the abdomen) known as the *sigmoid colon* which in turn empties into the rectum.

INFLAMMATORY BOWEL DISEASE (IBD) Though less common than the other two bowel problems to be discussed, IBD is potentially far more serious. IBD exists in two major forms:

(1) Crohn's disease: Named after the doctor who first described it, Crohn's disease is characterized by thickening and inflammation

332

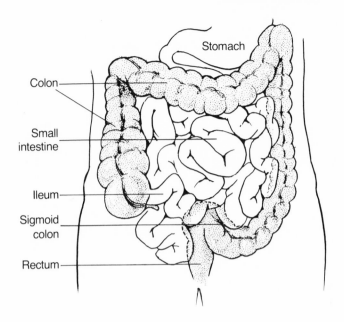

that tends to involve the full width of the wall of the intestine. When Crohn's disease is found in the last segment of the small intestine (the ileum), it is called *terminal ileitis,* or if other regions of the small intestine are involved, *regional enteritis.* Since the ileum is located in the right lower abdomen, symptoms (pain and tenderness) are often felt there during an attack of ileitis. The colon can also be affected by Crohn's disease, and the term "granulomatous colitis" (which refers to microscopic abnormalities) has been used interchangeably with Crohn's disease of the colon.

(2) Ulcerative colitis: In this form of IBD, the inflammation typically consists of ulcerations confined to the innermost lining of the colon; the small intestine is healthy. At times, the lining of the entire colon becomes inflamed; in cases of more limited involvement, the sigmoid and rectal areas are usually affected and discomfort is experienced in the lower left part of the abdomen. Rectal bleeding is common in ulcerative colitis, but may occur in Crohn's disease as well.

While these two variants of IBD are generally thought to be separate diseases, they share many features. In some cases of IBD of the colon, it may be impossible for a pathologist to be absolutely certain whether the underlying process is ulcerative colitis or Crohn's disease. There are other similarities as well:

(1) Cause: The bottom line for both Crohn's disease and ulcerative colitis is that "the cause is unknown." Each tends to occur most often in younger people and to display some familial tendency—though "inherited" would be far too strong a word to describe this pattern. Both diseases can produce specific problems outside the intestine (skin changes, arthritis, eye inflammation) suggesting a "body-wide" process. While viruses and bacteria are being investigated as possible causes, there is no evidence that either ulcerative colitis or Crohn's disease is contagious. Despite the fact that persons with severe complications of IBD are often affected emotionally, few would seriously contend that emotions are the initiating cause. The same patients often return to excellent spirits after their illness improves.

(2) Treatment: The course of IBD can be quite variable—with periods of activity alternating with quiescence. However, when the disease flares, treatment expertise is required to select the proper anti-inflammatory medications (steroids and sulfasalazine are the mainstays) and to handle complications such as abscess formation, fistulas (unwanted pathways from the intestine to other organs such as the bladder), and bowel obstruction. These complications occur mainly in Crohn's disease and often require surgery. The latter is usually done to alleviate the complications; surgery cannot be regarded as curative for Crohn's disease. Even after removal of affected portions of bowel, the disease tends to recur in intestine that remains. On the other hand, surgical removal of the entire colon will almost always restore a person who has long suffered from active ulcerative colitis to normal health; the "trade-off" is an ileostomy, by which the small intestine empties directly into a disposable bag attached to the abdominal wall. Chronically ill patients usually accept this in exchange for a return to good health, and most lead very normal lives thereafter. A newer surgical procedure—the so-called continent ileostomy—does not require a drainage bag to be attached, but the operation is trickier and later surgical revisions are often necessary.

(3) Cancer risk? This is a real concern, especially for persons with ulcerative colitis involving the entire colon for more than ten

years. They are clearly at a high risk for the development of colon cancer; the risk has been quoted as high as 2% per year—or 20% over each succeeding decade. Until now, one of the compelling reasons for removing the colon in such persons—aside from symptom relief—has been the prevention of possible cancer. Current efforts are being directed at improving methods of screening for cancer in ulcerative colitis patients, using colonoscopy and multiple biopsies of tissue to look for warning changes that would argue for surgery. While cancer of the small intestine is extremely rare, persons with ileitis are apparently at increased risk for this form of cancer—but this problem is not as great as the cancer risk in longstanding ulcerative colitis.

Much more could be said about inflammatory bowel disease. For those who wish further information, brochures are available from the National Foundation for Ileitis and Colitis, 295 Madison Avenue, New York, NY 10017.

DIVERTICULOSIS   As many as a third of all persons over age fifty in Western countries will develop sac-like outpouchings of the large intestine (colon) known as diverticula; this condition is called diverticul*osis*. The majority of persons so affected will never experience any symptoms or complications—and will find out about their diverticula only because they show up on a barium enema examination obtained for an often unrelated complaint. In other words, the mere presence of diverticula is not a "disease" but an anatomical "fact of life." However, approximately 15% of persons with diverticula will eventually develop inflammation within them—a condition known as diverticul*itis*.

There is great current interest in the possible role of dietary fiber in preventing the formation of diverticula. Studies have documented a lower incidence of diverticulosis in populations with higher fiber intake than that of Western countries. Some experts have postulated that fiber reduces the amount of pressure inside the colon required to evacuate feces—and lowering the pressure might, in turn, result in a decreased tendency to "push out" diverticula. Also, the development of inflammation in existing diverticula may be caused by impacting fecaliths—hard masses of feces that become trapped within the outpouchings; high dietary fiber may prevent fecaliths from forming. Current advice for persons with diverticula is to try to increase "roughage" (such as bran, wholegrain bread, and whole fruits), versus former recommendations that favored low-roughage diets.

The following complications may occur in persons with diverticula:

(1) Inflammation: As mentioned above, some persons with diverticula will develop inflammation in areas of outpouching. This occurs more commonly in men than in women—and more often on the left side than on the right, which is why diverticulitis is sometimes described as "left-sided appendicitis." Indeed, the symptoms may be similar—crampy or steady pain with local tenderness. Many attacks are mild and resolve without treatment.

(2) "Free" perforation: Just like an inflamed appendix, an inflamed diverticulum can also burst and give rise to an inflammation of the entire abdomen cavity, called "generalized peritonitis," a situation requiring surgery.

(3) Bleeding: About 25% of inflammatory attacks are associated with minuscule bleeding. Heavy bleeding—usually from the erosion of a large blood vessel in the diverticular sac—is uncommon but may require surgery if medical treatment is unsuccessful. A new approach to diverticular bleeding involves angiographic techniques that permit the insertion of a hollow tube (under x-ray guidance) into the vessel responsible for bleeding—followed by the injection of materials which obstruct or constrict the vessel, thereby stopping the bleeding.

(4) Abscesses and fistulas: Sometimes inflammatory changes produce areas of walled-off infection (abscesses) or abnormal anatomic pathways (fistulas) into nearby organs such as the bladder or vagina. Here again, surgical correction is often necessary.

(5) Obstruction: Inflammation can also lead to a narrowing of the width of the colon, resulting in partial or complete obstruction. Apart from obvious mechanical problems posed by obstruction, it is important to distinguish such changes—as they appear on x-ray—from similar ones that might be caused by cancer of the colon. Indeed, since both the symptoms and the anatomical changes of colon cancer and complicated diverticulitis can be similar, it is occasionally necessary to resort to such techniques as colonoscopy or exploratory surgery to distinguish between the two.

In short, diverticula are harmless changes most of the time, but they can cause serious complications and even confusion with cancer of the colon.

IRRITABLE BOWEL SYNDROME   This condition turns out to be the most common chronic abdominal disorder seen by physicians and is known by many colorful and descriptive names—spastic colon, nervous bowel, mucous colitis, or, as the British sometimes put it, "intestinal hurry." Unfortunately, some physicians have described this syndrome to their patients as a "touch of colitis"—thus unnecessarily confusing it with the more serious disease, ulcerative colitis. And that confusion is easily abetted by the fact that the initial symptoms of the two conditions may be similar—abdominal pain, diarrhea, uncomfortable defecation. However, in terms of ultimate course and consequence, they are quite different.

In brief, the irritable bowel syndrome primarily refers to a disturbed state of intestinal contractions for which no anatomic cause can be found. In other words, the patient with irritable bowel syndrome has real symptoms—typically crampy abdominal pain, often with accompanying gassiness, diarrhea, or constipation—but a diagnostic search for cancer, diverticulitis, ulcerative colitis, or Crohn's disease fails to turn up the anatomic deformities characteristic of these problems. What is often found—or at times only suspected—is an abnormal pattern of motility—the muscular contractions of the intestines which propel food and feces along. Excessive spasm may be seen on a barium enema or by sigmoidoscopy; more sensitive techniques for measuring colon contractions are available only in highly specialized laboratories. As mentioned, the problem is essentially disordered motility.

So here comes the question some of you have been waiting for: *Is the irritable bowel syndrome a real disease?* If you insist that a disease must have anatomic changes that can be seen on x-ray or under the microscope, the answer may be "no." But if you are willing to accept that motility problems can be just as real as deranged anatomy, then the answer must be "yes." There is little doubt that emotional factors play a role—sometimes a strong one—in this syndrome. Therefore, psychotherapy—or at least some humane understanding—can be very important in the treatment of this problem. Dietary manipulations and drugs to "settle" the intestine may also be useful. But patience—and careful explanation of the underlying problem—are probably the most important components of therapy for persons with an irritable bowel.

MILK AS A CAUSE OF BOWEL SYMPTOMS Abdominal cramps, bloating, excessive gas, and diarrhea are common symptoms that can also be caused by milk in a surprisingly high number of otherwise normal persons who have reduced levels of a single enzyme—lact*ase*—on the surface of their small intestines. Because of this, lact*ose* (the major sugar in milk) can't be properly absorbed; remaining within the intestine, the lactose eventually reaches the colon where bacteria metabolize it to products that can produce distention, cramps, gas, and loose bowel movements.

The enzyme lactase is found in high levels in newborns—for the obvious reason that the chief source of nutrition in early infancy is milk. But in childhood, enzyme levels mysteriously decline in most of the world's population, including 70–95% of persons of Mediterranean, Black, and Asian ancestry. On the other hand, lactase levels remain up in the majority of Caucasians. Persons who develop low levels of lactase do not uniformly experience symptoms, but some will complain of abdominal discomfort after as little as a single glass of milk. Other dairy products (cheeses, yogurt, ice cream) can do the same. When the symptoms are severe, they mimic an irritable bowel condition, and have often been diagnosed as such. The message: if bowel problems seem to come on (or get worse) after eating dairy products, it's worthwhile to check for lactase deficiency—which can be done by blood testing after drinking a lactose-containing solution.

Hepatitis and Cirrhosis

The liver is one of those vital organs—absolutely necessary for life—whose precise role is vague in the minds of most people. No brief phrase—akin to "pumps blood" for describing heart function—will suffice to describe all that the liver does. Hence, the purpose of this essay is to provide a better understanding of the liver and its ailments for those who regard it mainly as that which gets "pickled" from too much alcohol.

WHERE IT IS AND WHAT IT DOES   The liver is the largest organ of the body, weighing about three pounds and residing high up in the right side of the abdomen, protected by the lower ribs which surround it (see diagram). About a third of its blood supply comes directly from the heart, but the remainder reaches the liver only after it has passed through other digestive organs (for example, the stomach, intestines, and pancreas). A final basic anatomic fact is the connecting tube (bile duct) from the liver to the duodenum, which allows bile formed in the liver to flow into the intestines.

As might be expected of an organ that receives blood directly from the intestine, the liver plays a critical role in the handling of what we eat. In the case of glucose, for example, the liver converts most of this sugar into glycogen (which is really a bunch of glucose molecules stuck together chemically) and then stores the glycogen it has formed. By sequestering much of the glucose coming in from each meal, the liver prevents excessively high blood-sugar levels from occurring; during fasting periods, it combats hypoglycemia by releasing glucose from its reserve of glycogen. Similarly, the liver plays an intricate role in processing fatty acids and protein products (amino acids) from digested food. Fats are prepared by the liver for circulation to other organs and storage sites (for example, adipose

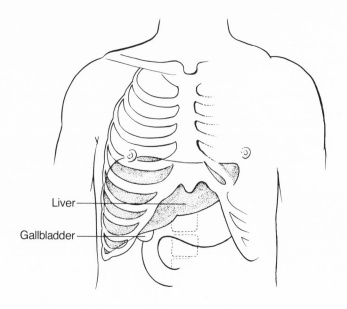

tissue, better known as "fat"). Amino acids are also channeled into the rest of the body, but more important, they are built into a great variety of proteins that are necessary for life, such as enzymes needed for metabolism, clotting factors to control bleeding, and albumin to regulate our blood volume. The liver is primarily responsible for metabolizing—and inactivating—most drugs as well as toxic chemicals that may be formed in our bodies or acquired from our environment. It also produces bile (which gets stored in the gall bladder) to help digest fatty foods. Bilirubin—the yellow pigment we form from the hemoglobin of red blood cells that die off—is taken up by the liver and sent out, along with bile, into the intestines. (Hence, the yellow color—jaundice—observed in patients whose livers cannot perform this task.) Other functions of the liver include hormone regulation, storage of vitamins, and participation in our defense system against invasive bacteria. In short, the liver is an incredible three-pound chemical factory. It is no wonder, then, that when liver disease hits, it can hit hard. And while many different liver diseases can occur, the two most important are hepatitis and cirrhosis—the subjects of the remainder of this essay.

HEPATITIS Hepatitis—meaning "liver inflammation"—can be caused by viruses, drugs, and chemicals (including alcohol), to name the most common offenders. In the minds of most people, though, it means a viral infection. Much has been learned about the viruses that cause hepatitis during the past decade, permitting an updated classification of viral hepatitis into several varieties.

(1) Type A hepatitis: Previously called "infectious hepatitis," hepatitis A is spread via contamination of food, clothing, toys, eating utensils, and other objects with feces; it is mainly a disease of children and young adults. Hepatitis A does not cause lasting liver damage, although its immediate symptoms of profound fatigue, nausea, loss of appetite, and generalized aching often produce several weeks of pure misery. But once the yellow starts to fade, complete recovery is the rule.

(2) Type B hepatitis: Formerly known as "serum hepatitis," hepatitis B *can* produce lingering liver inflammation—called chronic hepatitis—in up to 5% of its victims. Type B hepatitis is traditionally thought of as being spread by blood transfer (such as transfusions or shared needles among drug addicts), but the virus is now known to be present in various body fluids (tears, saliva, semen, and so on) which accounts for the fact that spread is also possible via intimate contact, including sexual activity. Unlike type A virus, which the body rids itself of by the time the jaundice fades, the B virus is not always eradicated; it can persist for years or even a lifetime. Persons who continue to harbor the active virus (about 10%) are not only at risk for chronic hepatitis (and even cirrhosis), but they also become hepatitis "carriers" who can transmit the disease to others, even when they seem to be in good health. Thus, although most persons who develop type B hepatitis recover completely, some will go on to have chronic liver inflammation and/or be infectious to others.

(3) "Non-A, non-B hepatitis": This is an unwieldy way of referring to cases of viral hepatitis that cannot be traced to the A or B viruses by our most sophisticated tests; they are believed to be caused by at least one and quite possibly several other viruses. Non-A, non-B hepatitis is clinically akin to the B variety in that it can go on to chronic hepatitis and is often spread by blood transfusion. Indeed, this version of hepatitis was recognized only when donor blood which had successfully passed screening tests for hepatitis B was found to produce hepatitis one to three months after being transfused.

Chronic hepatitis, meaning liver inflammation lasting longer than six months, can actually continue for decades. Although the symptoms of chronic hepatitis are generally milder than those of acute hepatitis, the danger is that continuing liver injury may lead to cirrhosis and irreversible liver failure. In addition to viruses, chronic hepatitis may also be due to certain drugs. Other patients with chronic hepatitis appear to be suffering from an unusual immunological attack by the body's defense system upon their livers. The diagnosis of chronic hepatitis may require a liver biopsy, which is obtained with a needle inserted through the upper abdomen after a local anesthetic has been injected. The purpose of the biopsy is not only to confirm the diagnosis that has been suggested by other means (the clinical history, physical exam, and blood tests) but to learn, by microscopic inspection, whether things are serious enough to warrant a trial of treatment with cortisone-like drugs (see below).

PREVENTION AND TREATMENT   We have learned enough about viruses to anticipate that a vaccine to provide lifelong protection against type B hepatitis should be available quite soon. In the meantime, though, certain other control methods make sense.

(1) Persons in close contact with a hepatitis patient (such as household members) should receive gamma globulin shots, which confer protection that lasts about four months. Such shots are strongly recommended for those traveling to countries where sanitation is poor. In addition to its known high potency against the A virus, recently produced gamma globulin has been found to confer modest levels of protection against the B virus. Special preparations of serum products extremely rich in antibodies to B virus are available for susceptible persons who are accidentally stuck with a needle contaminated by the B virus—a hazard of hospital workers.

(2) Blood banks should use volunteer donors whenever possible, as the incidence of transfusion hepatitis (even after screening out blood harboring the B virus) is much higher when commercial (paid) donors are used.

(3) Unfortunately, specific treatment for acute hepatitis, once it occurs, is not available; there is no effective drug to eradicate the virus and recovery is purely up to the body's defense systems. Advising rest is only recommending the obvious to a person stricken

with the fatigue and extreme weakness that typifies hepatitis. A reasonable nutritional intake should be encouraged by preparing those foods most desired by the patient, feeding them whenever appetite allows, and using medicines to control nausea. Forcing a high-calorie diet, though, makes no sense; the food-laden tray is more apt to provoke a wave of nausea and resentment than anything else.

(4) Treatment for chronic hepatitis is usually reserved for cases that are "active"—where there is much inflammation and scarring observed on expert review of the liver biopsy. This would give sufficient cause for concern that liver failure and/or cirrhosis might ultimately develop. In such instances, the use of cortisone-like drugs (for example, prednisone) for prolonged periods is recommended, despite the risks involved. The value of such treatment is most evident in chronic hepatitis *unrelated* to viral infection, but most experts will give steroids a try even when severe chronic hepatitis is linked to a virus.

CIRRHOSIS This word refers to an anatomically distorted, scarred, and sometimes shrunken liver—the end, irreversible result of chronic inflammation. While viruses can lead to cirrhosis, alcoholism is by far the most common cause. It is estimated that approximately 15% of all alcoholics develop cirrhosis. Why it is that "many are called but few are chosen" remains a mystery; although the total amount of alcohol consumed over the years seems to be the major influence, other factors (nutritional and genetic) may also play a role. The onset of cirrhosis is often "silent," with few specific symptoms to signal what is happening within the liver. Indeed, cirrhosis is compatible with a fairly normal existence if enough liver cells remain intact and able to perform the many jobs required of them. But as further scarring and destruction occur, some very predictable things begin to happen:

(1) *Yellow jaundice* occurs when the liver loses its ability to remove the yellow pigment bilirubin from the body.

(2) *Fluid accumulation in the legs* (edema) occurs because the liver cannot make enough albumin to keep fluid within the body's vessels; such fluid may also build up within the abdomen (where it is called "ascites") because of the low albumin coupled with a high pressure in certain deep veins, a consequence of liver scarring.

(3) Decreased clotting factors in the blood lead to easy, sometimes uncontrolled bleeding. Such bleeding frequently occurs from pressure-distended veins ("varices") at the lower end of the esophagus, a true medical (and often surgical) emergency.

(4) Susceptibility to drugs increases because cirrhotic patients cannot inactivate them; a small dose of a sedative can produce profound effects in such persons. Indeed, they may enter a comatose state from chemical depressants that are formed within our bodies naturally but disposed of quickly by healthy livers.

Although there are treatments for many of these complications, they work best when the cirrhosis is mild, and usually not at all when it is far advanced. While a cirrhotic liver can never return to normal, patients with alcohol-induced cirrhosis can begin to look and feel a lot better if they can get hooked on a prolonged program of abstinence and good nutrition before it is too late. When it comes to both prevention and treatment, the punch line is to avoid the punch.

Epilepsy

The following questions about epilepsy have been addressed to Dr. Edward R. Wolpow, Assistant Clinical Professor of Neurology, Harvard Medical School, and a member of our Advisory Board.

What is meant by "epilepsy," "seizures," and "convulsions" and what causes them?

Epilepsy is the tendency to have seizures—events in which control is lost over activity regulated by the brain. In a "generalized" seizure, consciousness is lost and there may be various sorts of involuntary body movements. In a "focal" seizure, only a small part of the brain is affected and the result may be an involuntary movement such as the twitching of a finger, or an altered state of consciousness (such as fear). If there is a great deal of abnormal movement, the seizure is called a convulsion. Most seizures last no more than a few minutes, but occasionally they persist for an hour or longer. Although "epilepsy" implies recurrent seizures, the person who has had only one seizure must still be considered at risk for having others, unless there is some unusual extenuating circumstance (such as the use of excitatory drugs, or a single seizure in a young child with a high fever).

A first seizure in an adult should prompt a series of medical tests to determine, if possible, its exact cause. Some seizures are due to irritation of the brain by tumors or infections (abscesses) for which specific therapy might be designed. Other seizures are due to abnormalities of the body's chemistry, such as low glucose, calcium, or sodium levels, and correction of these would prevent further seizures. Most seizures, though, occur in patients with no discernible structural or chemical abnormality of the brain. Various sorts of diagnostic x-ray examinations are often carried out after a first seizure, and a

345

central role remains for the electroencephalogram (EEG, or brain wave study) since this is the only test which measures the electrical activity which the brain produces.

Which medications are used and how effective are they?

No very effective medication was available until about 1915, when phenobarbital was found to be an excellent anticonvulsant. It is still widely used. Several other frequently prescribed anticonvulsants, including primidone (marketed as Mysoline) and mephobarbital (marketed as Mebaral), are chemically similar to phenobarbital. The potential for barbiturates to produce addiction, as well as their role in suicides, has led to efforts by some to attempt to ban by *law* all use of barbiturates. That extreme view is clearly unwarranted; when barbiturates are used as anticonvulsants and the dosages are carefully regulated by a physician, the risk of abuse or addiction is tiny and, in fact, there is often, after a period of adjustment, little or no sedation.

In 1938, phenytoin (marketed as Dilantin) became available. Phenobarbital and/or Dilantin made a very great difference in seizure control for most people with epilepsy; in many, seizures were stopped altogether. Dilantin is usually very well tolerated, although some individuals cannot use it because of allergy. In therapeutic doses, Dilantin does not have as great a sedating effect as phenobarbital. The last 10 to 20 years have produced other useful drugs, the most recent of which are carbamazepine (Tegretol), clonazepam (Clonopin), and valproic acid (Depakene). Currently, with the help of medications, epilepsy is fully controlled in a large proportion of patients who lead totally normal lives. Sadly, some studies show that employers rank epileptics in the category of individuals they would least like to hire—preferring criminals or persons with severe psychiatric illness. In fact, the work records of epileptics are excellent.

What about surgery for epilepsy?

In a very few patients who are poorly controlled with medications, epilepsy surgery may be useful. This surgery is of two types. First, if there is a single irritable area of the brain producing epilepsy, and this area can be removed by a neurosurgeon without producing a serious deficit, such removal can be attempted. In the operating room, the surgeon will record the electrical waves of the surface of the brain (the electrocorticogram) in various locations to be certain just which region of the brain to remove. In selected patients with focal epilepsy, results of this type of surgery can be excellent. More recently, interest has grown in the cerebellar stimulator, a device which is surgically placed on the surface of a part of the back of the brain called the cerebellum, with wires leading to an electrical stimulator that the physician or patient can control. When this stimulator is switched on, a weak electrical current is delivered to the cerebellum and there is a lessening of seizure activity. The long-term effectiveness of this type of therapy is still unclear.

What limitations should be placed on the activity of a person with epilepsy?

The regulations concerning motor vehicle operation vary from state to state. In ten states the physician is legally required to notify the motor vehicle bureau when he sees a patient with epilepsy. In the remaining forty, the physician advises the patient what he should do, but it is up to the patient to inform the motor vehicle bureau. In most states, an epileptic may legally drive an automobile if he has had no seizures for a certain period of time, such as a year. The same restrictions may apply to operating dangerous equipment. Many physicians recommend that their patients with epilepsy never drink alcohol since it might increase the chance of a seizure. Swimming is permitted, but never alone; someone who knows life-saving techniques should always be present and alert to the possibility of a seizure in the swimmer.

What first aid should be carried out if a person having a seizure is encountered?

First aid is required for "major motor" or "grand mal" seizures, in which the patient loses consciousness and stiffens or shakes all four limbs. The tongue may be caught between the teeth and badly bitten. The most important goal during a seizure (or when anyone is unconscious) is maintaining a clear breathing passageway. The patient should be placed down on the ground, either on his side or on his stomach, so that if vomiting occurs, inhalation of material into the lungs will be avoided. He should never be allowed to remain upright or to lie on his back. Even a heavy person lying on his back can easily be turned onto his side by standing at his feet and turning one leg over the other.

There is an ancient, tenacious myth that warns of the unconscious or seizing patient "swallowing his tongue." That can't happen, but attempts to reach into the mouth to "rescue" the tongue may lead to great damage to the patient and to bitten fingers. The only excuse for putting one's hand into the seizing person's mouth is to remove dentures, if that can easily be done.

Where can one get more information about epilepsy?

Information for patients and their families as well as others interested in this field can be obtained from the Epilepsy Society, 20 Providence Street, Boston, MA 02116.

Chronic Obstructive
Lung Disease

The phrase "chronic obstructive lung disease" (called C.O.L.D. for short) is probably foreign to most non-medical persons, but the two most common varieties of C.O.L.D.—chronic bronchitis and emphysema—are well-known villains. During the last decade, the mortality rate from these problems has shown the greatest rate of increase of any chronic disease; they are now sixth on the list of leading disease killers and result in over 50,000 deaths per year in the United States.

CAUSE AND EFFECT   The common denominator of the diseases leading to C.O.L.D. is obstruction of air flow either into or out of the lungs—or both (see diagram). As indicated above, two major processes—usually both, but often with one predominating—underlie most cases of C.O.L.D. Brief thumbnail sketches follow:

(1) Chronic bronchitis: Bronchitis refers to inflammation of the bronchi, the major breathing tubes leading into each lung. The typical symptom of bronchitis is a productive cough—meaning that thick greenish-yellow sputum (purulent sputum) is raised, signifying an underlying infection. Bronchitis is termed chronic when a productive cough exists for at least three months of the year for two successive years; once so established, chronic bronchitis usually becomes progressively worse until the cough is an almost constant companion. Biopsy studies of the lining of the bronchi of such persons demonstrate an increased thickness of the mucus-producing layer. It is not hard to imagine how this—along with the increase in secreted mucus—leads to obstruction of air flow. *Although air pollutants are receiving increased attention, smoking remains the most important cause of chronic bronchitis* and contributes to the problem in many ways—including a decreased effectiveness of the lung cells designed to destroy bacteria and a decrease in the number

349

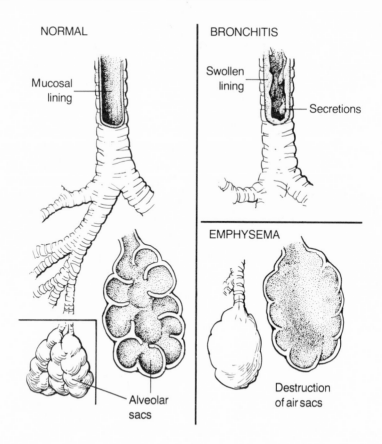

and activity of cilia, the hair-like structures lining the bronchi that sweep mucus and debris away from the lung.

(2) Emphysema: Most of us have known someone with emphysema and have recognized the resulting "air hunger"—the hard work of breathing requiring all available muscles of the neck, chest, and abdomen along with gasping sounds accompanying each breath, especially when exhaling. Autopsy studies of such persons classically demonstrate destruction of lung tissue where it most counts—in the small airways and the air sacs (alveoli) where gas exchange occurs. Because of this destruction, air gets trapped in the lungs, their "hyperinflation" often resulting in a "barrel-shaped" chest. In recent years scientists have been able to describe what apparently happens in the lungs of most persons afflicted with emphysema—namely, the *destruction of elastin,* a key component that normally gives re-

siliency to lung tissue. There are rare instances when a person is genetically predestined for emphysema because of a deficiency of an enzyme (alpha-1-antitrypsin) which acts to prevent the destruction of elastin. But again *the most important factor in the development of emphysema in most persons is smoking*. And while the link between smoking and emphysema is not fully understood, recent evidence indicates that inhaled tobacco smoke actually increases those body chemicals that destroy elastin.

As indicated earlier, both of these processes usually co-exist in an individual with C.O.L.D.—not surprising given the fact that smoking is the most important contributing factor in each. And again, the net effect of both diseases is an obstruction of air flow which, in turn, leads to reduced oxygen in the bloodstream and, ultimately, oxygen starvation of all body tissues.

DIAGNOSIS   It is important to detect these destructive processes before any permanent damage to the lungs has occurred. Unfortunately, this is not easily or routinely possible—but there are ways of identifying these diseases at an early stage when they can at least be arrested, if not reversed:

(1) Obviously, *an increasingly persistent and productive cough* must be taken seriously as a signal of impending chronic bronchitis. However, many smokers do not notice—or tend to deny—the slippage from a mild "smoker's cough" into a more serious state of chronic bronchitis. Fortunately, even after such a state has been reached, the cessation of smoking—at least in early stages—can often result in reversal of bronchitis. Unfortunately, permanent destruction of air sacs (characteristic of emphysema) can occur without any warning symptoms—and these changes are not reversible, though the process can at least be halted by quitting smoking.

(2) Since the major problem in C.O.L.D. is airway obstruction, several rather simple *tests have been designed to detect relatively early stages of obstructive lung disease*. The classic test—spirometry—measures the rate and amount of air that can be forced out of the lungs on maximal effort. One "home test" to measure obstruction of air flow involves measuring the time it takes to exhale the air inhaled during a maximally deep breath. Normally, this should take

no more than three seconds; if this "emptying time" is more than five seconds (as timed with a stop watch), significant obstruction of air flow is already likely to be present.

(3) Finally, it should be stressed that chest x-rays are inadequate in detecting bronchitis or emphysema in their early stages (although they are helpful in diagnosing complicating problems such as pneumonia). By the time changes characteristic of emphysema show up on an x-ray, extensive and permanent damage has already occurred; the comment that "your lungs look clean" on an x-ray can be very misleading to an emphysema victim.

In short, the diagnosis of these obstructive lung conditions is typically made after the fact, when serious and often permanent damage has already occurred.

PREVENTION AND TREATMENT All of the above logically points to only one conclusion concerning treatment—namely that "the best treatment is prevention." In this instance, the best prevention is clearly the avoidance of inhaled tobacco smoke. But there are other important aspects of prevention and treatment that should be emphasized:

(1) Increasing stress is being appropriately placed on forms of *air pollution* other than the intensive form of self-pollution called smoking. Bronchitis especially is worsened by high levels of nitrous and sulfur dioxides characteristic of urban air pollution. Specific occupational air pollution hazards—cotton dust, certain plastic vapors, welding fumes, and smelter gases (especially combined with cigarette smoking)—are now known to contribute to C.O.L.D., and even home aerosol sprays have been incriminated.

(2) Since *actual infection* often underlies chronic bronchitis, every effort should be made to protect persons with C.O.L.D. from further damage from infections by treating vigorously those that develop. Antibiotics taken at the earliest sign of an infection can be useful. Bronchodilators may help those with reversible bronchial constriction. Liquefying sticky mucous secretions (drinking water is the best and cheapest way) is helpful, as are physical therapy and postural drainage techniques in some cases of unusually thick secretions. Breathing exercises may also be useful for patients with advanced emphysema.

(3) Yearly *flu shots* should be administered, and *the new vaccine against pneumococcal bacteria* (the most important cause of bacterial pneumonia) should be offered to persons with C.O.L.D.

IN SUMMARY   Given the insidious onset of obstructive lung disease and the difficulty in treating established bronchitis or emphysema, the final word must be directed to the importance of "no smoking."

Arthritis

Many people assume that all severe joint symptoms are caused by rheumatoid arthritis and that little can be done to treat this disease. Both assumptions are false. There are over 100 recognized causes of arthritis (literal definition: "inflammation of a joint"), many of which are temporary or curable. And even if the diagnosis turns out to be rheumatoid arthritis, most cases can be managed so as to preserve reasonable function. The message is clear: *any chronic joint problem that limits function or requires pain medication deserves the attention of a physician skilled in the diagnosis and treatment of joint diseases.* (Note: An *acute* joint flare-up—swollen, hot, red, painful, and often associated with fever—constitutes a medical emergency and should be evaluated immediately.) While there are many causes of joint problems, the following essay will discuss the two most common types of chronic joint disease.

RHEUMATOID ARTHRITIS   The cause of rheumatoid arthritis (RA)—which affects about 5 million people in this country—is unknown. There is no solid evidence to support suggestions that RA is caused by germs or by dietary problems. While RA is a disease that can affect many parts of the body (a *systemic* disease), its course in any given individual can be quite variable; periods of decreased symptoms may occur without any treatment—thus making the use of copper bracelets and similar "cures" impossible to evaluate apart from careful comparison studies. Most important, the majority of patients with RA can be helped to lead near normal lives; severe crippling is the exception, not the rule.

There is no simple blood test that can definitely diagnose RA, though blood tests may be helpful in confirming the diagnosis or eliminating other possibilities. X-rays are useful in evaluating the status of affected joints and sometimes in actual diagnosis. Very often, a "joint aspiration" (taking fluid from a joint for chemical and microscopic study) is important for proper diagnosis. Ultimately, a diagnosis is made by the total picture—history, physical examination, and lab studies—as interpreted by a competent physician.

There are four basic elements in the treatment of RA:

(1) *Rest:* While some studies question the value of rest, the majority of experts strongly recommend both physical and emotional rest during periods of active disease.

(2) *Physical therapy:* A wide range of aids—exercises, heat treatments, joint splinting—can be used. Unfortunately, most patients and some doctors have little knowledge of or interest in these techniques. One indication of a physician's competence in the treatment of serious rheumatoid disease is careful attention to physical therapy.

(3) *Drugs:* While often thought of as initial treatment, drugs should only be used *in addition* to rest and physical therapy. *Aspirin* is still considered to be the mainstay of drug treatment. Several other drugs are available as substitutes for aspirin (for example, Motrin, Naprosyn, Clinoril); they are largely promoted as having fewer side effects. Although such drugs may indeed be useful in people who cannot tolerate aspirin, most experts feel they are usually no more effective than aspirin while costing much more. For example, a ten-day supply of these drugs costs approximately six dollars, versus less than two dollars for aspirin. *Steroids* (cortisone-like drugs) are often inappropriately used in this and other chronic diseases. Most authorities feel that steroids should be used only on a short-term basis when symptoms are particularly severe. Injections of steroids into a joint may be useful on occasion. However, there is evidence that repeated injections may contribute to joint damage. *Gold* injections, *chloroquine,* and *penicillamine* (not to be confused with the antibiotic penicillin) are the only drugs currently available that may *arrest* the progression of rheumatoid disease. Therefore, most experts recommend that patients with *active* disease be tried on one of these drugs, which have potentially serious side effects and should be given only under the supervision of a knowledgeable physician.

(4) Surgery: An important development in the treatment of crippling disease has been joint repair and replacement therapy. Hip and knee replacements, as well as plastic inserts to correct severe finger-joint deformities, are now available on a routine basis in many hospitals. Procedures such as "synovectomies"—the removal of inflamed joint lining—can produce considerable improvement for wrists and hands that are badly affected by rheumatoid arthritis. Joint surgery for arthritis requires special skills and should *not* be done by surgeons who undertake such operations only occasionally.

DEGENERATIVE JOINT DISEASE   While the underlying cause of DJD—also referred to as "osteoarthritis"—is not clear, most experts believe this common problem (over 10 million people affected in this country) is due to a mechanical wear-and-tear effect. Thus, avoiding joint injury, protecting joints from excess stress, and losing excess weight may reduce DJD. However, DJD seems to be a part of the "normal" aging process in many people. In fact, most elderly people will show anatomical signs of joint degeneration on x-ray, but most of them will have no symptoms and should not worry about an x-ray diagnosis of osteoarthritis. Diagnosis and treatment of DJD is to some extent similar to that described above for RA. However, since inflammation is not a part of this disease, drug therapies are limited to relief of symptoms. Surgery can be very useful in advanced cases; most cases of hip replacement are for DJD.

IN SUMMARY   Something *can* be done for people with chronic arthritis. Treatment may improve function and prevent further damage. At times the skills of a rheumatologist—the specialist of internal medicine trained in joint diseases—may be required. Further information concerning joint disease can be obtained by writing the Arthritis Foundation, 3400 Peachtree Road, N.E., Atlanta, Georgia 30326.

Some Problems of Aging

MYTH 5

Tooth decay is the major cause
of tooth loss in adults.

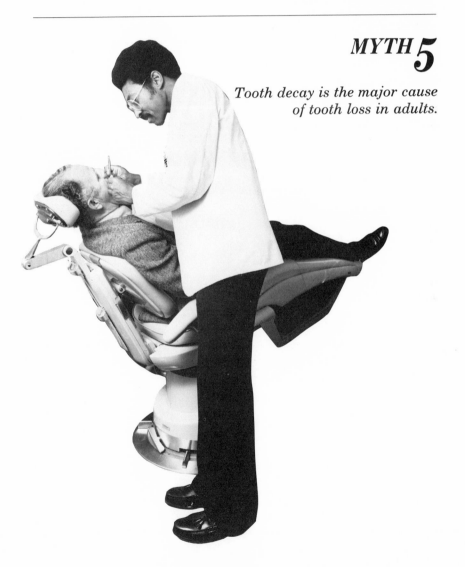

Cataracts

Given that over 200,000 cataract operations are performed each year in this country and the current confusion about various types of such surgery, we have asked Dr. B. Thomas Hutchinson, Surgeon at the Massachusetts Eye and Ear Infirmary and a member of our Advisory Board, to answer questions that might bring some of the issues "into focus."

What are cataracts and how does one know if he has a cataract?

A cataract is an opacity or clouding of the normally transparent lens, which is located within the eyeball, just behind the pupil and iris. Such clouding often prevents the proper focusing of light onto the retina. This opacity results in the principal symptom of a cataract—blurring of vision that is often influenced by light and glare. Because there may be other reasons for visual blurring, one should have an examination by an eye physician to ensure that glaucoma, inflammation, retinal detachment, or other diseases are not present within the eye, since these might require more prompt attention and treatment than a cataract. Certainly, any person who has a new visual deficit should be examined by an ophthalmologist.

What are the reasons for removing a cataract?

The major indication for cataract surgery is poor vision that significantly interferes with a person's enjoyment of life. Fortunately, with the current safety and effectiveness of cataract surgery, one need not wait many months or even years until a cataract is "ripe"—a term

359

used for a cataract so dense that nothing can be seen through it. Obviously, the desire and need for surgery will vary from person to person, depending upon his visual requirements. Early cataracts, causing little or no visual blurring, usually are not removed and they require no attention beyond a periodic examination by an eye physician. People with particular visual requirements, such as draftsmen, truck drivers, and watchmakers, might well require cataract surgery long before a person who is not bothered by slight visual blurring. In rare instances, a cataract may be associated with another disease in the eye and require removal even though the opposite eye might provide adequate vision.

What causes cataracts to form?

Cataracts may be present at birth as a result of either inheritance or faulty development of the embryo, as might be caused by german measles during the first part of pregnancy. After birth, cataracts may form in early childhood as a result of a variety of metabolic problems, injuries, or other eye diseases such as tumors, parasitic infections, and inflammation. Although medications, radiation, endocrine imbalances, diabetes, and injuries may cause cataracts to develop in adults, the most common type of cataract found today is the "senile" cataract, an inappropriate term implying "cataract of older age groups" and having nothing to do with mental senility.

Do any treatments other than surgery work?

Surgery remains the only definitive treatment for cataracts. Although pills, drops, and ointments have been promoted to arrest or dissolve cataracts, none are effective. In a few instances, patients may be helped to see slightly better by dilating the pupil with drops, allowing them to "look around" their central cataract.

How are cataracts removed and how safe are these operations?

Although there are many different techniques for cataract removal, *all* require an incision into the eye, *all* require a period of several weeks for complete healing, and *all* have potential risk, such as infection, bleeding, and anesthetic complications, for the individual.

Fortunately, these complications are rare and cataract surgery is successful in 95% to 98% of the cases. There are two basic types of cataract surgery. In the method employed most frequently, *intra-capsular extraction,* the entire lens is removed. Often a freezing probe is used to extract the cataract through an incision into the eye near the margin of the iris. The *extracapsular extraction* method involves the removal of the central portion of the lens via a suction device. The "back" of the lens capsule, ordinarily clear, is left within the eye. This type of surgery is generally used in children and young adults but may also be used in the elderly. Occasionally, a small second operation is necessary to cut open the back part of the capsule at a later time if it becomes cloudy.

Phacoemulsification, a special type of extracapsular cataract operation, requires a smaller incision. The cataract is sucked out through a special needle whose tip vibrates at high frequency, fragmenting the cataract as it is removed. Some types of cataracts, especially in the young, may be simply sucked out through a small, blunt needle tip. Contrary to popular belief, the laser, which may be used for the treatment of other eye diseases, is *not used* for cataract removal.

The different techniques for cataract extraction each have particular advantages for special circumstances. The most common form of cataract surgery today provides the patient with a rapid convalescence and low risk because of new instrumentation and suture material. The decision as to which operation is best in a given patient will certainly depend upon individual considerations. The age of the patient, the type of cataract, and the presence of coexisting eye disease will often dictate the best type of operation. Where options exist, the ophthalmologist is obliged to discuss them and to point out the relative hazards as well as possible advantages of each technique. Fortunately, any cataract operation, as routinely performed today, has an extremely high success rate—almost always producing an improvement of vision when no other eye disease is present.

Much has been written recently regarding contact lenses as well as artificial lenses implanted within the eye, instead of the thick, "coke bottle" glasses often worn by patients who have had cataract surgery. What is the current status of these devices?

Since the eye's own lens has been removed or destroyed in cataract surgery, some other method of focusing light upon the retina must be used. Glasses, contact lenses, and intraocular lenses (IOL) are the three methods of providing this focusing power to the eye.

Spectacle lenses, because of their thickness and extra power, cause objects to appear to be significantly larger and closer than the normal eye's vision. If an individual has had a cataract operation in one eye only, this difference in image size, approximately 30%, prevents the patient from using both eyes simultaneously. Thus, he may wear a spectacle correction for *either* the operated eye or his unoperated eye but *he cannot fix an object with both eyes simultaneously,* as the brain cannot bring the two disparate images together into a single three-dimensional picture. However, if a contact lens is placed on the surface of the cornea of the operated eye, the image disparity between the two eyes will be reduced from the 30% level to approximately 8%, a difference that can be merged into a single, three-dimensional image. Also, the contact lens allows the perception of the environment as "normal sized" as compared to the thicker lens that is placed in a spectacle frame. Contact lenses have been so improved over the past few years that almost all patients can, with proper instruction, use them. In fact, the eye that has had cataract surgery often tolerates the contact lens better than the eye that is fitted to a contact lens for purely cosmetic reasons. Quite recently, contact lenses have been developed that may be worn not only for days but for weeks or months without removal.

Another new and somewhat more controversial method of correcting vision after a cataract operation is the *intraocular lens* (IOL). The IOL is a small, plastic lens that is placed *within* the eye to restore the focusing power previously provided by the patient's lens before the cataract formed. This would seem to be the perfect solution, as there is no need for either a contact lens or glasses after cataract surgery. The intraocular lens would, therefore, seem to be ideal for those aged or infirm patients who cannot manage the contact lens or maneuver well with the spectacle glasses. Indeed, many elderly patients are extremely pleased with the often dramatic improvement of vision afforded by these artificial implants. Although the IOL has received extensive news coverage too often suggesting universally good results, the fact is that there are well-recognized complications caused by placing the artificial material within the eye. On a national average, the frequency of these complications is greater with IOL implantation than are the risks and failures of cataract surgery alone. Although there are many "models" of intraocular lenses, none are ideal and free of complications. Generally, IOLs are not used in eyes with other diseases or in individuals who have only one eye. *In summary, when these lenses work well, they are fantastically effective—but when they work poorly, they may be catastrophic to the vision and even to the eye itself.* Obviously the decision for an intraocular lens should not be made lightly, either by the patient or the ophthalmologist.

Glasses, contact lenses, or the intraocular lens? Again, it is necessary that the patient and his eye physician discuss thoroughly the relative advantages and disadvantages for these different methods of optical correction. All are usually successful!

Glaucoma

Glaucoma can be simply described as an increase in pressure within the eyeball sufficient to damage the optic nerve that carries images from the eye to the brain. Approximately 60,000 Americans are blind because of glaucoma; an estimated 2 million Americans are afflicted—and 25% of them are not aware of it! The most common form of glaucoma (over 90% of cases) causes damage to the eye without any warning symptoms until visual loss occurs—which is tragic because the damage is permanent and could have been prevented by early diagnosis and treatment.

TYPES OF GLAUCOMA   A complete classification for glaucoma includes over thirty different types. Glaucoma can occur in infancy or childhood but more commonly it is a disease of middle and older age groups. While everyone agrees that increased eye pressure is the underlying problem in glaucoma, there are many reasons why such increases may occur. Glaucoma can result from injury, cataracts, or inflammation within the eye. In predisposed eyes, even medical treatment with steroids or certain drugs which dilate the pupil can cause glaucoma. The vast majority of adult cases, however, are typically described as either *chronic* (open angle) or *acute* (closed angle). Acute glaucoma is relatively uncommon, but at its onset it can represent a true emergency since permanent visual loss may occur within hours! Fortunately, this type of glaucoma almost always produces symptoms pointing to serious trouble: blurring of vision, colored rings or haloes around lights, plus severe eye pain and redness. (These symptoms should not be dismissed as conjunctivitis—"pink eye"—in which such discomfort and visual changes do not occur.) A competent eye physician (ophthalmologist) should be consulted at once. Although medical treatment may initially be effective for acute glaucoma (and is actually the treatment of choice for chronic glaucoma), surgery is generally recommended as a permanent cure for the acute, painful variety. Unfortunately, the much more common type of glaucoma—chronic or open angle—has no dramatic warning symptoms, and it is this type that will be the focus of the rest of this discussion.

SCREENING AND DIAGNOSIS   Since vision lost from glaucoma *cannot be regained,* it is imperative that the diagnosis be made early, before such loss has developed. Although several different methods of examination are used, the following are the most important:

(1) Measuring the eye pressure—tonometry: Most eye physicians recommend that people over 40 be screened for increased eye pressure periodically (approximately every two years). Those with a family history of glaucoma, or with a known history of previous eye injury or disease, should begin their regular check-ups earlier and be re-examined somewhat more frequently. The instrument most commonly used by physicians other than medical eye specialists is the Schiotz tonometer, which is placed directly on the front surface of the eye after anesthetic drops have been instilled. Ophthalmologists typically use a method known as "applanation tonometry," in which a pressure probe is applied to the front surface of the eye, also in a painless manner after anesthetic drops. This technique is more accurate than Schiotz measurement, but is not widely available for screening purposes. Another device increasingly used for glaucoma detection by technicians and non-medical eye specialists is the "air-puff" tonometer which measures the eye pressure with a small painless burst of air against the eyeball.

(2) Examination of vision and the eye: When glaucoma is suspected, an ophthalmologist will wish to examine many aspects of eye function and structure. Not only is the "central vision" measured by a reading chart, but the peripheral portion of the visual field will be inspected for evidence of hidden areas of damage. If glaucoma is present, this measurement of "side vision" that surrounds central reading vision is monitored periodically to ensure that no further damage occurs to the eye while the patient is under treatment.

Each of the patient's eyes are then thoroughly examined in a painless manner. *Gonioscopy* involves the use of special lenses and lights to examine the internal drainage system of the eye. This examination will tell whether the pressure increase in the eye is due to angle closure (in which case surgical treatment might be necessary) or whether the drainage system is open; appropriate treatment is based on what is revealed by gonioscopy.

The complete examination will also include an examination of the "back of the eye" after dilating the pupils. In particular, the eye physician will be looking for possible damage to the optic nerve and will often be able to correlate the area of visual loss with the appearance of the optic nerve and surrounding tissues. The blood vessels of the eye and the retina will also be examined to be sure that no additional disease is responsible for potential visual loss.

As is the case with high blood pressure—which, incidentally, bears no direct relationship to eye pressure—it is important not to label someone as having glaucoma on the basis of a single pressure reading. This is particularly true when the Schiotz or air-puff tonometer is used. Since a diagnosis of glaucoma almost automatically leads to treatment, it is important to confirm it by additional tests administered by an ophthalmologist.

TREATMENT   The vast majority of people with chronic glaucoma can be successfully treated with daily medications. There are several classes of drugs that are designed either to increase fluid drainage from the eye or to decrease the amount of fluid produced by the eye. (Fluid leaves the eyeball through small veins on the surface and is in no way associated with tears or fluid external to the eye.)

(1) Drugs that constrict the pupil (miotics): Until recently, the most widely used drugs for the treatment of chronic glaucoma have been those that improve the drainage system in the eye. Pilocarpine, the most frequently used miotic in the United States, usually causes no significant side effect, although it may be associated with visual blurring—especially in young people and in older people with cataracts—since it makes the pupil small. In addition, the small pupil lets in less light to the back of the eye, which may cause "darker vision" in poorly lit surroundings. Pilocarpine drops are used three to four times daily, usually a matter of only slight inconvenience to the patient on a day-to-day basis.

(2) Drugs that dilate the pupil: Epinephrine, another eye drop often used to treat glaucoma, reduces the fluid produced in the eye, as well as slightly improving the drainage system capacity. This drug, too, may affect the pupil size—characteristically dilating or widening the pupil, making vision slightly blurred and perhaps unduly bright. It has the advantage of longer action, often requiring use only once or twice daily. Although epinephrine is usually well tolerated, some patients develop allergic or irritative reactions to this medication; because the drops may be absorbed into the circulation, heart palpitations or nervousness are sometimes experienced.

(3) Timolol maleate: This drug, approved by the Food and Drug Administration in 1979, is a "beta blocker" that is believed to decrease fluid production within the eye. The majority of those who have used the drug thus far find it comfortable, effective, and without significant visual side effects. As with all beta-blocker drugs, care must be used in people with a history of heart disease, asthma, or lung disease. As with the other eye drops, some patients will show great improvement of pressure and others will have little reduction in pressure. Interestingly, the medication will sometimes lose its effectiveness after several weeks. Many eye specialists now use timolol as the "drug of choice" for the initial treatment of glaucoma even though it is more expensive than the other eye drops.

(4) Carbonic anhydrase inhibitors: Drugs such as acetazolamide (Diamox), taken by mouth, act to decrease eye-fluid production. Because of long-term side effects such as kidney stones, weakness, lethargy, and gastrointestinal disturbances, these medications are usually reserved for those in whom drops do not adequately control the intraocular pressure.

(5) Surgery: In the vast majority of cases, the chronic type of glaucoma can be adequately controlled with the above drops and pills, taken either singly or in various combinations; vision will not deteriorate if the eye pressure is kept in a range protective to the optic nerve. Fortunately, for patients not adequately controlled with medication, surgery is very effective and visual loss can be arrested with an appropriate operation. As with the medications, there are several types of glaucoma operations, all having the common purpose of lowering the pressure in the eye to a level that will protect the vision. These operations, like any surgery, carry certain risks, but they have a very high success rate.

IN SUMMARY   The basic meaning of glaucoma is an elevation of the pressure within the eyeball sufficient to damage the optic nerve. In *acute* glaucoma there are usually symptoms of pain, blurred vision, and "haloes," the result of very high pressures within the eye that can produce major damage in a matter of hours or a few days. Surgery to improve fluid drainage from the eye is almost always warranted in acute glaucoma. The more common, *chronic* type of "open-angle" glaucoma is a leading cause of painless, progressive blindness, despite the fact that techniques for its detection and treatment are well established. In brief, the loss of vision to glaucoma is especially tragic in that it is, except in rare circumstances, completely preventable!

Periodontal Disease

When a tooth loosens in childhood, we know there's another one below the surface to replace it. Such is not the case in adulthood, a reason why we should have healthy respect for periodontal disease. Dr. Paul Goldhaber, Dean of the Harvard School of Dental Medicine, has been asked about the essentials of this very common problem.

What is periodontal disease and who should worry about it?

Periodontal disease is a process that damages tissue surrounding a tooth and eventually erodes the bone that forms its socket (see diagram). It is the major cause of lost teeth after the age of thirty or thirty-five.

Dental caries (tooth decay), when treated with modern techniques, can progress pretty far and yet a working tooth can be saved. However, if supporting tissues are destroyed by periodontal disease, even a good tooth may be lost. As periodontal disease begins, the gum turns from its natural pink to red, and then a little space forms between the gum and the tooth. At this stage, the gum disease (technically termed "gingivitis") is not necessarily painful. Gingivitis may linger on for many years without progressing, but as a rule it goes on to periodontitis (meaning "inflammation around the tooth"). At this stage, the gum peels away from the surface of the root and crown of the tooth to leave deep pockets where bacteria accumulate and destroy the socket of bone that supports the tooth. This infection may also penetrate the space between the tooth and its socket. Once there, it destroys the fibers (or ligaments) that anchor tooth to bone. After the tooth has been loosened and its supports eroded, it cannot be kept in place.

369

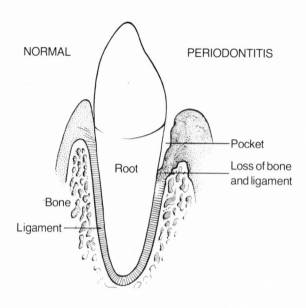

If the open end of a pocket becomes sealed off, an abscess, or enclosed infection develops. Such *gum* abscesses are entirely distinct from the *root* abscesses of dental caries, and they are not preceded by pain or sensitivity to hot and cold as root abscesses are. But once gum abscesses form, they are painful indeed.

How can periodontal disease be prevented? How is it treated?

Like caries, periodontal disease is caused by bacteria (although of a different type) so all accepted forms of prevention are aimed at preventing the accumulation of bacteria adhering to teeth and of the gelatinous material that covers them. Removing these "plaques" is what brushing and flossing are all about. Both are mechanical efforts to remove bacteria from the gum margin. Even with a fairly good program of home care, though, some plaques form and with time become calcified. This material (called either "tartar" or "calculus") should be removed by a dental hygienist at regular intervals. It was once thought that mechanical irritation from the tartar was the principal cause of gingivitis, but the bacteria themselves are now thought to be the main problem; housed in and upon the tartar they have made, they attack the gum tissue.

Established periodontitis—with its pockets of infection and areas of weakened bone—defies home treatment. There are two standard approaches to the problem:

(1) With surgery, a periodontist or dentist cuts open the pocket to expose the area of infection. Now able to see directly, he or she then thoroughly cleans out the diseased material and removes all evidence of infection. The gum is then put back in place, usually with the gum line somewhat closer to the root than it was, so that the pocket is now shallower. When results are good, this procedure allows a patient to keep the disease under control with the usual home-care methods (brushing and flossing).

But sometimes problems persist. Very deep pockets cannot always be eliminated, and they may develop again. Thus, the area may need to be cleaned by the dentist at fairly frequent intervals, and surgery may again be required, even though the procedure was expertly done the first time.

(2) An alternative to surgery is a procedure known as "deep scaling." At frequent intervals—perhaps as often as every two to three months—the patient must have pockets curetted (scraped) by a dentist or a hygienist working with a dentist. It is important for the dentist or periodontist to make sure that the deepest areas have been properly cleaned each time. If the base of the pockets can be reached, and if the procedure is done frequently enough, surgery can be avoided, but even the most experienced periodontists may have difficulty cleaning out deep pockets.

Of these two approaches, surgery is more likely to provide a long-term solution. But patients may refuse surgery because it frightens them. Or if periodontal disease is located near the front teeth, surgery—which is likely to expose the roots of the teeth—may be avoided for the sake of appearance. Deep scaling, done skillfully and frequently enough, is then an acceptable alternative to surgery.

Can we look forward to improvements in prevention and treatment?

Current research is aimed at finding ways to reduce or eliminate the need for surgery. Because bacteria are the cause of periodontal disease, a good deal of attention has been focused on ways to kill the offending organisms.

Scrupulous oral hygiene should be the cornerstone of prevention. Unfortunately, many people find it difficult or impossible to keep up adequate motivation for proper home care. Periodic cleaning by a dental hygienist, thus, is very important. Although a period of six months between cleanings is the standard recommendation, the frequency of visits should be a matter of individual need. But it is also apparent that we must look for other approaches to prevention.

Mouthwashes containing antimicrobials (substances that kill bacteria) have been tried and they show reasonable promise in the treatment of gingivitis. In principle, this approach is a good one, but there are practical problems. For example, chlorhexidine, one of the more effective agents, stains teeth if it is used for long periods of time. As yet, the Food and Drug Administration has not approved any mouthwash for use in this country, but studies conducted abroad have been encouraging. Material impregnated with a drug and then stuffed into the pockets of infection can deliver antimicrobials to the site of bacteria. Research on this approach is in progress.

In general, it is more practical to give antibiotics as pills. But if they must be given for long periods, as is likely in cases of periodontitis, questions of dosage, side effects, and possible resistance of bacteria become important. So far, the most promising drug is the antibiotic tetracycline, which has already been shown to be safe for the long-term treatment of acne. But many questions must be resolved before it can be accepted as a standard therapy for periodontitis.

At present, it seems unlikely that a vaccine can be developed for periodontal disease because a variety of different bacteria cause it. Caries, on the other hand, is caused by just one species, and so there is hope of developing a vaccine for that disease.

Can the gums be affected by other diseases?

Yes. Just one interesting example is "trench mouth." Formally known as "acute necrotizing ulcerative gingivitis," this condition tends to affect people in their mid to late teens or early twenties. The disease is sudden in onset and very painful; it can be highly destructive to gum tissue and even lead to deformities of the gum. Remarkably enough, trench mouth seems to be precipitated by emotional stress—usually as a result of separation from a lover or spouse. There is no evidence that trench mouth is contagious, although bacteria do play a role, and the disease responds beautifully to antibiotics. Apparently the emotional stress interferes with natural resistance to infection, but little is known about the way this process is triggered.

Gallstones

The gallbladder is primarily an organ for storage—a fact that is easy to infer from its sac-like shape. Lying along the back side of the liver, it collects and concentrates bile juices that are produced in the liver and continually flow into it through a system of ducts (see diagram). Following a meal, chemical signals stimulate the gallbladder to contract; stored bile is then discharged into the duodenal portion of the small intestine to help digest fat. However, the presence of a gallbladder is not vital to good health. In millions of persons who have had theirs removed, bile passes directly from the liver to the intestine without apparent detriment to eating habits or digestion. So, unlike the appendix, the gallbladder serves a known—but non-essential—function. Like the appendix, though, it causes more abdominal havoc than its existence would seem to justify: more than 15,-000,000 Americans have stones in their gallbladders; 800,000 new cases are diagnosed each year; 500,000 patients with gallstones are hospitalized each year and more than half of them have their gallbladders (stones and all) surgically removed—an operation called a *cholecystectomy.*

The past decade has brought an explosion of knowledge about how abnormal bile contributes to gallstone formation. Most important, it is now known that in the case of cholesterol-containing gallstones—which are far and away the most common kind—the stones form because the bile juice contains too much *cholesterol* as compared to its other major ingredients *(bile salts* and *lecithin).* The excess cholesterol cannot remain in solution, and it precipitates out—as "stones." Because *bile salts* help make cholesterol more soluble—and thus serve to dissolve precipitated cholesterol—their use in the treatment of gallstones has been extensively investigated. There is no direct relationship between the cholesterol content of our blood

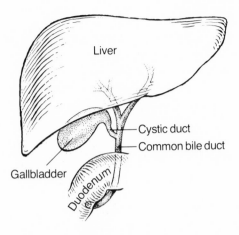

Liver

Cystic duct

Common bile duct

Gallbladder

Duodenum

and that of bile—and we can't prevent gallstones by cutting down the cholesterol in our diet (though that kind of modification is, of course, recommended for prevention of coronary artery disease). Estrogen treatment predisposes bile to form stones, and the increased incidence of gallstones in women—especially those who have had frequent pregnancies—is also attributed to estrogens.

THE SYMPTOMS   The hallmark of an acute gallbladder attack is pain in the upper abdomen, often more pronounced on the right side and sometimes traveling through to the back under the right shoulder blade. The pain develops suddenly—frequently after a meal— and usually maintains a peak intensity for several hours. It is not worsened by moving about, and patients experiencing gallbladder attacks are often restless in their agony. In addition to pain, other symptoms (fever, chills, vomiting, and even jaundice) may occur— depending on the location of the stones and the duration of the attack.

In most cases the symptoms occur when a stone that had previously floated freely in the gallbladder is pushed out of the contracting gallbladder and becomes wedged in the cystic duct. (This duct is the tube that carries bile from the gallbladder to the common duct, which leads to the small intestine.) Sometimes a stone passes all the way to the common duct and lodges there. In this instance, there is a blockage of *all* bile flow (from the liver as well as the gallbladder) and jaundice—a yellow discoloration of the skin and eyes—appears. Continued stone blockage of either the cystic or the common duct can lead to infections, with worsening pain and fever as the chief symptoms. Occasionally, gallstones can cause inflammation of the pancreas when they advance down to the lowest part of the common duct. Some pass all the way through to the intestine, and the obstruction is then relieved naturally.

It is very important to stress that less dramatic symptoms of dyspepsia—belching, bloating, fatty food upsets, and so on—are seldom caused by gallbladder disease. Studies have demonstrated that the simultaneous occurrence of gallstones and indigestion is usually a matter of chance. In one report, for example, only 24 of 142 women who complained of chronic indigestion had gallstone disease when studied. Because gallstones are so common, they may indeed be found in dyspeptic persons, but this does not constitute proof that the stones are responsible for the symptoms—a fact that can sadly become evident when symptoms remain in the aftermath of "successful" removal of the gallbladder and its stones. Therefore, *it is critically important to establish that gallstones are the culprit behind the symptoms before surgery is considered.*

DIAGNOSIS   The symptoms of gallstone disease are often unmistakable, but in other cases the diagnosis is far less certain. In *no* instance should gallstones be considered the culprit without one or more of the following diagnostic studies to prove their presence:

(1) X-rays of the abdomen performed without any preparation (so-called plain x-rays) will detect gallstones in only about 15% of cases. Therefore, in the past an *oral cholecystogram* (x-rays taken after the swallowing of tablets containing a dye which outlines the gallbladder as well as any stones present) was almost routine in anyone with suspected gallstone disease. A diseased gallbladder might function poorly and fail to concentrate the dye sufficiently to show on the x-ray study. Such "non-visualization," if occurring after repeat examination, was taken as positive evidence of gallbladder disease—*if* the tablets had been taken properly and there was no other problem interfering with the normal routing of dye to the gallbladder.

(2) Ultrasound uses sonar-like waves that bounce off internal body structures (including gallstones) to form an image of these structures. The advantage of this technique is its excellent detection

rate without risk or discomfort. Ultrasound is increasingly used as the initial examination for gallstones—in place of the oral cholecystogram. It is also very useful in evaluating those persons whose gallbladders don't visualize with the dye used for a cholecystogram.

(3) Injection of dye directly into the bile duct system can be accomplished by inserting a thin needle directly into the liver or by filling the common bile duct with dye after it has been identified through a flexible fiber-optic tube (endoscope) inserted through the mouth down to the first part of the small intestine (duodenum). These procedures require special skills and carry a slight risk, but they are becoming commonplace in many centers. They are the most useful in situations when jaundice is believed to be caused by bile duct blockage.

The point to be stressed is that diagnostic conclusions and treatment decisions—especially the one to operate—should not be made until one or more of the studies described above have been completed.

TREATMENT   Some persons with an acute gallbladder attack (cholecystitis) will experience severe and prolonged symptoms indicative of impending gangrene and perforation. Emergency surgery is clearly the treatment of choice in such situations. Most patients, however, get over their attacks and are free of symptoms within a matter of hours.

The question of surgery becomes difficult for persons who recover from a gallbladder attack and then feel fine. They understandably question the need for major surgery. However, the vast majority of experts agree that "elective" removal of the gallbladder—that is, under symptom-free and non-emergency conditions—is advisable in a person who has had even a single attack of clearly diagnosed gallbladder disease. The basis for this recommendation is the fact that once an attack has occurred, further ones are likely and each one carries the possibility of serious complications and the resulting need for emergency surgery—always more dangerous than elective surgery. The risk of an elective operation is *very* low when performed by a competent surgeon in a good hospital.

Another question involves the accidental discovery of gallstones (during x-ray studies for other reasons) that have not caused symptoms—so-called "silent stones." Most experts feel less comfortable in having any standard policy about surgery here, but prefer to individualize the recommendation for each patient. The same is true when gallstones occur with very minor symptoms that are uncharacteristic for gallstone disease.

The development of *pills to dissolve gallstones* has attracted increasing attention in recent years as a future alternative to surgical treatment. The following points summarize current information about gallstone treatment with chenodeoxycholic acid (CDA), the pill that is undergoing extensive trials in this country and is in actual use in Italy:

(1) CDA will dissolve approximately 70% of cholesterol gallstones that are *uncalcified* and *less than 2 centimeters in diameter*. It is ineffective for larger stones and those that are judged by their x-ray appearance to contain calcium.

(2) The length of treatment time required to dissolve stones usually ranges from 6 to 30 months and would therefore preclude pill treatment for emergency situations.

(3) The recurrence rate of stone formation is as high as 30% during the first year after CDA treatment is stopped. Thus, continued treatment—probably for a lifetime—would seem necessary to keep stones from reforming.

(4) Although baboons develop potentially serious liver injury from CDA, humans do not. The main side effect is diarrhea, which is present to some degree in up to 50% of patients taking CDA. (A "second generation" drug to dissolve gallstones—*ursodeoxycholic acid*—has the apparent advantages of effectiveness at dosages lower than CDA and freedom from the diarrhea.)

CDA will probably be eventually approved for use in treating at least some types of gallstone disease. It would appear best suited for the treatment of gallstone sufferers who are high surgical risks, but it will not be a general panacea for reasons mentioned above—failure to dissolve some gallstones, the need for chronic treatment that might last a lifetime, the side effect of diarrhea, and, probably, the expense of long-term treatment.

IN SUMMARY   Gallstones are one of the most common afflictions of the human race. There is little, if anything, one can do to prevent their formation or the resulting acute attacks. Fortunately, we can live without our gallbladders, and surgical removal is an effective and relatively safe form of treatment *in accurately diagnosed cases.* Pill treatment to dissolve certain kinds of gallstones should be available in the future, but its ultimate role in therapy remains to be determined.

Prostate Ailments

First, a spelling lesson. We humans, accidentally or otherwise, may assume a prost*r*ate position—but we do not have a gland spelled in that manner. Male members of the human race do, however, have a prostate gland—and with or without a second "r," this walnut-sized gland all too often spells trouble. The prostate's potential for trouble is directly related to its position in life. As shown in the diagram, the prostate gland surrounds the urethra—the tube that emerges from the bladder and carries urine, via the penis, to the outside world. Little imagination is needed to understand how infection or enlargement of the prostate can interfere with the act of urination. The diagram also illustrates how close the prostate gland is to the front wall of the rectum—thereby making much of the gland accessible to the physician's finger during a rectal examination. Finally, it should be noted that the prostate surrounds the final passage of sperm (via the ejaculatory ducts) into the urethra; during ejaculation, the prostate gland squeezes fluid into the urethra to aid in the transport and nourishment of sperm. Given this strategic location, one might expect the prostate to perform essential—even heroic—functions. But, in fact, apart from its contribution to semen, the gland's major role seems to be to cause trouble. (In recent years, a group of physiologically active substances known as *prostaglandins* have become the object of intense interest. Though initially found in the prostate, they are actually widespread throughout the body and not at all unique to the prostate.) This essay will survey the three major disorders associated with the prostate gland.

INFECTION Fortunate is the male who makes it through life without at least one bout of prostatitis. Unfortunately, some men also become the victims of so-called chronic prostatitis—recurring,

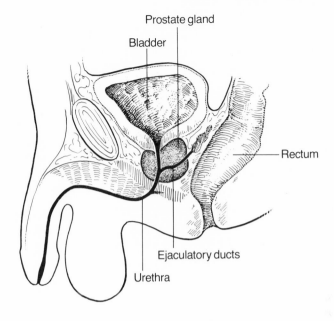

low-grade infections which are difficult to treat and which, while not life-threatening, cause considerable discomfort and annoyance.

Acute prostatitis is characterized by the rather abrupt onset of fever, pain at the base of the penis, and painful urination; uncontrolled dripping of cloudy fluid from the urethra may also occur (a problem associated with some venereal diseases as well). Usually, an infecting bacterial organism can be identified from urine specimens and the infection treated with antibiotics. In older men, prostate infections may be associated with gland enlargement which may require surgery. When there is persistent inflammation of the prostate, it may be necessary to use x-ray dye studies and direct inspection via the penis (through a cystoscope) to rule out underlying anatomical problems.

As mentioned, *chronic prostatitis* is usually a more difficult problem. Often no bacteria can be identified as the certain cause. In recent years, newly identified forms of microbial life—some requiring special antibiotics—have been implicated in chronic prostatitis. But, quite frankly, physicians frequently resort to rather blindly trying various—often "broad spectrum"—antibiotics in the hope that one will alleviate symptoms. Some experts who believe that emotions can play a role in chronic prostatitis may use tranquilizers as well. (Caffeine-containing beverages, decreased sexual activity, prolonged sitting, and many other factors have been associated in popular myth with prostate infections, but scientific evidence does not support these as significant causes.)

BENIGN PROSTATIC ENLARGEMENT   The exact reasons for enlargement of the prostate are unclear—though presumably they are related to hormonal changes associated with aging; about 10% of males aged forty already have some degree of enlargement, and by age 60 prostate enlargement is almost universal.

When the prostate increases in size, it may impinge on the urethra—thereby narrowing the passageway for urine flow. This, in turn, causes a set of symptoms known as *prostatism*—difficulty in starting the flow of urine, decreased force of the urinary stream, dribbling of urine after voiding is felt to be completed, and increased frequency of urination, especially during the night ("nocturia"). Prostatism usually develops gradually but may, in advanced stages, produce a sudden and complete blockage to the flow of urine—obviously requiring emergency treatment. Even lesser stages of blockage can lead to serious infections of the urinary tract caused by the back-up of urine.

Benign enlargement is caused by an overgrowth of glands associated with the urethra but located inside the prostate gland. The usual form of surgery to alleviate the blockage is a transurethral resection (TUR). The excessive tissue is extracted via the urethra using a special type of cystoscope and electrical cutting device which removes the central portion of the gland. Thus, much of the original prostate gland—which was pushed to the outside—remains after surgery. Therefore, even after such surgery, the prostate must be checked periodically for further growth or the development of cancer. The decision for surgical removal and the type of surgery to be done depend ultimately on the discomfort of the individual and the judgment of a competent urologist. Whether there are symptoms or not, surgical removal may be necessary because of an associated urinary tract infection that threatens kidney damage or changes in the bladder, which is forced to work extra hard to expel urine through the penis. Most surgical procedures done for benign enlargement do not result in any degree of impotence; they may, however, cause retrograde ejaculation—meaning that semen is passed back into the bladder during intercourse. *At present, there are no agents scientifically proven to cause shrinkage of the prostate gland.*

CANCER OF THE PROSTATE   While less common than benign enlargement, cancer of the prostate gland is a far more serious problem given the fact that it is one of the major causes of cancer deaths in men—about 20,000 per year in this country. Most cancers of the prostate—especially in older men—grow at a slow pace and are not likely to spread excessively or cause death; indeed, the majority of males over age 80 probably have small amounts of this type of cancer. When prostate cancer is established by microscopic study to be of this indolent type, most experts advise no treatment other than annual check-ups and transurethral (through the penis) removal of the obstructing tissue.

When the prostate cancer is a more aggressively spreading kind, various treatment measures can be employed. For example, radical prostate surgery—more extensive than simple tissue removal for enlargement—has often been used. However, recent studies indicate that the results of radiation treatment *may* be comparable to those of surgery in some of these cases. In short, the exact form of treatment that should be used in any given case will depend on the stage of the disease, the age of the patient, the latest information from studies comparing treatment methods, and, most important, the skill and judgment of an experienced urologist.

The most critical theme concerning prostate cancer is the *importance of annual rectal exams in males over age 50.* If a prostate cancer can be detected in early stages before spread has occurred, chances for cure are considerably improved. Most prostate cancers occur in the rear part of the gland, which can be easily felt during a rectal exam. *Therefore, any male over 50 who does not receive a rectal exam as part of a routine physical exam is getting short-changed.* Unfortunately, by the time a cancer can be felt, it may have spread beyond the gland—making a cure much less likely. Thus, there is enormous interest in current research to develop a simple blood test to detect chemicals from the prostate gland that indicate early cancer. Such tests are in advanced stages of refinement, but there is still considerable uncertainty as to how they should be used—given that results showing elevations may signify an indolent cancer that should not be treated. As with all screening tests, results become important only if there is a clear strategy for responding effectively to positive findings.

IN SUMMARY   The prostate gland seems to cause an inordinate amount of trouble. However, most of these troubles are not life-threatening, and the prostate's unique location permits early detection of cancer *if* annual rectal exams are done routinely in men over age 50.

Senility

The dictionaries coolly define senility as "the sum of the physical and mental changes occurring in advanced life" or as "the physical and mental infirmity of old age." But for the more than two million Americans over age 65 who suffer from the ravages of intellectual decline—and for the families who care for them—the word often signifies deep despair. In recent years, medical and social scientists have become more precise about the mental problems of aging—and, more important, more aggressive about the possibilities of reversing or even "curing" some problems of aging formerly dismissed as "simple senility." The purposes of this essay are to describe these developments and to highlight the more common "reversible" causes of senility.

DEFINITIONS The more precise word for the condition most people label as senility is *dementia*—the usually gradual development of widespread intellectual impairment including failing attention, loss of memory, decreased ability to handle numerical calculations, and loss of orientation for time and place. Personality changes (irritability, loss of humor, etc.) usually accompany the actual intellectual deficits. In addition, some elderly persons may experience a mental state more accurately described as *delirium*—the usually more sudden development of dramatic changes including confusion, hallucinations, and rather sudden alterations in the degree of alertness. Delirium is more likely to have reversible causes—such as sudden medical illness or alcohol withdrawal—though it may also be superimposed on the process of gradual intellectual deterioration. Whatever the word used, however, the practical questions remain the same: What is causing the problem? Can anything be done to reverse the situation?

385

CAUSES   While exact statistics are hard to come by, it is generally estimated that about 80% of all dementia in persons over age 65 is caused by two irreversible disorders. *Alzheimer's disease*—by far the most common—is a disease of unknown cause associated with progressive dementia leading to death within five to ten years; at autopsy, the brain shows characteristic microscopic abnormalities in the cerebrum—the largest, "intellectual" part of the human brain. Though many tantalizing research leads are under exploration, *there is as yet no treatment for this condition proven to be effective.* The other major cause of irreversible dementia among the elderly is a phenomenon usually known as *multi-infarct dementia*—meaning many small strokes that destroy small areas of brain tissue. Theoretically, the treatment of existing high blood pressure might help in preventing further "mini-strokes"—but the treatment of hypertension in the elderly can be very tricky since "over-treatment" can also lead to brain damage due to insufficient blood flow.

That's the bad news. The relatively good news is that approximately 10–20% of persons over 65 with mental deterioration have underlying causes that may be partially or completely reversed—including the following:

(1) Inappropriate drug ingestion: This "cause" is put at the top of the list to emphasize the increasing recognition of the phenomenon of excessive and inappropriate drug use by the elderly. Some of this use stems from the problems of dementia itself (forgetfulness as to when the last dose was taken, confusion about how long medication should be taken) or a tendency to try something suggested by a friend. However, much of the blame must be laid at the doorstep of physicians who too readily prescribe drugs without careful checking as to what the person is already taking, or who spend too little time to consider (and explain) the special problems that many common drugs might cause older people. Indeed, one of the first steps in evaluating the development of dementia in anyone is to review all drug use carefully—including non-prescription drugs. In some cases it may be necessary to check the medicine cabinet at home rather than rely on the verbal report given. The discontinuation of drugs should be done under the supervision of a knowledgeable physician, since serious withdrawal problems can occur.

(2) Unrecognized depression: As with persons of any age, seri-

ous underlying depression may be missed in the midst of intellectual deterioration. But there is a special danger of this happening to an elderly person—given the easy explanation of "senility" for such deterioration and the erroneous assumption that elderly persons are not likely to become depressed. Indeed, during depression they are more likely to deny mood changes and instead focus on bodily complaints. But depression is being increasingly identified as the basis for impaired mental function in elderly people, and proper treatment can lead to striking improvement.

(3) Underlying physical disease: This category is all-inclusive and runs the gamut from alcoholism to infection to low thyroid function to an unrecognized blood clot next to the brain. A recent task force sponsored by the National Institute of Aging listed fifty "reversible causes of mental impairment." The important issue, of course, is that these causes must be considered if they are to be discovered. And it is still too easy to dismiss changes in mental function or status in someone chronologically advanced as a matter of "growing older."

Which brings us to the all important question of when and where to seek evaluation for someone with changing mental function.

DIAGNOSIS AND TREATMENT   There is obviously a fine line between doing too much and too little for those we love—between frantically seeking further opinions and possible cures for a situation that is beyond medical help, versus too quickly assuming that nothing can be done. Ultimately the best answer to this dilemma is to find a qualified person or institution that takes a special interest in evaluating problems relating to the elderly. In the past, such resources were often lacking in many communities—and even in many major medical centers. Today, however, there is a great interest in the training and teaching of physicians in the special medical and social problems of the elderly, and expertise will be increasingly available in the near future. Wherever help is ultimately sought, the medical evaluation is likely to include the following elements:

(1) A careful history of past and current problems with special emphasis on tendencies to depression and a survey (including home check, if necessary) of all drug use.

(2) A thorough physical exam with special emphasis on abnormalities of the nervous system and tests of mental function.

(3) A thoughtful set of laboratory examinations which will typically include not only familiar studies (such as blood and urine) but almost always a so-called CAT (computerized axial tomography) scan for structural abnormalities of the head and brain. Indeed, because of its safety and effectiveness, the CAT scan is one of the most important advances of the past decade for evaluating intellectual impairment in the elderly.

The above investigations may lead to other tests or considerations. Avoiding unnecessary tests is also important for the patient and family. But given the legitimate hope that reversible causes of dementia might be found, the emphasis today should be on thorough initial evaluation rather than casual dismissal of the problem as "old age."

Hydrocephalus in the Elderly

Fluid is normally produced by the brain to serve as its cushion for blows to the head. Hydrocephalus ("water in the head") refers to situations in which *excessive* fluid accumulates in the spaces of the brain and skull. Such accumulation can be caused by many conditions in which either increased fluid is produced or insufficient amounts are reabsorbed.

In infants, excessive fluid usually leads to expansion of the growing skull. However, in adults such expansion is not possible and brain tissues are more quickly compressed. While less common in adults, hydrocephalus can occur—particularly in the elderly where symptoms may be confused with degenerative brain diseases that cannot be treated.

This type of hydrocephalus, called "normal pressure hydrocephalus"—or NPH for short—is characterized by normal spinal fluid pressure combined with rather specific symptoms: mental changes of senility, difficulty in walking, and loss of urine and bowel control. Each of these symptoms is common in the elderly. However, when they occur together, it is important to think of the possibility of NPH, because surgical shunting (creating a pathway for fluid to escape from the brain) may dramatically improve the patient—especially if accomplished during the early phase of deterioration.

Today, NPH is diagnosed by the presence of characteristic symptoms plus studies (such as CAT-scan pictures of the brain) to confirm increased fluid in the brain. The message: think of the possibility of normal pressure hydrocephalus when an older person develops "senile" behavior, walking difficulties, and inability to control urination.

Bunions,
Varicose Veins,
Etc.

BUNIONS   The question: What causes bunions? The answer: There are numerous causes that range from the shape and bone structure of the foot that one is born with to joint disease, such as rheumatoid arthritis. One cause of bunions is shoes with pointed toes, especially when the shoes are too short and have high heels. The net result of wearing such shoes is to force the big toe (more elegantly referred to as the "great" toe) toward the outer side of the foot, thereby putting abnormal pressure on the inner side of the joint where the big toe joins the rest of the foot. The response to such long-term pressure is a partial dislocation of the toe joint, along with a build-up of surrounding soft tissue and underlying bone; resultant swelling, redness, and tenderness produce what is popularly known as a bunion.

Most bunions cause little more than cosmetic problems—provided the shoes worn are soft, wide, and roomy. However, bunions make shoe fitting difficult and stylish footwear impossible. Disabling pain may be controlled by anti-inflammatory drugs, but surgical correction of the deformity is sometimes necessary for relief. However, surgery for purely cosmetic reasons is likely to be disappointing. In the absence of significant deformity and pain, the pros and cons of surgical treatment should be weighed very carefully before deciding to operate. It is cheaper and safer to get shoes that fit the feet than to try to make the feet fit conventional shoes surgically.

VARICOSE VEINS   The words "varicose veins" refer to any veins that are abnormally swollen or prominent due to increased pressure inside them. For practical purposes, however, most people have in mind those cosmetically distressing swellings of the veins just under the skin of the lower leg when they talk about "varicosities." So, for those of you who want to know more about them, the following is a "one-minute-read" summary of what everyone should know about varicose veins:

(1) The problem with varicose veins is mainly appearance. They seldom signify serious underlying disease of the deeper veins, though there are times when further tests should be performed to exclude this possibility. (A rash or ulcers on the skin are two such signals.) Since the problem is largely a matter of looks—and since surgical removal of the veins is not always successful—many physicians feel that surgery should be a treatment of last resort, to be considered only when the effect on appearance is quite drastic.

(2) Various commonsense maneuvers may help prevent—or treat—varicose veins. These measures include avoiding stationary standing or sitting (which obviously contributes to the pooling of blood in the veins); regular movement of the lower legs (which helps to squeeze the blood up from the lower legs); elevating the legs above heart level whenever possible (which is not only relaxing but improves blood return to the heart); and wearing elastic stockings (which can admittedly be homely but some of the newer types aren't so bad looking).

There are no foolproof methods of preventing varicosities—especially in those apparently destined by inheritance to have them. But the above measures can usually help.

INTERMITTENT CLAUDICATION   These fancy medical words describe a problem that most sufferers will immediately recognize as pain that develops in the calf muscles of one or both legs after walking a certain (usually consistent) distance. The pain is relieved within minutes by resting. The cause of this pain is almost always a partial blockage (by atherosclerotic plaques) of the major artery in the upper leg (the femoral artery), resulting in an inadequate blood supply to the lower leg during exercise. Although vascular reconstructive surgery (cleaning out the artery or bypassing the block) is often recommended as a definitive treatment, such surgery is usually not needed. At other times, surgery may be technically impossible because of the extent of the blockage within relatively small vessels that are beyond easy reach.

Recently, another technique—transluminal angioplasty—has been increasingly used for this problem. Known as "balloon surgery," this procedure allows vessels to be dilated by threading a balloon to the appropriate area and inflating it (see p. 258). Angioplasty has the advantages of not requiring general anesthesia or a prolonged hospitalization. The long-range outcome of this more expedient technique remains to be studied. Maneuvers short of invasive procedures (surgery or angioplasty) that may be helpful include stopping smoking (often resulting in dramatic improvement), reducing excess weight, and participating in graduated walking-exercise programs. The widely promoted use of vasodilating drugs (to widen blood vessels) has no proven value in this condition—and may even worsen problems. Thus, while intermittent calf pain is an annoying condition, it is seldom life-threatening and non-surgical treatment can often be beneficial.

A NEW DRUG FORMULATION FOR PARKINSON'S DISEASE   The recent release of a new formulation of Sinemet—the most widely used drug for Parkinsonism in this country—prompts this brief review of the treatment of Parkinson's disease—so-named for the British physician Dr. James Parkinson, who first described the disease in 1817. Today, we understand that the symptoms of Parkinsonism—slowness of muscle activity, rigidity, and tremor— are often caused by a deficiency of an important brain chemical, dopamine. And based on this understanding, an important breakthrough in treatment for Parkinsonism was achieved in the 1960s by the use of a drug, levodopa (or L-dopa) which increases brain levels of dopamine. However, L-dopa alone also often results in elevated *body* levels of dopamine that cause undesirable side effects. Therefore, the next development in drug therapy for Parkinsonism was to combine L-dopa with carbidopa (which inhibits the formation of dopamine outside the brain) in the combination drug known as Sinemet. And, as mentioned above, a new formulation of this combination is now available—giving doctors several varieties of Sinemet to work with in arriving at a combination that is best for a given patient.

Several other effective drugs for treating the symptoms of Parkinsonism are available when Sinemet is not thought to be the appropriate treatment. Indeed, people with mild forms of the disease may not be started on levodopa since it sometimes has a limited span of effectiveness in a given person. When therapy is started with Sinemet or other drugs, side effects often occur, and it is important for the initial stages of treatment to be carefully supervised by an expert. But the good news is that most people with Parkinsonism can be helped—which is a statement that could not be made twenty-five years ago.

A NOTE ON SAFETY CAPS   The Poison Prevention Packaging Acts have mandated the use of child-resistant containers for nearly all prescribed drugs, as well as aspirin and iron products. However, these containers are often difficult for the elderly to open, as emphasized recently by a group of New York physicians—who stress that the elderly can obtain any drug in non-resistant containers merely by asking the pharmacist for them.

DIMINISHED VISION AND POOR LIGHT   In this age of complicated medical problems—and equally complicated solutions—it is refreshing to come across answers that are simple and direct. A recent issue of a British medical journal, *The Lancet,* contains an intriguing article entitled, "Visual Disability and Home Lighting." In it, researchers from St. Bartholomew's Hospital in London describe the results of checking lighting in the homes of 63 elderly patients (average age of 76) in their low-vision clinic. What they found seems remarkable: the average lighting in the home was one-tenth that found in the hospital—and the average reading light was one-seventh that in a comparable hospital setting. Even more striking was the result of their "treatment" program: the use of "augmented" lighting at home (in the form of a 60-watt bulb in a small adjustable lamp) produced an improvement in vision in 82% of these patients. While this is only a single report, it does raise the possibility that a number of older persons who seek medical attention for diminished vision could achieve distinct benefit by shedding some light on their problem.

You and the Doctor

MYTH *6*

A chest x-ray is a good way
to detect lung cancer in time
for a cure.

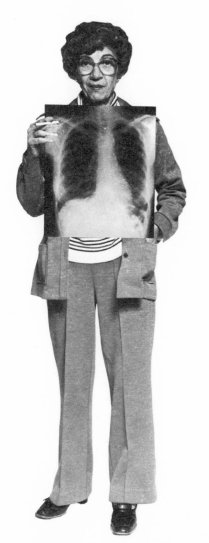

Choosing a Doctor

Like most important questions, "Who should I have for my doctor?" is not easily answered. Your preference for a man or woman doctor, for one who is older or younger, or for a particular personality type will naturally affect your choice. A particular medical need, such as bowel problems, allergies, or arthritis, may lead you to a doctor with special interest and experience in that area. But these are fairly natural and obvious aspects of making a choice. To select and evaluate your "primary" physician—the one you turn to first for medical help and the one you rely on to help you prevent illness—questions are worth asking. Health care is complex, and doctors are only human; so you should not expect across-the-board perfection. But it's fair to have standards and expect your doctor to meet them. Here are some suggestions for things to consider.

BACKGROUND   Good training lays the foundation for everything that follows—and it is relatively easy to learn how a doctor has been trained. The American Medical Association publishes *The Directory of Medical Specialists* and other directories which are available in most local libraries. It is important to know that your doctor has graduated from a fully accredited medical school (as the overwhelming majority now have), but going beyond that—to find out whether it's a "prestige" school—is usually unimportant. And high class standing (which may be evidenced by membership in the Alpha Omega Alpha honor society) does not correlate all that well with later performance as a physician.

Post-graduate training ("residency") probably has more influence on the quality of a doctor's work than basic schooling. For several decades it has been standard to expect that primary physicians would acquire three full years of training after medical school, whether as internists or as family practitioners. At the end of this period the doctor must pass an examination to become "board certified" or a "diplomate" in a specialty (including family practice). Someone who finishes the training but has not yet taken or passed the examination is known as "board eligible." Physicians over age 50 often have not gone through the formal process of certification; younger physicians in practice normally have done so, and it's worth checking.

A doctor's hospital appointments—the places where he or she is authorized to admit patients—also tell you something about qualifications and professional standing. Most hospitals carefully screen the physicians appointed to their staffs; the better a hospital, the better qualified its physicians are likely to be.

KEEPING UP   The superstar young physician of 1960 would be worse than mediocre today without a continuing effort to keep abreast of medical progress. There are lots of ways to do this. Reading is important. If books are around a doctor's office, see whether they are of relatively recent vintage instead of dusty with disuse and tattered with age. If there are medical journals, at least some of them should be the renowned and substantial ones—the *New England Journal of Medicine, Lancet, Annals of Internal Medicine, American Journal of Medicine, JAMA (Journal of the American Medical Association)*—not *Medical Economics, Diversion,* or other magazines sent free of charge as a vehicle for drug advertising.

Attending courses at a medical school, meetings of a specialty society, or weekly "rounds" at a hospital is an important means of keeping up with recent advances. Teaching in a nearby hospital or medical school is both an excellent means of keeping the teacher informed and an indication that his or her ability is recognized by these institutions.

Many specialty boards have recognized that "certification" early in a career means little in respect to competence for a lifetime, and they are now offering *re*certification at intervals. Such examinations remain voluntary for internists, but the Board of Family Practice now requires periodic recertification.

REPUTATION   Much as when deciding to purchase a particular car, you may find it's worthwhile to ask someone who's "used one."

The experience of a single person in a doctor's practice may not be representative, but a consensus from several can be a useful guide to strengths, weaknesses, and idiosyncrasies. You can tap into the general opinion in the medical community by asking other doctors or nurses, pharmacists, hospital secretaries, and the like.

ACCESSIBILITY   To be any good at all, primary medical care has to be available in time of need. A good primary physician responds to truly urgent problems by fitting the patient into his or her schedule, returns calls, and sees to it that there is ample coverage when he or she is away or off duty.

PRACTICE PATTERNS   An orderly office, defined office hours, equipment in good working condition, a secretary who knows where to find the doctor, overall cleanliness, and correspondence that is at least as punctual as the billing—these are nuts-and-bolts indications of a well-run practice. A willingness to discuss billing practices, and possibly adapting them to your needs, might also be desirable.

When you sit down with the doctor, he or she should give you a chance to describe the problem initially in your own words without a barrage of yes-or-no questions before you get two sentences out of your mouth (though yes-or-no questions, *later on,* can be important in clarifying things). The physical examination should be performed carefully and with due consideration for your modesty (but not at the expense of neglecting rectal and genital examinations). If you come in with what seems to be a minor complaint and many expensive tests are ordered, an explanation should be provided.

An emphasis on using the "latest" drugs may be misplaced. While a few really important new drugs become available each year, most are just more expensive versions of the older ones—with the disadvantage that their side effects aren't as well known as those of the older ones. Prescribing drugs by "generic" names rather than "brand" names is, as a rule, a good way of protecting your pocketbook as well as treating your ailments.

Your primary physician should be prepared to refer you to competent specialists when serious or complicated problems come up. It is crucial to have additional expert help when the need arises. On the other hand, the doctor who refers routine, minor complaints (trivial rashes, mild headaches of long standing, brief digestive disturbances) to specialists is just running up your bills. Such over-re-ferring sometimes occurs in large fee-for-service, "multi-disciplin-ary" group practices; at the other extreme, a "prepaid health plan" may be exceedingly cautious about referrals.

RELATIONSHIP TO YOU   Ask yourself whether you feel your doctor is really listening to you. He or she may be harassed and dis-tracted by the problems of others, but that's small solace when *you* need attention. You should feel free to ask the important questions on your mind and not be made to feel ashamed because you don't have a medical degree. There are several points to consider at the end of a visit:

(1) Have you received an explanation that *you* can understand?

(2) Do you know what *you* are supposed to do—exactly—when you get home?

(3) Is there some provision for follow-up, especially if you have been given a treatment or a prescription? Do you know what you're supposed to do if you don't get better—and when?

(4) Is the doctor ordering a whole slew of tests and brushing off your questions rather than counseling you on the nature of the problem and how to deal with it?

(5) Is the doctor willing to tell you what to expect, to the best of his or her ability to predict?

(6) If there is something you don't understand when you get home, do you feel free to call back and get clarification?

If the answers to these questions are mainly no, you may feel you are being cheated—and you may very well be right.

THE DOCTOR'S DEMEANOR   Perhaps the most desirable atti-tude in a doctor is *confidence without dogmatism*. A sense of humor and deep warmth would certainly add to this, but more important is an ability to knowledgeably discuss options and alternatives without making pronouncements. And he or she should welcome a "second opinion" when a difficult decision is at hand.

IN SUMMARY   You can't be *sure* that a doctor is the right one for you until you've had a chance to "settle in" together, although a little homework can tell you a surprising amount. By the same token, when personal "chemistry" prevents a relationship from working, nobody is obliged to stick it out. It is possible and even desirable to part company, with all due respect, and try again. This should be as true in a clinic or group practice as it is with a solo practitioner.

It is predicted that a surplus of physicians will appear in the next decade. The term "glut" is even being used. One consequence is that all of us will have a wider range of choices as we seek the "right" doctor for ourselves and our families.

Periodic Check-Ups

The decade of the 70s produced—among many other progeny—a new emphasis on personal responsibilty for keeping healthy, rather than fatalistically waiting for illness to strike without notice. But with this more aggressive individual pursuit of sustained health has come an increased questioning of such practices as the complete head-to-toe check-up—an annual ritual still enacted by many doctors and patients despite the criticism of too much, too soon. The favored alternatives to the complete check-up—selective health examinations—are comparable to automobile maintenance inspections: only specific high-risk parts are checked for hidden faults to ascertain whether a breakdown is likely in the months ahead. Attention is directed to the crucial areas with the goal of preventing a major mishap, whereas other items (upholstery, windows, paint) are generally ignored as a matter of convention.

Many considerations underlie the shift in emphasis from routine, complete exams to more selective health screening practices—including the following:

(1) Cost and risk versus benefit: While almost any test or examination will occasionally uncover an important abnormality, careful study indicates that the cost (or even the risk) of many traditional procedures far outweighs the rare benefit derived when they are done routinely on healthy persons. If cost were no consideration, some medical tests might be defended on the basis that even a slim chance of benefit seems worthwhile in the absence of risk. But medical resources are simply not unlimited; cost constraints have become necessarily prominent in decision making—both at a societal and a personal level. If more time and money go into examining healthy people, less of each is available to treat the sick.

(2) Testing errors: No test is foolproof. So-called false-positive test results—those which are erroneously abnormal—occur frequently in a healthy population. Such results can pose a danger (aside from needless anxiety) in that they commit the physician to more expensive and invasive studies (such as angiography, biopsies) to pursue the "abnormality." Therefore, even simple tests carry the risk that an incorrect readout will lead to potentially dangerous tests at unnecessary cost.

(3) Variability of personal factors: Increasingly, both science and common sense point to the importance of individualizing health assessment according to special needs posed by *age* (very frequent checks on height and weight are key checkpoints of health during the first year of life, but not in adulthood), *family history* (a strong family history of breast cancer should influence the frequency of mammography examinations), *personal life-style* (an alcoholic requires more scrutiny than someone who does not abuse alcohol), and *specific work exposures* (frequent hearing tests to detect early deafness makes sense in noisy work settings).

(4) Importance of timing: Often the routine annual approach encourages a false sense of security ("everything was OK at my last check-up") that can lead to minimizing new symptoms that should be investigated immediately—such as rectal bleeding or the onset of chest pain after exertion. In short, much more important than an annual physical is the investigation of significant symptoms whenever they occur.

A PHILOSOPHY   Given the above, most thoughtful physicians willing to ignore their own income considerations and the expectations of many patients would agree that much of the "comprehensive" annual health examination makes little sense. Income considerations are, however, often real—based on the unfortunate tendency to reward health care professionals (and institutions) for "doing" rather than "thinking" or "caring"—for performing a procedure rather than exploring the total health profile and practice of a given patient. For example, it is far more important to the majority of American adults to discuss issues of life-style, nutrition, alcohol and tobacco consumption, work history, seat-belt use, feelings of depression, family problems, and sexual concerns than to do an electrocardiogram or sigmoidoscopy. But the latter are readily reimbursed—whereas the former are not, even though they are more apt to reveal information that has a major bearing on future health. There are growing attempts to challenge the traditional payment systems for health care—such as encouraging prevention and reducing hospitalization costs in HMO (health maintenance organization) enrollment plans or adjusting health and life insurance costs according to personal life-style. And increasingly, both medical evidence and financial considerations are pointing in the direction of emphasizing health education, life-style changes, and selective (versus routine) testing—rather than ritualistic, non-directed, annual check-ups for healthy persons.

In short, visiting one's physician periodically, perhaps every two or three years in adult life, remains reasonable; at the very least, the visit sustains a useful doctor–patient relationship. A review of personal habits and health practices should occur, and selected portions of a physical exam can be performed (as well as taught) to encourage frequent self-examination—for example, of the breasts or testicles. But extensive testing (blood collecting, x-rays, electrocardiograms) should not automatically occur as part of each visit for the well person.

DIAGNOSTIC TESTS FOR THE HEALTHY PERSON—SOME SELECTIONS Having presented the issue in general terms, we must now face the practical question about what tests make sense—and when. Ultimately, many of these choices are matters of judgment because important data are still lacking. Our Advisory Board generally agreed on the relative importance accorded to the different tests, and the stage of life when each test should play a role. However, how often a specific test should be given remains a debatable issue; we've still tried to put down a reasonable response in most cases.

We have listed the tests roughly in order of their value as compared to their expense; the tests at the top are more likely to be beneficial in relation to cost and/or risk than those at the bottom. Remember, we're considering the healthy person; any test may assume greater priority if specific symptoms bring you to a doctor's attention. So here goes—our version of the "top 15":

(1) Immunizations: Though not tests so much as procedures, there are no medical practices more justified by cost, preventive im-

pact, and relative safety than the routine immunizations of childhood—or those which are sensible in adult years (tetanus boosters and, for senior citizens or those with chronic illnesses, the pneumonia vaccine and flu vaccine, for example).

(2) Infant screening for metabolic disorders: The pay-off from discovering a metabolic disorder (such as an underactive thyroid) at birth in an infant who would be retarded for life without early treatment is potentially enormous.

(3) Blood pressure measurement: The evidence is so clear as to the value of treating high blood pressure—which is usually symptom-free until its catastrophic complications occur—that the simple act of checking blood pressure yearly should be high on anybody's list of important tests.

(4) Stool checks for "hidden blood": Screening kits, available to check for hidden blood in stools, allow samples to be sent directly to a physician or laboratory for testing. This is a useful, inexpensive way to screen for cancer and other bowel problems. The test should be given at age 40 and repeated every two years thereafter.

(5) Pap smear: While scientific evidence supports the recent American Cancer Society recommendation of a Pap smear every three years in *women between 20 and 40 who have had two previous negative Pap tests a year apart,* there is concern that the extended time intervals may result in women dropping the periodic Pap habit altogether. Obviously, a yearly Pap smear is better than none at all.

(6) Tests for venereal disease: These tests have assumed even greater importance for those who engage in sex with a number of partners, often casual acquaintances. The blood test for syphilis and swab tests (vagina, urethra, rectum) for gonorrhea are simple and inexpensive; we feel they should be done every two or three years in all sexually active persons—including teenagers.

(7) Skin test for tuberculosis: The value of periodic skin testing (every five years until age 35) for tuberculosis is that when "conversion" from prior negative tests to a positive one occurs, it means that tuberculosis bacteria have invaded the body in the interim. Treatment of recent "conversions" is not always a matter of routine, but there should be a search for evidence of clinical tuberculosis (for example, a chest x-ray) as a minimum response.

(8) Screening for vision and hearing: Most of us remember checks on visual and hearing acuity during our schooldays. There may also be good reason for occasional periodic checks (every five

years) past age 60, a time when many correctable problems are not otherwise brought to medical attention.

(9) Tonometry: Glaucoma—increased pressure within the eye which can lead to permanent visual loss—has no early warning signals in most cases; tonometry is a painless procedure to check for elevated pressure that should be employed every two to three years past age 40 or annually if there is a family history of glaucoma. Reducing the pressure with medicine prevents the loss of vision that might otherwise occur.

(10) Mammography (for breast cancer): The fact that this is number 10 on our list does not mean we think it is a bad test. Indeed, in the high risk woman (strong family history of breast cancer in particular), the benefits of possible early detection far outweigh the minimal risk of radiation. And given the decreased amount of radiation used in most mammography procedures today—versus even five years ago—this risk is probably less than originally thought. However, we agree with the usual recommendation that, in the absence of risk factors, routine mammography (every two to three years) is not needed until age 50.

(11) CBC (complete blood count) and urinalysis: These low cost tests seem to be a part of everybody's list. The blood count is essentially a screen for anemias (that require additional tests for specific diagnosis), while the urinalysis checks for certain kidney and bladder problems (including silent infections) and diabetes. Our recommended frequency of testing is every three to five years.

(12) Multiple blood screening tests: While the large number of tests that can be done inexpensively on a small sample of blood by modern technology can lead to undue concern about "abnormalities" that later prove to be unimportant or erroneous, there are reasons to obtain particular blood tests to screen for specific health problems: *cholesterol* levels correlate with the risk for atherosclerosis; an elevated *blood sugar* may mean early diabetes; a *blood urea nitrogen* is a good check for kidney function; and a *calcium* level tests for overactivity of the parathyroid glands. Once every five years is reasonable.

NOTE   We're reaching the bottom of our list now. You'll find three fairly conventional practices that we feel should be used only sparingly, for the reasons mentioned.

(13) Sigmoidoscopy: Examining the last 10 inches of the large bowel by a sigmoidoscope is extremely important in a patient with bowel symptoms or whose stool contains blood as well as in a person with a strong family history of bowel cancer. But the discomfort and expense of this test do not recommend it as highly as a primary technique to screen for bowel cancer in the general population. (It's only fair to say that some would dispute the low priority we've given it here.) Frequency: if used, every three years after age 40.

(14) Electrocardiogram (ECG): The *resting ECG* is probably overused to screen for coronary artery disease. An *exercise cardiogram* will certainly increase the diagnostic accuracy, but even this test will miss 20% of existing coronary disease; it is also expensive. While a single ECG at age 35 will give a "baseline" pattern with which to compare subsequent deviations, annual cardiograms in the absence of chest pain make more dollars than sense. Once every decade is probably enough.

(15) Chest x-ray: Many will be surprised to find this common test at the very bottom of the list. While the chest x-ray is an outstanding tool for evaluating patients with chest symptoms, the simple fact is that it has rather little "payoff" when used in the absence of symptoms. Lung cancer is rarely detected by chest x-ray early enough to affect the eventual outcome; smokers can take no comfort in relying on chest x-rays to pick up cancer at a stage that is early enough.

Diagnostic Testing

Some have estimated that the cost of diagnostic testing in this country amounts to 16 billion dollars per year—and rises at an annual rate of 15%. The question of "How much is enough?" has been raised repeatedly. Dr. Stephen Goldfinger provides his views on appropriate diagnostic testing.

Does a doctor really sit down and think about the tests he's going to order, or is it just a reflex action on his part?

Much of the time there's a fair amount of thought, although some tests do seem to be ordered instinctively, such as an electrocardiogram for the patient with severe chest pain. The key consideration is whether the test can produce any information that will make a difference in the care of the patient. If not, the reason for obtaining the test should be seriously challenged. A second important matter is the cost of each test and whether even an abnormal finding is worth the price. Finally, it's vital to ask whether the test itself can harm the patient. Taking a blood sample is trivial. But other studies may require the passage of needles or tubes to deeper areas of the body and these are potentially dangerous.

When might you think of withholding a test on the basis of expense alone?

It's usually not expense alone that's the issue, but rather the value of the money spent. Here's an example that almost every doctor has faced at some time. A patient develops new back pain that is most likely not important, but that could be the first symptom of cancer of the pancreas. The chance of this is very slim, and the testing to rule it out would be both expensive and uncomfortable. But even if the tests were to pick up a cancer, it is virtually always too advanced to be cured if the first symptom is back pain. In this example, expensive tests that identify a disease result primarily in earlier anxiety and depression for the patient. How far should the doctor go to make the diagnosis early? Would the cancer victim understand, months later, why the diagnosis was not pursued at the time symptoms first occurred? Might the doctor's "unaggressiveness" even be the basis for a lawsuit?

Have physicians been sufficiently trained to think in terms of the cost-benefit of tests in the past?

No, but things are changing. Every physician must ultimately recognize the impact of his individual decision on the health dollar. Depending upon how he orders tests, the bill can be very large or quite modest. The most compulsive physician who wants to explore every possibility may be acting wastefully, and this is the great dilemma. But it's one that is being increasingly discussed—if not solved—at every level of medical education.

What about the patient who often wants "the best and the latest and the biggest"? How do we try to change the public's belief that more tests mean better medicine?

Honest information is the only way I know. Doctors must be willing to take the time to explain that the tests themselves are not flawless. In some situations, test results even tend to confuse the issue and lead to other tests that become costly or dangerous and may still not provide decisive information. It is also important to make people aware that, in many circumstances, it is perfectly appropriate to live with a problem that has not been completely diagnosed. Very few of the many minor symptoms we all have represent an early, curable cancer that requires prompt delineation. Some of the best physicians I know frequently settle for the "test of time"—simple observation to see whether a symptom develops into a significant problem. In part, excellent clinical judgment can be defined on the basis of the tests a doctor doesn't order.

Some physicians, usually of an older generation, say that the modern era of extensive testing has really de-humanized medicine and detracted from good patient care. Is this possible?

Yes, when testing and technology dominate the scene. All would agree that newer tests have enabled excellent care to occur in a manner that wouldn't otherwise be possible. But a doctor who spends time with a patient only for the sake of knowing which tests to order—rather than to provide a full evaluation and explanation—is not offering the kind of care that I'd wish to have.

Are new tests studied with the same care for safety and effectiveness as are new drugs when they are introduced?

There is increasing concern about how good any new test really is in terms of its sensitivity and its specificity. In other words, how often will a test fail to show the disease when it's really present? How many times will it report that a disease is present when it really is not? And then there are the *equivocal* findings. So the accuracy of the test has to be weighed along with its cost and danger. The FDA is now requiring a comprehensive review of many new tests, such as those proposed for cancer screening. But it's probably true that if all the old tests were subjected to such review, some would surely be rejected—just as many time-honored drugs would probably fail to get FDA approval if they were now to be reviewed in the same way that new ones are.

Some feel that tests are ordered to line the pockets of those who order them. Is this a potential danger?

It is, at times. One should be most concerned when doctors have their own laboratories, x-ray machines, and the like, and each office visit winds up with extensive tests for seemingly minor complaints. Surely, there are times when frequent tests are necessary, as in following a patient with chronic kidney disease. But I'm talking about patients who get too many cardiograms, x-rays, and blood tests on a repeated basis for symptoms that are mild and stable. Even if insurance companies or the government is paying for them, all of us ultimately pay in our insurance premiums and taxes.

Ghost Surgery

We have asked Dr. Andrew Warshaw of our Advisory Board, an active general surgeon at the Massachusetts General Hospital and Associate Professor of Surgery at Harvard Medical School, to comment on the subject of so-called "ghost surgery."

Does ghost surgery occur—at least to the degree that the public has come to suspect?

Let's start by defining two different circumstances. One is the situation in which the person in training—the surgical resident—is performing an operation that was supposed to be performed by an attending surgeon who is nowhere near the operating room. This is, in my experience, extremely uncommon and unjustifiable, except in a very unusual emergency. However, it's not really the central issue that we're dealing with. The issue that has to be faced is whether or not residents should be doing part or all of an operation under the direct supervision of the attending surgeon who is present, but not actually holding the scalpel. For this kind of phenomenon is common and is, in fact, a necessary mainstay of surgical training.

What does supervision really mean?

Answering that question requires explaining that surgery is a team effort. Most operations cannot be carried out by a single person. We need a team, which includes not only the surgeon, but surgical assistants, nurses, and, of course, the anesthesiologist. All of these individuals have a responsible role to play in the operation; holding the scalpel is only one part. In fact, I can think of many situations where I can be more effective by assisting and holding retractors to provide the best possible view of the operative area while my assistant does

412

the actual cutting. I would be making the operation simpler, easier, and safer than if our roles were in the usual reversed fashion. Of course, the next question concerns how much supervision the responsible surgeon can provide if his assistant is the one who is holding the scalpel. The answer to that requires judgment, not only about the resident's level of training and personal capabilities, but also about how difficult the given operation is. If the attending surgeon is both responsible and knowledgeable, he can guide a resident through an operation with essentially the same surgical result because each of the steps (incisions, sutures, and so on) will be the same as he would have provided. I consider that to be my ultimate responsibility if I am going to supervise a resident. Basically, I have to guarantee the end result to be the same as if I had done the entire operation.

Isn't it legally and morally necessary for the patient to be told exactly who is going to do what, or is this impossible in some circumstances?

In the past, surgeons have taken for granted that what went on at the operating table was entirely up to them and that all they had to do was to defend the result. In the present environment, I think most of us realize that this is no longer true. It is important for us to be as thorough as the patient wishes in explaining what is going to happen at surgery—and that includes an explanation of the duties of the various members of the surgical team. Some patients cannot accept the idea that a resident would do *any* of the surgery. In this circumstance, the surgeon has the obligation to abide by the patient's wishes. There are other patients who, having picked their surgeon on the basis of what they believe to be his skill and his good judgment, accept the possibility that he may help the resident perform part of the surgery, with the net effect being a positive one.

Describe for us the typical training of a surgeon—something that doesn't happen overnight, obviously.

Initially, a surgical trainee has to become familiar with real live human anatomy, and with the basic techniques and maneuvers that are employed in the operating room. So most of what he does at first is to assist and watch. As he becomes familiar with the basics, he becomes more of an active participant, whether it's clamping, cutting, tying, suctioning, or some other procedure in an operation. Over a period of months and years, he becomes very skilled at all of these techniques. In time, he will be fully prepared to put them all to use as the "primary" surgeon—while the attending surgeon takes on an interesting role. He becomes the resident's assistant "manually"— but remains his guide and mentor for the general direction and decision making of the operation. The goal is to bring the resident to the point that he no longer requires guidance because of the competence he's acquired. This is important. After all, if all he ever did was to watch or only assist, then the first time he is responsible for doing an operation would be away from his training center. It would occur without supervision. Nobody would be present to prevent or correct his mistakes.

Why do hospitals have residents, and are there disadvantages to choosing a hospital that doesn't have them?

The major purpose of a resident's being in a hospital is, of course, his own training. But in addition he makes many contributions to patient care. The residents are the doctors "on the scene" 24 hours a day and are readily available if an emergency arises in the days before and after surgery. They are there to help the patient with little as well as big problems, even when the attending surgeon is busy elsewhere or out of the hospital. They thereby provide the patient with a real measure of security and care throughout his hospitalization over and above that provided by the attending physician. A more subtle benefit is the fact that residents put an obligation on the attending staff to be as up-to-date as they can possibly be. In other words, there's an element of intellectual stimulation that should give the patient a better brand of medical care. To put it bluntly, residents help keep us "on our toes."

Would you hesitate to have residents involved in your own case if you needed surgery?

If I trusted my doctor and the hospital I was at, I would have no hesitation in having residents involved both inside and out of the operating room. In fact, I would welcome them.

Placebos and Hypnosis

Patients often view treatment in terms of pills, surgery, diets, and the like. Yet, dramatic relief can sometimes be achieved by other means. In the following interview, Dr. Herbert Benson, Associate Professor of Medicine and Director of the Division of Behavioral Medicine at Harvard Medical School, discusses the mysterious "placebo effect"; then we will comment briefly on another method of therapy, hypnosis.

What do you mean by the placebo effect? Aren't placebos just a way to fool patients with medically worthless substances?

The term "placebo" comes directly from the Latin word meaning "I will please." A standard dictionary definition is "a medicine given merely to humor the patient; especially, a preparation containing no medicine but given for its psychological effect." Indeed, the placebo effect can be achieved, in part, with such substances as sugar pills or injections of sterile water. For two reasons placebos have come to be ridiculed or belittled as part of medical practice. First, they have sometimes been used with the intention of "fooling" a patient into feeling better. Second, whenever a new drug is tested, it is compared with a placebo. If the new drug cannot be shown to improve on results obtained with the placebo, the drug is put back on the shelf because the placebo is regarded as the equivalent of "nothing."

But the dictionary definition is too narrow, and it is misleading to think of placebos as just a means of deception. Under certain circumstances placebos have alleviated pain, healed ulcers, improved the electrocardiogram, and enhanced exercise performance. They have also provided relief from hay fever, coughing, and hyperten-

415

sion. On the negative side, placebos have caused headaches, rashes, palpitation, and various intestinal upsets.

Then how should we think of placebos?

Placebos are really much more than sugar pills or injections of water. The term can be used to cover all the nonspecific aspects of treatment, for example, the presence and attitude of a doctor and the setting in which treatment takes place. They contrast with such specific effects as the ability of penicillin to kill bacteria or of a surgeon to repair a heart defect. The placebo effect, in general, embraces three elements: the patient's beliefs and expectations, the physician's beliefs and expectations, and the psychological interaction between the two people. In the past, various useless agents were believed to be effective against disease: lizard's blood, crushed spiders, putrid meat, crocodile dung, bear fat, fox lungs, eunuch fat, and moss scraped from the skull of a hanged criminal. Likewise, cupping, blistering, plastering, and leeching had their day. When *both* physician and patient believed in them, these remedies could indeed have been helpful some of the time.

The placebo effect is one of the best examples of a mind–body interaction, in which thoughts and beliefs are translated into body changes. Although these mind–body interactions are still poorly understood, we are learning more about them. It is now known, for example, that the brain produces its own pain-killing substances, the endorphins, which resemble morphine. In a recent experiment, placebo pills were given to patients after a tooth was pulled. Many of these patients felt relief of pain thanks to the placebo. If they then received naloxone, a drug which interferes with the action of endorphins, the pain came back. In other words, *the placebo helped them to produce their own pain-killers* (*endorphins*), and the naloxone then blocked the action of these endorphins.

Does the placebo effect have any role in treating patients today?

For ages placebos and the placebo effect have been *most* of what healers had to offer their patients. It is only in the last sixty years that specific therapy has become a substantial part of medicine. Specific treatments are beneficial regardless of whether one believes in them, and they do not depend on a sound doctor–patient relationship. Vitamin D cures rickets, penicillin cures pneumonia, and insulin improves diabetes in skeptical as well as believing patients, and whether the doctor is sympathetic or not. In the face of these potent specific agents, the importance of the placebo effect has come to be minimized. Because new drugs have been awesomely and consistently successful by comparison with the rather modest efficacy and unpredictability of traditional approaches, the worthwhile elements of nonspecific treatment have often been abandoned and its users ridiculed.

Our justifiable faith in the tools of modern medicine has led to an almost complete reliance upon pills, procedures, and operations—even though they are often not completely effective. Use of placebos could easily enhance and supplement our potent modern approaches.

Are you suggesting that sugar pills should be used more often?

No. We shouldn't think of the placebo effect as being achievable only by pills. Deception undermines the doctor–patient relationship. More to the point, there is no need to use placebo pills, because the beneficial aspects of the placebo effect can be obtained without misrepresentation. A good "bedside manner" and a warm, sympathetic, trusting doctor–patient relationship will evoke a positive placebo effect. This effect can be translated into healthy changes in the body. For example, anesthetists usually discuss the experience of surgery with a patient before the operation. If the anesthetist is enthusiastic and confident in describing what to expect, the patient is likely to have a much easier time during recovery. In one study, patients who had the positive discussion needed only half the pain-relieving medication required by those who had no such encounter. The patients with this enhanced doctor–patient relationship were also discharged earlier—by an average of more than two and a half days.

So the doctor–patient relationship is much more than a nicety. A sound, meaningful interaction helps promote better medical results. When specific drugs are not clearly indicated, wise physicians recognize that they can often practice an excellent form of medicine by giving a dose of themselves. Such physicians often spend time giving reassurance and support to their patients, who should recognize the worth of this process and not assume that giving drugs is the only proper way to practice medicine. If a patient has difficulty relating to his or her physician and there is little mutual trust, the patient might do well to talk about the problem with the physician. If there is still little communication, perhaps the patient should seek another doctor.

Many medications that are sold without a prescription act primarily by a placebo effect. Through advertising, people are led to believe that many naturally occurring unimportant aches and pains should be eliminated as quickly as possible. Then they are instructed that the remedy being advertised offers the best relief. The advertising makes full use of the placebo effect by creating the problem and then offering the solution. In truth, when people recognize that many symptoms are unimportant and will disappear of their own accord, there may be little need for these substances. Of course, unusual, alarming, or persistent symptoms should be checked out with a doctor.

The nineteenth century French physician Armand Trousseau allegedly remarked: "You should treat as many patients as possible with new drugs, while they still have the power to heal." He meant that new drugs usually have an extra dose of the placebo effect. In general, we should be wary of new preparations; their benefits may be borrowed from the placebo effect and their hazards not yet recognized.

The placebo effect is a potent therapeutic tool, which can be used ethically, without deception, to enhance the benefits of modern medicine. Although far from understood, it has withstood the test of time, and it continues to be both safe and inexpensive.

Hypnosis—Legitimate or Not?

Now that hypnosis is being more widely employed in medical and dental practice, it is frequently asked whether hypnosis is "safe" and "legitimate." The general answer to this question is "yes"—with certain qualifications:

(1) Hypnosis should never be used as a method to treat something outside the practitioner's area of expertise. For example, it is quite legitimate for a family doctor to use hypnosis to deal with smoking. In the same way, a dentist may skillfully use hypnosis for pain relief. But it would be illegitimate for either one to use hypnosis to explore deep psychological conflicts—which would be apt to lie beyond their expertise.

(2) Hypnosis should not be used to "cover up" something that has not been fully evaluated through other means that might lead to permanent cure. For example, it would be dangerous to treat pain with hypnosis until the underlying cause—such as a treatable cancer—has been properly sought.

While the definitions of hypnosis vary widely, most experts describe it as a technique that promotes heightened concentration. Hypnosis does not result in a state of unconsciousness that allows sinister manipulation. Within the guidelines described above, it can be a valuable method of therapy, and it is being utilized increasingly by various branches of the healing professions.

Dying

One side effect of medical progress has been to prolong the period of "dying" for many people—the time after a fatal disease is diagnosed and before death. Caring for these patients presents difficult challenges. We asked Dr. Melvin J. Krant, an expert on cancer, Professor of Medicine at the University of Massachusetts School of Medicine, and Director of the Palliative Care Unit at the University's hospital in Worcester, to talk about care of the dying.

Do dying patients need special places to die in?

I am often called by people who ask if there isn't some special place where a relative with a fatal disease can go to live out his or her life quietly. The question usually reflects desperation arising from a situation that is falling apart or a romanticized idea that dying should be a time of peace and enlightenment without bodily difficulty. Of course, places where a patient can die exist; they include homes, hospitals, nursing homes, and "hospices." But the important point is usually not *where* somebody spends the last weeks or months of life so much as *how* their care is organized.

The principles for shaping care of the dying are not really anything new; many individuals have followed them for a very long time. But they are now being made more explicit and adapted to institutional settings. I would personally stress the following:

The patient and family need to be helped together. As the dying person becomes disabled, the family is called upon to provide both physical and emotional support. Professionals have to consider the patient and family together in order to provide the best possible environment for dying. Family members may need counseling and emotional help to carry out their mission.

Families should not have to go it alone. As problems arise, they need around-the-clock support from professionals who can answer questions and help with arrangements. An individual rarely takes responsibility for helping with a dying relative more than once or twice in his or her own lifetime. Assistance from people with more experience is needed if panic and frustration are to be minimized.

The patient and family need to take an active part in making decisions. But they should never have to bear final responsibility for reaching medical judgments; that is an unfair demand to place on them.

Patient and family both have the right to expect that the patient's symptoms, such as pain and nausea, will be carefully and thoroughly controlled. This is an area where providers of health care are sometimes criticized for being too cautious with medication.

A strong tie to a physician or hospital is essential if the dying person is to receive optimal care. When crises occur, both patient and family should have access to appropriate staff who are familiar with the patient and can help with crises.

Hospital care is often criticized as being too technological, as treating the disease and not the patient.

High technology can be—and is—used to spare patients discomfort or limitation that they would otherwise suffer. Romantic fantasies that dying should be a graceful, gentle process are highly unrealistic. Many complications can occur before the end comes, and they need to be treated. For example, a person with cancer attacking the thigh bone may be helped by an operation to pin the bone so that it can still be used for walking. The alternative would be to lie in bed with sandbags bracing the leg—a low-technology alternative that is much less desirable when surgery is possible. Another person may contract a urinary infection and lapse into feverish delirium. Simple treatment with antibiotics can spare the patient considerable discomfort; morphine is not necessarily a better choice. Yet another person may be protected from weakness and disorientation by receiving blood transfusions. The point of these treatments is not, as some critics sometimes maintain, to "prolong the agony." Quite the reverse: without altering the time it takes a person to die, the therapy can provide comfort, support, and an opportunity to remain more active and self-sufficient.

Has it become impossible to die quietly at home?

Nobody can guarantee that dying will be peaceful. Dying, like living, has its ups and downs. Of course, in the last few days, dying can usually be made peaceful, but the long period before the very end can be a succession of crises requiring thoughtful care.

The majority of people with late-stage cancer (and it is primarily they whom we are talking about when we say "dying patients") can die at home, if that is what they and their families want. But where the person is at the moment of death is much less important than where the period of failing vitality is spent. The principal advantage of home care is that it allows a patient to remain in familiar and friendly surroundings. But there are potentially major disadvantages. As yet, insurance policies frequently do not pay for the same services at home as in a hospital; money remains an enormous issue for families who want to keep a patient at home. Physical care of a dying patient can be exceedingly burdensome. Most families need help with it. A professional homemaker or home health-care aide, who can assist with the day-to-day tasks of managing the household, can make a great contribution in this setting. Unfortunately, such people are scarce, and funds to pay them can be even scarcer.

Serious medical crises are one reason for taking patients to a hospital. Another equally valid one can simply be the need of family members for a period of recuperation; their energies can be drained by the job required of them, and a period without the pressure can be essential. Unfortunately, hospitals are often not in a position to allow admissions on these grounds alone.

What about other facilities, such as hospices and nursing homes?

The nursing home can be a very helpful institution when the needs of a dying patient outstrip the resources of family members. Often there is nothing ennobling or beautiful about the physical care required by a dying patient. Family members may be taxed by it to the point that they lose out on the really important contribution they can make: showing their love and helping the patient with emotional needs. In this situation, a nursing home can provide a highly valuable service. Admittedly, the nursing home industry in this country has deficiencies, and conditions are sometimes deplorable. *But they do not have to be,* and families should not automatically assume that this is an unacceptable alternative.

"Hospice" is a relatively new use of an old term. It is now applied to facilities that are focused entirely on care for dying patients. The hospice philosophy is in many ways similar to the one that I have outlined, but it is often associated with a bias against hospital care that may narrow options prematurely. Although the hospice movement has generated a lot of enthusiasm, few hospices have been established in the United States, and they differ from one another in style and organization. Many community hospitals are developing a palliative-care (hospice) mode of service to help with home care, as well as to provide a hospital setting when needed. In such a setting, many patients die in a hospital but spend the major part of the last months at home in considerable comfort supported by a staff dedicated to maximizing living during the time of dying.

Evaluating Medical
Information

One of the problems of modern society is how to evaluate the mass of information that pours out of the media. And when health information is involved, that problem becomes more personal and pertinent. Since this book is intended to provide guidance through the maze of health information, we would like to suggest the following guidelines for you to use when evaluating medical information:

(1) In general, the kind of medical information that deserves attention comes from studies published in reputable journals for scrutiny by other scientists. The purpose of a study—versus a story—is to remove personal bias from the conclusions. Personal bias rarely takes the form of intentional distortion resulting from financial or ego involvement. More often, bias stems from honest errors of observation, undue optimism, or limited evidence. Proper studies attempt to remove these and other sources of error. When you encounter new information, *ask yourself if it goes beyond personal observation and whether it has stood the test of criticism by other scientists.*

(2) A major theme of medical information is the *effectiveness* of new treatments. Proof of effectiveness must depend on more than individual, anecdotal "stories" about how someone (or even many) got better doing this or that. *Proof of effectiveness requires controlled studies which compare the treatment under discussion to other treatment—or to no treatment.* As described above, such studies must be done with proper controls to remove bias, in large enough numbers to be statistically valid, and in a manner that makes the results available for examination. When you encounter a claim of effectiveness, *ask yourself if the treatment in question was compared either to other treatments or to "doing nothing."*

(3) Another major issue in medical information is the *safety* of new (or old) treatments. The question, in our complex and techno-

logical age, is not *absolute* safety (even staying in bed is risky) but *relative* safety. All of life—including medical treatment—involves some risk. The question becomes whether the risk is justified when compared to alternatives. Studies to determine risk usually require large numbers of observations over long periods of time, though occasionally an intolerable danger becomes apparent very early in a study. When you encounter information about "safety," *ask yourself—"safe compared to what?"*

(4) One should be especially wary of enthusiastic claims for unusual remedies for chronic or incurable diseases—such as crippling arthritis or terminal cancer. There are, unfortunately, some people who deliberately profit from the understandable desperation of others.

In short, when evaluating medical information, remember that *the burden of proof rests with those who recommend doing or giving something*—especially if it involves a remedy or procedure not well established in medical practice.

ACKNOWLEDGMENTS

We would like to extend our deep gratitude to the many people who have provided assistance in the preparation of the *Harvard Medical School Health Letter* and *The Harvard Medical School Health Letter Book,* especially Lynn Brown Kargman, Christina Knapp, Susan Wallace, and William Bennett.

G. Timothy Johnson
Stephen E. Goldfinger

Index